T0015524

The 36-Hour Day

A Johns Hopkins Press Health Book

Nancy L. Mace, MA, is retired. She was a consultant to and member of the board of directors of the Alzheimer's Association and an assistant in psychiatry and coordinator of the T. Rowe and Eleanor Price Teaching Service of the Department of Psychiatry and Behavioral Sciences at the Johns Hopkins University School of Medicine.

Peter V. Rabins, MD, MPH, is professor emeritus in the Departments of Psychiatry and Medicine at the Johns Hopkins University School of Medicine. The author of *Is It Alzheimer's? 101 Answers to Your Most Pressing Questions about Memory Loss and Dementia,* he was the founding director of the Division of Geriatric Psychiatry and Neuropsychiatry and the first holder of the Richman Family Professorship in Alzheimer Disease and Related Dementias.

The 36-Hour Day

7th Edition

A Family Guide to Caring for People
Who Have Alzheimer Disease
and Other Dementias

Nancy L. Mace, MA
Peter V. Rabins, MD, MPH

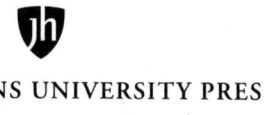

JOHNS HOPKINS UNIVERSITY PRESS

Baltimore

Note to the Reader: This book is not meant to substitute for medical care of people who have Alzheimer disease, other dementias, or memory loss, and treatment should not be based solely on its contents. Instead, treatment must be developed in a dialogue between the individual and their physician. Our book has been written to help with that dialogue.

© 1981, 1991, 1999, 2006, 2011, 2017, 2021 Johns Hopkins University Press
All rights reserved. Published 2021
Printed in the United States of America on acid-free paper
9 8 7 6 5 4 3 2

Johns Hopkins University Press
2715 North Charles Street
Baltimore, Maryland 21218-4363
www.press.jhu.edu

Library of Congress Cataloging-in-Publication Data

Names: Mace, Nancy L., author. | Rabins, Peter V., author.
Title: The 36-hour day : a family guide to caring for people who have Alzheimer disease
    and other dementias / Nancy L. Mace, MA, Peter V. Rabins, MD, MPH.
Other titles: Thirty-six hour day
Description: Seventh edition. | Baltimore : Johns Hopkins University Press, 2021. |
    Series: A Johns Hopkins Press health book | Includes index.
Identifiers: LCCN 2020045438 | ISBN 9781421441702 (hardcover) |
    ISBN 9781421441719 (paperback) | ISBN 9781421441726 (ebook) |
    ISBN 9781421441733 (paperback, large print)
Subjects: LCSH: Alzheimer's disease—Patients—Home care—Popular works. |
    Senile dementia—Patients—Home care—Popular works. | Large type books.
Classification: LCC RC523 .M33 2021 | DDC 616.8/31—dc23

A catalog record for this book is available from the British Library.

Special discounts are available for bulk purchases of this book. For more information, please contact Special Sales at specialsales@jh.edu.

To everyone who gives a "36-hour day"
to the care of a person with a dementing illness

Contents

Foreword

For two generations this book has provided coherent support, helpful direction, and much comfort to families and friends of people afflicted with Alzheimer dementia. Acclaimed by many as the most accessible and comprehensible guide for home care of people with this progressive illness, it now, with this seventh edition, passes another milestone in an illustrious publication record. I'm proud to remember how I played a small role in launching this book back in 1981, and I have witnessed, with pleasure, what it has done for its readers in earlier editions over all these years.

We all can acknowledge that the central problem today remains much as it did when the first edition of this book appeared. We still do not know how to prevent or cure this distressful disorder, even though perhaps we can recognize it more certainly and can slow its progress significantly. But we have learned much together about helping people to care for and protect their afflicted kith and kin.

As before (and now with information about the latest advances in research), this edition describes the place and utility of medications that slow the progression of the disorder and medications that relieve some of its more distressful symptoms. But the book still places these medicinal matters into a context of care that is comprehensive and reflective of more everyday concerns. In this sense, its frame of reference remains the same: how to see the person within the disorder and how to sustain that person in harmony with life despite the progress of the affliction.

I believe we can identify something even more significant in the history of this little book and the help it has provided. The illness represents a personal problem that, like many other aspects of life, may follow a better or worse path depending on contexts and circumstances forged by the mediations of family and friends. This book has successfully enhanced the mediating powers of these interested parties by identifying and resolving problems that emerge at various points of transition in the course of this illness. In the process of working effectively in this way, the authors and readers have demonstrated just how much more of life—abiding friendships, shared experiences, daily encounters, trusting relations—remains to be enjoyed by people who have dementia and by their family members despite this illness and its tribulations.

With that spirit, authors and readers have contributed thoughts and experiences to this latest edition, and I salute its appearance both for what it represents as a product of past collaborations and for what it, as an invigorated new version, will bring to render effective the "36-hour-day" labors of new readers.

We can now see with even more confidence that present-day contributions to loved ones in the form of effective and suitable care lead ultimately to a future where cure and prevention will emerge. Because these patients have committed champions, Alzheimer dementia is not a neglected field of study but rather one in which scientific investigation is moving rapidly ahead. As we can foresee the likelihood of a major advance in our powers of treatment and prevention before the next edition will be conceived, we can also recognize how much of the energy spurring such progress should be attributed to the readers of this book and their caregiving commitments to patients as valued people.

Paul R. McHugh, MD

Director, Department of Psychiatry and Behavioral Sciences, 1975–2001

Johns Hopkins University School of Medicine

Preface

The publication of this seventh edition of *The 36-Hour Day* provides an opportunity for us to thank the many people and organizations that have contributed to the book since its first publication in 1981 and to its predecessor, *The Family Handbook*. In 1979, *The Family Handbook* was written, with the help of Jane Lucas Blaustein, at the behest of the family members who founded the Maryland Chapter of the Alzheimer's Association.

Many of the caregiving suggestions in *The 36-Hour Day* have come from people who were experiencing the symptoms of dementia, from the caregivers of people with dementia, from health care professionals across the country, and from advocates such as the staff of the Alzheimer's Association. We thank them and continue to admire both their perseverance and their willingness to share their experiences and thoughts.

The idea underlying the book—that much can be done to improve the lives of people who have dementia and of those caring for them—came directly from our teachers, Paul McHugh and Marshal Folstein. The first edition would not have come about without their support, advocacy, and intellectual input.

In the first edition we identified colleagues Jeanne Floyd, Janet Bachur, and Jane Blaustein as contributing ideas and time. Since then, many other colleagues have taught us through their examples and direct suggestions and have inspired us by their dedication. We particularly thank Martina Lavrisha, Rebecca Rye, and Mary Ann Wylie for their help and input over the years.

Financial support for the writing of the first edition was provided by the T. Rowe and Eleanor Price Foundation, and this support has allowed us to teach others what we have learned in subsequent years. More recently, The Richman Family Chair in Alzheimer Disease and Related Disorders has supported the research and clinical efforts of Peter Rabins and contributed to the last several revisions.

Karen Rabins has carefully read every edition and provided editing and proofreading expertise. Our editors at the Johns Hopkins University Press—Anders Richter, Wendy Harris, Jacqueline Wehmueller, and Joe Rusko—have contributed their expertise and support. We thank them for their advice and suggestions.

As Paul McHugh writes in his foreword, a worldwide effort of clinicians, researchers, family members, advocacy organizations, and government agencies has transformed how people who have dementia and their families are cared for. The bravery and dedication of those struggling with these diseases and of their caregivers underpin the continued search for treatments and preventions. Until total prevention is achieved, compassionate care will remain central to the treatment of dementia.

Peter V. Rabins
Nancy Mace

The 36-Hour Day

CHAPTER 1

Dementia

For two or three years, Mrs. Windsor had known that her memory was slipping. First, she had trouble remembering the names of her friends' children, and one year she completely forgot the strawberry preserves she had put up. She compensated by writing things down. After all, she told herself, she was getting older. But then she would find herself groping for a word she had always known, and she worried that she was developing Alzheimer's.

Recently, when talking with a group of friends, Mrs. Windsor realized that she had forgotten more than just an occasional name—she had lost the thread of the conversation altogether. She was able to compensate for this, too: she always gave an appropriate answer, even if she secretly felt confused. No one noticed, except perhaps her daughter-in-law, who said to her best friend, "I think Mother is slipping." It worried Mrs. Windsor—sometimes depressed her—but she always denied that anything was wrong. There was no one to whom she could say, "I am losing my mind. It is slipping away as I watch." Besides, she didn't want to think about it, didn't want to think about getting old, and, most importantly, didn't want to be treated as if she were senile. She was still enjoying life and was able to manage.

Then in the winter Mrs. Windsor got sick. At first she thought it was only a cold. She saw a doctor, who gave her some pills and asked her what she expected at her age, which annoyed her. She rapidly got much worse. She went to bed, afraid, weak, and very tired. Mrs. Windsor's daughter-in-law got a telephone call from Mrs. Windsor's neighbor. Together they found Mrs. Windsor semiconscious, feverish, and mumbling incoherently.

During the first few days in the hospital, Mrs. Windsor had only an intermittent, foggy notion of what was happening. The doctors told her family that she had pneumonia and that her kidneys were working poorly. All the resources of a modern hospital were mobilized to fight the infection.

Mrs. Windsor was in a strange place, where nothing was familiar. People, all strangers, came and went. They told her where she was, but she forgot. In strange surroundings, she could no longer compensate for her forgetfulness, and the delirium caused by the acute illness aggravated her confusion. She thought her husband came to see her—a handsome young man in his war uniform. Then when her son came, she was surprised that they would come together. Her son kept saying, "But Mom, Dad has been dead for twenty years." But she knew he wasn't, because he had just been there. Then when she complained to her daughter-in-law that she never came, she thought the woman lied when she said, "But Mother, I was just here this morning." In truth, Mrs. Windsor could not remember the morning.

People came and poked and pushed, and shoved things in and out and over her. They stuck her with needles, and they wanted her to participate in physical therapy. Walking on the treadmill became part of her nightmares; she dreamed she was on a forced march to an unknown place. She could not remember where she was. When she had to go to the bathroom, they told her that she had to have someone go with her. Embarrassed, she cried and wet herself.

Gradually, Mrs. Windsor got better. The infection cleared and the dizziness passed. Only during the initial, acute phase of her illness did she imagine things, but after the fever and infection had passed, the confusion and forgetfulness seemed more severe than before. Although the illness had probably not affected the gradual course of her memory loss, it had weakened her considerably and taken her out of the familiar setting in which she had been able to function. Most significantly, the illness had focused attention on the seriousness of her situation. Now her family realized she could no longer live alone.

The people around Mrs. Windsor talked and talked. No doubt they explained their plans, but she forgot. When she was finally released from the hospital, they took her to her daughter-in-law's house. They were happy about something that day, and they led her into a room. Here at last were some of her things, but not all. She thought perhaps the rest of her things had been stolen while she was sick. They kept saying they had told her where her things were, but she couldn't remember what they said.

This is where they said she lived now, in her daughter-in-law's house—except that long ago she had made up her mind that she would never live with her children. She wanted to live at home. At home she could find things. At home she could manage—she believed—as she always had. At home, perhaps, she could discover what had become of a lifetime of possessions. This was not her home: her independence was gone, her things were gone, and Mrs. Windsor felt an enormous sense of loss. Mrs. Windsor could not remember her son's loving explanation—that she couldn't manage alone and that bringing her to live in his home was the best arrangement he could work out for her.

Often, Mrs. Windsor was afraid, with a nameless, shapeless fear. Her impaired mind could not put a name to or provide an explanation to her fear. People came, memories came, and then they slipped away. She could not tell what was reality and what was memory of people past. The bathroom was not where it was yesterday. Dressing became an insurmountable ordeal. Her hands forgot how to button buttons. Sashes hung inexplicably about her, and she could not think how to manage them or why they hung there.

Mrs. Windsor gradually lost the ability to make sense out of what her eyes and ears told her. Noises and confusion made her feel panicky. She couldn't understand, they couldn't explain, and often panic overwhelmed her. She worried about her things: a chair and the china that had belonged to her mother. They said they had told her over and over, but she could not remember where her things had gone. Perhaps someone had stolen them. She had lost so much. What things she still had, she hid, but then she forgot where she hid them.

"I cannot get her to take a bath," her daughter-in-law said in despair. "She smells. How can I send her to the adult day care center if she won't take a bath?" For Mrs. Windsor, the bath became an experience of terror. The tub was a mystery. From day to day she could not remember how to manage the water: sometimes it all ran away, sometimes it kept rising and rising, and she could not stop it. The bath involved remembering so many things. It meant remembering how to undress, how to find the bathroom, how to wash. Mrs. Windsor's fingers had forgotten how to unzip zippers; her feet had forgotten how to step into the tub. There were so many things for an injured mind to think about that panic overwhelmed her.

How do any of us react to trouble? We might try to get away from the situation for a while and think it out. One person may go out for a beer; another may weed the garden or go for a walk. Sometimes we react with anger. We fight back against those who cause, or at least participate in, our situation. Or we become discouraged for a while, until nature heals us or the trouble goes away.

Mrs. Windsor's old ways of coping with trouble remained. Often when she felt nervous, she thought of going for a walk. She would pause on the porch, look out, drift out, and walk away—away from the trouble. Yet the trouble remained and now it was worse, for Mrs. Windsor felt constantly lost and nothing was familiar: the house had disappeared, the street was not the one she knew—or was it one from her childhood, or where they lived when the boys were growing up? The terror would wash over her, clutching at her heart. Mrs. Windsor would walk faster.

Sometimes Mrs. Windsor would react with anger. It was an anger she herself did not understand. But her things were gone; her life seemed gone. The closets of her mind sprang open and fell shut, or vanished altogether. Who wouldn't be angry? Someone had taken her things, the treasures of a lifetime. Was it her daughter-in-law, or her own mother-in-law, or a sister resented in childhood? She accused her daughter-in-law but quickly forgot the suspicion. Her daughter-in-law, coping with an overwhelming situation, was unable to forget.

Many of us remember the day we began high school. We lay awake the night before, afraid of getting lost and not finding the classrooms the next day in a strange building. Every day was like that for Mrs. Windsor. Her family began sending her to an adult day care center. Every day a bus driver came to pick her up in the morning, and every day her daughter-in-law came to get her in the afternoon, but from day to day Mrs. Windsor could not remember that she would be taken home. She had trouble finding her way around the building. Sometimes she went into the men's bathroom by mistake.

Many of Mrs. Windsor's social skills remained, so she was able to chat and laugh with the other people in the day care center. As Mrs. Windsor relaxed in the center, she enjoyed the time she spent there with other people, although she could never remember what she did there well enough to tell her daughter-in-law.

Mrs. Windsor loved music; music seemed to be embedded in a part of her mind that she retained long after much else was lost. She loved to sing old, familiar songs. She loved to sing at the day care center. Even though her daughter-in-law could not sing well, Mrs. Windsor did not remember that, and the two women discovered that they enjoyed singing together.

The time finally came when the phys-
ical and emotional burden of caring for
Mrs. Windsor became too much for her
family, and she went to live in a nursing
home. After the initial days of confusion
and panic passed, Mrs. Windsor felt secure
in her small, sunny bedroom. She could
not remember the schedule for the day,
but the reliability of the routine comforted
her. Some days it seemed as if she were still
at the day care center; sometimes she was
not sure. She was glad the toilet was close
by, where she could see it and did not have
to remember where it was.

Mrs. Windsor was glad when her
family came to visit. Sometimes she re-
membered their names; more often she
did not. She never remembered that they
had come last week, so she regularly
scolded them for abandoning her. They
could never think of much to say, but
they put their arms around her frail body,
held her hand, and sat silently or sang old
songs. She was glad when they didn't try
to remind her of what she had just said or
that they had come last week, or ask her
if she remembered this person or that one.
She liked it best when they just held her
and loved her.

•

Someone in your family has been diagnosed as having dementia. This could
be Alzheimer disease, vascular dementia, or one of several other diseases (see

Chapter 17). Perhaps you are not sure
which condition it is. Whatever the
name of the disease, a person close to
you has lost some of their intellectual
ability—the ability to think and remember. They may become increasingly forgetful. Their personality may appear to
change, or they may become depressed,
moody, or withdrawn.

Many, although not all, of the disorders that cause these symptoms in
adults are chronic and irreversible.
When a diagnosis of an irreversible
dementia is made, the person who
has dementia and their family face the
task of learning to live with the illness.
Whether you decide to care for the
person at home or to have them cared
for in a nursing home or an assisted
living facility, you will find yourself
facing new problems. You will also be
coping with your feelings about having
someone close to you develop an inca-
pacitating illness.

This book is designed to help you
with that adjustment and with the
day-to-day management of a family
member who has dementia. We have
found that there are questions many
families ask. This book can help you
begin to find answers, but it is not a
substitute for the help of your doctor
and other health care professionals.

What Is Dementia?

You may have heard different
terms for the symptoms of forgetfulness and loss of the ability to reason

and think clearly. You may have been
told that the person has "dementia" or
"Alzheimer's." You may also have heard

the terms "neurocognitive disorder," "delirium," or "chronic brain syndrome." You may have wondered how these conditions are different from "normal aging."

Doctors use the word *dementia* in a specific way. *Dementia* does not mean crazy. It has been chosen by the medical profession as the least offensive and most accurate term to describe this group of illnesses. *Dementia* describes a group of symptoms that can be caused by many diseases; in this way it is an umbrella term that applies to many disorders and is not the name of a disease that causes the symptoms. *Neurocognitive disorder* is a newer term that some clinicians and researchers use instead of *dementia*. It has the same meaning as *dementia*.

There are two major conditions that begin in adulthood and cause the symptoms of mental confusion, memory loss, disorientation, intellectual impairment, or similar problems. These two conditions may look similar to the casual observer and can be confused with each other. The first is dementia. The second condition, *delirium*, is discussed on page 305. You will want to familiarize yourself with delirium because occasionally a treatable delirium will be mistaken for a dementia. Sometimes people who have Alzheimer disease or another dementia develop a delirium as well and have symptoms that are worse than the dementia alone would cause.

The symptoms of dementia can be caused by many different diseases. In Chapter 17, we summarize some of the diseases that can cause dementia. A few of these diseases are treatable; most are not. Thyroid disease, for ex-

ample, may cause a dementia that can be reversed with correction of a thyroid abnormality.

Alzheimer disease is the most frequent cause of irreversible dementia in adults. The intellectual impairment progresses gradually from mild forgetfulness to total disability. There are structural and chemical changes in the brains of people who have Alzheimer disease. At present, physicians know of no way to stop or cure it. However, much can be done to diminish the patient's behavioral and emotional symptoms and to give the family a sense of control of the situation.

> *Dementia* describes a group
> of symptoms that can be
> caused by many diseases

Vascular dementia is believed to be the second or third most common cause of dementia. It usually results from a series of small strokes within the brain but can be due to other diseases that affect arteries in the brain. Strokes are sometimes so tiny that neither you nor the afflicted person is aware of any change, but many small strokes added together can destroy enough bits of brain tissue to affect memory and other intellectual functions. This condition used to be called "hardening of the arteries," but autopsy studies have shown that it is stroke damage rather than inadequate circulation to the brain that causes the problem. In some cases, treatment can reduce the possibility of further damage.

Alzheimer disease and vascular dementia sometimes occur together.

Today, doctors believe that brain blood vessel abnormalities and small strokes trigger or contribute to the brain changes that are characteristic of Alzheimer disease.

Alzheimer disease usually occurs in elderly people, but about one-third of older people suffer from dementia caused by another disease. Before age 65, about half the cases of dementia are caused by Alzheimer disease and half by other diseases. This book addresses general principles for the care of people with any of the diseases that cause dementia.

People who have dementia may also have other illnesses, and their dementia may make them more vulnerable to other health problems. Other illnesses or reactions to medications often cause delirium in people who have dementia. The delirium can make the person's mental functions and behavior worse. It is vital for the person's general health, and to make their care easier, to detect and treat other illnesses promptly. It is important to choose a doctor who is able to spend the time to do this with the person who has dementia.

Depression is common in older people, and it can be the cause of memory loss, confusion, or other changes in mental function. The memory of a person with depression sometimes improves when the depression is treated. A person who also has an irreversible dementia can develop depression, and depression should always be treated.

Many uncommon conditions cause dementia. These are discussed in Chapter 17.

The diseases that cause dementia know no social, ethnic, or racial lines: the rich and the poor, the wise and the unwise are affected. There is no reason to be ashamed or embarrassed because a family member has dementia. Many brilliant and famous people have developed diseases that cause dementia.

Severe memory loss is *never* a normal part of growing older

Severe memory loss is *never* a normal part of growing older. According to the best studies available, 10 to 12 percent of older people have a severe intellectual impairment, and another 10 to 15 percent have milder impairments. The diseases that cause dementia become more prevalent in people who live into their 80s and 90s, but 50 to 70 percent of those who live to age 90 never experience significant memory loss or other symptoms of dementia. Difficulty recalling names or words is common as we age but usually is not enough to interfere with our lives. Most of us know older people who are active and in full command of their intellect in their 70s, 80s, and 90s. Pablo Picasso, Nancy Reagan, Nelson Mandela, Antonin Scalia, and Maya Angelou were all still active in their careers when they died: all were past 75; Picasso was 91.

As more people in our population live into later life, it becomes even more crucial that we learn everything we can about dementia. It has been estimated that more than 5 million people in the United States have developed some degree of intellectual impairment.

According to the Alzheimer's Association, dementia cost the United States $240 billion in 2019. This translated to a cost of $53,700 per person per year.

The Person Who Has Dementia

Usually the symptoms of dementia appear gradually. Sometimes the afflicted person may be the first to notice something wrong. The person who has mild dementia is often able to describe their problem clearly: "Things just go out of my mind. I start to explain and then I just can't find the words." Family members may not notice at first that something is wrong. The person who has dementia has difficulty remembering new information, although they may be skillful at concealing this. You may observe that their ability to understand, reason, and use good judgment is impaired. The onset and progression of the condition depend on which disease has caused the condition and on other factors, some of which are unknown. Sometimes the onset of the trouble is sudden: looking back, you may say, "After a certain time, Dad was never himself."

People respond to their problems in different ways. Some become adept at concealing the difficulty. Some keep lists to jog their memory. Some vehemently deny that anything is wrong or blame their problems on others. Some people become depressed or irritable when they realize that their memory is failing. Others remain outwardly cheerful. Usually, the person who has mild to moderate dementia is able to continue to do most of the things they have always done. Like a person who has any other disease, they are able to participate in their treatment, family decisions, and planning for the future.

Early memory problems are sometimes mistaken for stress, depression, or even mental illness. This misdiagnosis creates an added burden for the person and the family.

•

A wife recalls the onset of her husband's dementia, not in terms of his forgetfulness but in terms of his mood and attitude: "I didn't know anything was wrong. I didn't want to see it. Charles was quieter than usual; he seemed depressed, but he blamed it on people at work. Then his boss told him he was being transferred—a demotion, really—to a smaller branch office. They didn't tell me anything. They suggested we take a vacation. So we did. We went to Scotland. But Charles didn't get any better. He was depressed and irritable. After he took the new job, he couldn't handle that either; he blamed it on the younger men. He was so irritable, I wondered what was wrong between us after so many years. We went to a marriage counselor, and that only made things worse. I knew he was forgetful, but I thought that it was caused by stress."

Her husband said, "I knew something was wrong. I could feel myself getting uptight over little things. People thought I knew things about the plant that I . . . I couldn't remember. The counselor said it was stress. I thought it was something else, something terrible. I was scared."

In those illnesses in which the dementia is progressive, the person's ability to carry out usual activities gradually declines, and their troubles cannot be concealed. They may become unable to recall what day it is or where they are. They may be unable to do simple tasks such as dressing or putting words together in a way that makes sense. As the dementia progresses, it becomes clear that the damage to the brain affects many functions, including the ability to remember, organize information, plan, speak, and move (coordination, writing, walking). The person may have difficulty finding the right name for familiar things, and they may become clumsy or walk with a shuffle. Their abilities may fluctuate from day to day or even from hour to hour. This makes it harder for families to know what to expect.

Some people experience changes in personality. Many retain the qualities they have always had: the person may always have been sweet and lovable and remain so, or they may always have been a difficult person to live with and may become more so. Other people may change dramatically, from agreeable to demanding, from energetic to apathetic, or from cranky to good-natured. They may become passive, dependent, and listless, or they may become restless, easily upset, and irritable. Sometimes they become demanding, fearful, or depressed.

A daughter says, "Mother was always the cheerful, outgoing person in the family. I guess we knew she was getting forgetful, but the worst thing is that she doesn't want to do anything anymore. She doesn't do her hair, she doesn't keep the house neat, she absolutely won't go out."

Often little things enormously upset people who have dementia. Tasks that were previously simple may now be too difficult for a person, and they may react to this by becoming upset, angry, or depressed.

Another family says, "The worst thing about Dad is his temper. He used to be easygoing. Now he is always hollering over the least little thing. Last night he told our 10-year-old that Alaska is not a state. He was hollering and yelling and stalked out of the room. Then when I asked him to take a bath, we had a real fight. He insisted he had already had a bath."

It is important for those around the person to remember that many of their behaviors are beyond their control: for example, they may not be able to keep their anger in check or to stop pacing the floor. The changes that occur are not the result of an unpleasant personality grown old—they are the result of damage to the brain and are usually beyond the control of the person who has dementia.

Some people who have dementia experience hallucinations (hearing, seeing, or smelling things that are not real). This experience is real to the person experiencing it and can be frightening to family members. Some people become suspicious of others; they may hide things or accuse people of stealing from them. Often, they simply mislay things and forget where they put them and, in their confusion, think someone has stolen them.

•

A son recalls, "Mom is so paranoid. She hides her purse. She hides her money, she hides her jewelry. Then she accuses my wife of stealing them. Now she is accusing us of stealing the silverware. The hard part is that she doesn't seem sick. It's hard to believe she isn't doing this deliberately."

•

In the final stages of a progressive dementia, so much of the brain has been affected that the person may be confined to bed, unable to control urination, and unable to express them-selves. In the last stages of the illness, many people require skilled nursing care.

The behavior changes that occur are the result of damage to the brain and are usually beyond the control of the person who has dementia

---

The course of the disease and the prognosis vary with the specific disor-der and with the individual person. For this reason, not all these symptoms will occur in the same person. Your family member may never experience some of these symptoms or may experience others we have not mentioned.

Where Do You Go from Here?

You know or suspect that someone close to you has dementia. Where do you go from here? You will need to take stock of your current situation and then identify what needs to be done to help the person and to make the burdens on yourself bearable. There are many questions you must ask. This book will get you started with finding the answers.

The first thing you need to know is the cause of the disease and its progno-sis. Each disease that causes dementia is different. You may have been given different diagnoses and different expla-nations of the disease, or you may not know what is wrong with the person.

You may have been told that the person has Alzheimer disease when they have not had a thorough diagnostic exam-ination. However, you must have a diagnosis and some information about the course of the disease before you or the doctor can respond appropriately to day-to-day problems or plan for the future. It is usually better to know what to expect. Your understanding of the illness can help to dispel fears and worries, and it will help you plan how you can best help the person who has dementia.

Early in your search for help, you may want to contact the Alzheimer's Association (www.alz.org) or your local dementia support organization. They can refer you to resources and offer you support and information.

We can continue to love a person even after they have changed

Even when the disease itself cannot be stopped, *much can be done to improve the quality of life of people who have dementia and their family members.*

Dementing illnesses vary with the specific disease and with the individual who is ill. You may never face many of the problems discussed in this book. You may find it most helpful to skip through those chapters and read only the sections that apply to you.

The key to coping is common sense and ingenuity. Sometimes a family is too close to the problem to see clearly a way of managing. At other times there is no one more creative at solving a difficult problem than the family members themselves. Many of the ideas offered here were suggested by family members who have called or written to share their ideas with others. These ideas will get you started.

Caring for a person who has dementia is not easy. We hope the information in this book will help you, but we know that simple solutions are not yet at hand.

This book often focuses on problems. However, it is important to remember that confused people and their families do still experience joy and happiness. Because dementing illnesses develop slowly, they often leave intact the person's ability to enjoy life and to enjoy other people. When things go badly, remind yourself that, no matter how bad the person's memory or how strange their behavior, they are still a unique and special human being. We can continue to love a person even after they have changed drastically and even when we are deeply troubled by their present state.

CHAPTER 2

Getting Medical Help for the Person Who Has Dementia

This book is written for you, the family. It is based on the assumption that you and the person who has dementia are receiving professional medical care. The family and the medical professionals are partners in the care of the person who has dementia. Neither should be providing care alone. This book is not meant to be a substitute for professional skills. Many health care professionals are knowledgeable about the diseases that cause dementia, but misconceptions about dementia still exist. Not all physicians or other health care professionals have the time, interest, or skills to diagnose or care for people who have dementia.

> **When possible, one physician should coordinate the person's care and monitor all tests and treatments**

What should you expect from your physician and other professionals? The first thing is an accurate diagnosis. Once a diagnosis has been made, you will need the ongoing help of a physician and perhaps other professionals to manage the dementia, to treat concurrent illnesses, and to help you find the resources you need. This chapter is written as a guide to help you find the best possible medical care in your community.

When possible, one physician should coordinate the person's care and monitor all tests and treatments.

In the course of an illness that causes dementia, you may need the special skills of a consulting physician such as a neurologist, geriatric psychiatrist, or geriatrician in addition to a primary care doctor, neuropsychologist, social worker, nurse, geriatric care manager, and recreational, occupational, or physical therapist. Each is a highly trained professional whose skills complement those of the others. They can work together, first to evaluate the person who has dementia and then to help you address ongoing care needs. However, you should insist that one physician keep track of all tests and treatments and coordinate care.

The Evaluation of the Person with a Suspected Dementia

When people have difficulty thinking, remembering, or learning or show changes in personality, it is important that they undergo a thorough evaluation. A complete evaluation tells you and the doctors several things:

- the exact nature of the person's illness

- whether the condition can be reversed or treated

- the nature and extent of the disability

- the areas in which the person can still function successfully

- whether the person has other health problems that need treatment and that might be making their thinking and behavior problems worse

- the social and psychological needs and resources of the person with a suspected dementia and of the family or caregiver

- the changes you can expect in the future

Procedures vary depending on the physician and hospital, but a good evaluation includes a medical and neurological examination, consideration of the person's social support system, and an assessment of their remaining abilities. You may not have a choice of physician or other service, but you can learn what is important in an evaluation and insist that the person receive a complete workup.

The evaluation may begin with a careful examination by a physician. The doctor will take a *detailed history* from someone who knows the person well and from the person themselves if possible. This will include how the person has changed, what symptoms they have had, the order in which the symptoms developed, and information about other medical conditions. The doctor will also perform a *physical examination*, which may reveal other health problems. A *neurological examination* (checking a person's strength and sensation, asking them to balance with their eyes closed, tapping their ankles or knees with a rubber hammer, and other tests) may reveal changes in the functioning of the nerve cells of the brain or spine.

> It is important that any person with possible memory or other thinking problems be thoroughly evaluated by a knowledgeable clinician

The doctor will also do a *mental status examination*, which consists of questions about the current time, date, and place. Other questions test the ability to remember, to concentrate, to do abstract reasoning, to understand and use words, to perform simple calculations, and to copy simple designs. Each of these questions can reveal problems of function in different parts of the brain. The scoring of the test takes into consideration the person's education and the fact that the person may be nervous.

The doctor will order *laboratory tests*, including a number of blood tests. The *CBC* (complete blood count) can detect anemia (low red blood cell count) and evidence of infection, either of which can cause or complicate a dementing illness. *Blood chemistry tests* check for liver and kidney problems, diabetes, and various other conditions. A *vitamin B12 level test* checks for a vitamin deficiency that might cause dementia. *Thyroid studies* evaluate the function of the thyroid gland. Thyroid problems are among the more common reversible causes of dementia. Tests for HIV and the bacteria that cause Lyme disease and syphilis are ordered if the person's symptoms and history raise them as possibilities. The *VDRL test* can indicate a syphilis infection (syphilis was a common cause of dementia before the discovery of penicillin), but a positive result does not necessarily indicate that the person has ever had syphilis. Blood tests involve inserting a needle into a vein, which is no more unpleasant than a pinprick.

The *lumbar puncture* (LP), also called a spinal tap, is done to obtain a sample of the fluid that surrounds the spinal cord and brain. Testing of the spinal fluid can rule out infection in the central nervous system (for example, Lyme disease, syphilis, or tuberculosis), measure proteins that indicate the presence of Alzheimer disease or frontotemporal dementia, and reveal abnormalities

that suggest other uncommon causes of dementia. It is done after a local anesthetic has been injected into the back. The lumbar puncture is done only when there is a reason to suspect those conditions for which it can provide diagnostic information. While it sounds frightening to many people, it is safe. Headache and a continuing leak of spinal fluid are occasional side effects.

The *EEG* (electroencephalogram) records the electrical activity of the brain. It is done by attaching thin wires to the head with a gel or paste-like material. It is painless but may confuse the person who is forgetful. It aids in the diagnosis of delirium and seizures and can offer evidence of abnormal brain functioning. The EEG may be normal early in the course of some dementias.

The *CT scan, MRI, PET scan*, and *SPECT scan* are radiological (imaging) techniques that help the physician identify changes in the brain that indicate strokes, Alzheimer disease, and many other conditions that can cause dementia. An MRI or CT scan should be part of the initial evaluation of everyone with possible dementia. Because PET and SPECT scans are expensive and may not provide useful information, the doctor will order one only when it might provide information crucial for an accurate diagnosis. These imaging tests are described in more detail on page 320. They involve lying on a table and placing one's head next to an object that looks like a very large hair dryer or inside a large open metallic donut. They are painless tests but may be noisy and can confuse a person with a cognitive impairment. If so, a mild sedative can be prescribed to help the person relax.

If an injection is part of the test, there can be minor pain associated with the injection.

For some procedures, such as the lumbar puncture and imaging tests, the person (or their substitute decision maker, if necessary) will be asked to sign an informed consent form. This form lists all the possible side effects of the procedure. Reading it can make the procedure seem alarming and dangerous, but, in fact, these are relatively safe procedures. The radiation exposure from CT, PET, and SPECT scans is significant but within safe limits. If you have any concerns about possible side effects, ask a doctor to explain them to you.

The clinical history, the physical and neurological exams, and the laboratory tests will identify or rule out known causes of dementia. Other evaluations in addition to the medical assessment are done to understand the person's abilities and to help you plan for the future.

A *psychiatric and psychosocial evaluation* is based on interviews with the person and their family. This provides the basis for the development of a specific care plan for the person. It may be done by a doctor, nurse, or social worker. It includes helping family members evaluate their own emotional, physical, and financial resources, the home in which the person lives, the available community resources, and the person's ability to accept or participate in making plans for the future.

The physician must determine whether the patient is depressed. Depression can cause symptoms similar to dementia, and it can make an existing dementia worse. Whenever there is the possibility of depression, a psychiatrist experienced in geriatrics should see the patient. Depression is quite common and often improves with treatment.

An *occupational therapy evaluation* helps to determine how much people are able to do for themselves and what can be done to help them compensate for their limitations. It is done by an occupational, rehabilitation, or physical therapist. These therapists are important members of the health care team. Their skills are sometimes overlooked because in the past they were consulted only in cases where there was the potential for physical rehabilitation. However, they are able to identify the things that the person is still able to do, and they can devise ways to help the person remain as independent as possible. Part of this assessment is an evaluation of *ADLs* (activities of daily living). The person is observed in a controlled situation to see if they can manage money, fix a simple meal, dress themselves, and perform other routine tasks. If they can do part of these tasks, this is noted. These therapists are familiar with a variety of devices that can help some people.

Neuropsychological testing (also called cognitive function testing or psychometric testing) may be done to determine which areas of the person's mental function are impaired and which are still working well. This testing takes several hours. The tests evaluate such abilities as memory, reasoning, coordination, writing, judgment, expressing oneself, and understanding instructions. The testing psychologist will be experienced in making people feel relaxed and will take the person's education and interests into consideration.

The final part of the evaluation is your *discussion with the doctor* and perhaps with other members of the evaluating team. The doctor will explain the findings to you and the person with dementia if they are able to understand at least part of what is happening. The doctor should give you a specific diagnosis (or explain why a specific diagnosis is not possible at that time). The doctor should also give you a general idea of the person's prognosis (again, they may not be able to tell you exactly what to expect). The findings of other procedures, such as the ADL evaluation, the psychological tests, and the psychosocial history, will also be explained to you. You should be able to ask questions and come away with an understanding of the findings of the evaluation. The doctor may recommend medications or refer you and the person with dementia to community support services (or to someone who can advise you about such services). You, the doctor, and the person with dementia may identify specific problems and set up a plan to cope with them.

A complete evaluation may take more than one day. You may want to arrange to spread the evaluation over more than one day so that the person with a suspected dementia will not become too tired. It usually takes several days for laboratories to report their findings and for the doctor to put all these data together into a report.

Evaluations are almost always done on an outpatient basis. Sometimes family members and occasionally professionals advise against "putting a confused person through the 'ordeal' of an evaluation." We believe that every person with problems in memory and thinking should be adequately evaluated. An evaluation is not an unpleasant ordeal. Staff accustomed to working with people who have dementia are usually gentle and kind. Making the person as comfortable as possible ensures that the staff can determine the person's best performance.

You may want to arrange to spread the evaluation over more than one day so that the person will not become too tired

---

As we have said, there are many reasons why people develop the symptoms of dementia. Some of these are treatable, and a small number are fully reversible. If a treatable problem is not detected because an evaluation was not done, the afflicted person and their family may suffer unnecessarily for years. Certain causes of dementia can be treated if identified promptly but can cause irreversible damage if they are neglected.

Even if the evaluation finds that the person has an irreversible dementia, it will give you information about how best to care for the person and how best to manage their symptoms. It gives you a basis on which to plan for the future. Finally, by getting the evaluation, you will know that you have done all you can for them—and that is important too.

Finding Someone to Do an Evaluation

In most areas of the country, a family can find someone to do a thorough evaluation of a person with a suspected dementia. Your family physician may do the evaluation or refer you to a specialist who can. Your local hospital may give you the names of physicians who evaluate people with illnesses that cause dementia. The staff at teaching hospitals or medical schools in your area may know of professionals with a special interest in this field. The local Alzheimer's Association or other dementia service agency is a good place to inquire about knowledgeable physicians in your area. Dementia centers and "memory disorder clinics" have opened in some communities. If you hear of one, you may want to ask your physician about its reputation. Patients in managed care programs should expect—and receive—a full evaluation and explanation of the findings.

Before you schedule an evaluation, you can ask the evaluating physician what procedures they use and why. If you feel from this preliminary conversation that the doctor is not really interested in dementia, you should probably seek someone else.

How do you decide whether an accurate diagnosis has been made for someone in your family? In the final analysis, you must settle on a doctor whom you trust and whom you feel has done all they can, and then rely on their judgment. This is much easier when you are familiar with the terminology, the diagnostic procedures, and what is known about the diseases that cause dementia. If you have been given differing diagnoses, discuss this frankly with the doctor. It is important for you to feel certain that an accurate diagnosis has been made. Occasionally a physician will make a diagnosis of Alzheimer disease without doing a complete evaluation. It is not possible to make an accurate diagnosis without a complete assessment and tests that exclude other conditions. If this happens to you, we suggest you consider seeking a second opinion.

You may hear about people with similar symptoms who were "miraculously" cured, or you may hear statements like "memory loss can be cured." Considerable confusion has arisen because some of the causes of dementia are reversible and because dementia and delirium (see Chapter 17) are sometimes confused. There are also unscrupulous individuals who offer bogus "cures" for these illnesses. Chapter 18 discusses some of the things that have been promoted in the media as "treatments" for cognitive decline but whose benefits are unsubstantiated. An accurate diagnosis and a doctor you trust can help assure you that everything that can be done is being done. You can also keep informed about the progress of legitimate research through the websites of the Alzheimer's Association (www.alz.org), the National Institute on Aging at the National Institutes of Health (www.alzheimers.gov), and major research institutions.

The Medical Treatment and Management of Dementia

The illnesses that cause dementia require continuing medical attention. The availability of professional services varies. You, the caregiver, will provide much of the coordination of care. However, there are times when you will need the help of health care professionals.

The Physician

You will need a physician who can prescribe and adjust medications, answer your questions, and treat other, concurrent illnesses. The physician who provides continuing care will not necessarily be the specialist who carried out the initial evaluation of the person. They may be your family doctor, part of a geriatric team, or another doctor with a special interest in geriatric medicine. This doctor does not have to be a specialist, although they should be able to work with a neurologist or a psychiatrist if necessary. The doctor you select for continuing care must have the following attributes:

- be willing and able to spend the necessary time with you and the person who has dementia

- be knowledgeable about dementing illnesses and the special susceptibility of persons with dementia to other diseases, medications, and delirium

- be easily accessible

- be able to make referrals to physical therapists, social workers, and other professionals

Not all doctors meet these criteria. Some doctors have large practices and do not have the time to focus on your problems. It is impossible for any one person to keep up with all the advances in medicine, so some doctors may be knowledgeable about some fields of medicine but not be skilled in the specialized care of people who have dementia. Finally, some doctors are uncomfortable caring for people with chronic, incurable diseases. However, no physician should give you a diagnosis without following through with referrals to professionals who can give you the help you need. You may have to talk with more than one doctor before you find one who is right for you. Discuss your needs and expectations honestly with the doctor and talk over how you can best work with them. Doctors are required to keep patients' medical information confidential. Because of this, some doctors are reluctant to talk to other members of the family or may ask the person with dementia to sign a release form. There may be good reasons why you need to know about the person's medical conditions. Physicians who work with many families of people who have dementia find that conferring with the whole family is important. Discuss this problem frankly with doctors and ask them to be as open as they can be with the whole family.

The Nurse

In addition to the knowledge and experience of a physician, you may need the skills of a nurse who can work with the physician. The nurse may be the clinician you can reach most easily and can help coordinate the work that you, the doctor, and others do to provide the best possible care for the person who has dementia.

Nurses understand the difficulties of caring for a person with dementia at home. They can observe the person for changes in health status that need to be reported to the doctor and can give you support and counsel. After talking with you, the nurse can identify and help solve many of the problems you face and can teach you how to provide practical care for the person (for example, coping with catastrophic reactions, giving baths, helping with eating problems, managing a wheelchair). Nurses can teach you how and when to give medicine and how to know whether it is working correctly. A nurse may be available to come to your home to assess the person and offer suggestions for simplifying the person's environment and minimizing the effort you need to expend. Nurse practitioners can perform many of the functions of a physician, including prescribing medication. They often work closely with a primary care physician.

An advanced practice nurse, licensed vocational (practical) nurse, or physician's assistant may also be helpful to you. Your physician should be able to refer you to a nurse or physician's assis-

tant, or you can locate this help by calling your health department or a home health agency. Medicare or other health insurance pays for nursing services in specific situations if they are ordered by a physician (see pages 247–49).

In some areas, an occupational therapist or physical therapist may be available to help.

The Social Worker

Social workers have a unique combination of skills: they know the resources and services in your community, and they are skilled in assessing your unique situation and needs and matching these with available services. Some people may be unfamiliar with the help that social workers can provide. They are professionals whose ability to help you find resources can be invaluable. They can provide practical counseling and help you and your family think through plans. They can also help families work out disagreements over care.

Your physician may be able to refer you to a social worker, or if the person with dementia is hospitalized, the hospital social worker may be able to help. The local office on aging may have a social worker on staff who can help anyone over age 60.

Most communities have family service agencies staffed by social workers. To locate local social service agencies, look online for "social service organizations" for your state and local governments. You can also contact the national office of the Alliance for Strong Families and Communities (www.alliance1.org), which accredits private agencies and can provide you with the names of your nearest agencies.

Social workers work in a variety of settings. These include public social service agencies, nursing homes, senior citizen centers, public housing projects, and local offices of the state department of health. Sometimes these agencies have special units that serve elderly persons. There are also social workers in private practice in some communities. Some social workers will arrange supportive services for your relative who lives out of town. Social workers are professionally trained. In many states they must also be licensed or accredited. You should know the qualifications and training of the person you select.

Fees for social services vary depending on the agency, the services you need, and whether you are using other services of that agency (such as a hospital). Some agencies charge according to your ability to pay.

It is important to select a social worker who understands the illnesses that cause dementia.

The Geriatric Care Manager

The geriatric care manager helps people coordinate the complex services needed to care for ailing older adults. Many but not all geriatric care managers are knowledgeable about dementia, so it is important to get references or check with an agency such as the Alzheimer's Association to find out how they have helped others. You should directly ask the care manager about their knowledge level and experience in organizing care for people who have dementia, and you should ask for a fee schedule.

The Pharmacist

Increasingly powerful and effective medications are being prescribed for the management of dementia and the other illnesses that people who have dementia may experience. Be sure the pharmacist is aware of all the prescription and nonprescription drugs the person is taking so they can watch for potential drug interactions and alert you to potential side effects, especially when the person's prescriptions are ordered by multiple physicians.

CHAPTER 3

Characteristic Behavioral Symptoms in People Who Have Dementia

In Chapters 3 through 9 we discuss many of the problems that may occur in caring for a person who has dementia. Although as yet nothing can be done to cure some illnesses that cause dementia, *much can be done to make life easier for you and the person who has dementia.* The suggestions we offer come from our clinical experience and the experiences that family members have shared with us.

Each individual, each family, and each caregiver are different. You may never experience many of these problems. The problems you will face are influenced by the nature of the specific disease causing the dementia, by your personality, by the personality of the

person who has dementia, and, often, by other factors such as where you live. We do not want you to read through this section as if it were a list of what lies ahead of you. It is a comprehensive list of potential problem areas for you to use as a reference when a specific problem arises.

Do not read through this section as if it were a list of what lies ahead of you. It is a comprehensive list of potential problem areas for you to use as a reference when a specific problem arises. Much can be done to make life easier for you and the person who has dementia.

The Brain, Behavior, and Personality: Why People Who Have Dementia Do the Things They Do

The brain is a complex, mysterious organ. It is the source of our thoughts, our emotions, and our personality. Injury to the brain can cause changes in emotions, personality, and the ability to reason. The illnesses that cause dementia are biological: many of the mental functions and behavioral changes seen in dementia arise from structural and chemical changes in the person's brain. Most illnesses that cause dementia do their damage gradually, so the effects are not seen suddenly as they are when someone has a major stroke or head injury. Consequently, the behavior of a person who has dementia often seems puzzling. It is not always evident that many of the noticeable symptoms (changes in personality, for example) are the result of a disease, because the person often looks well. In contrast, the behavioral problems seen in a brain disease that begins suddenly are often easier to link to that condition.

You may wonder which behaviors are caused by the disease and which are deliberate or willful. Sometimes, family members disagree or even argue about this. In the following chapters we discuss some of the behavioral symptoms you may face and suggest ways you can respond. Understanding that the damage to the brain and an environment that is not adapted to the person's needs are common causes of behavioral symptoms will help you cope with them.

The brain is composed of billions of microscopic neurons, or nerve cells, and their many connections to other neurons is one reason the brain is a very complex organ. All the tasks of the brain—thinking, talking, dreaming, walking, listening to music, and hundreds of others—are the result of how these cells communicate with one another.

Different parts of the brain perform different tasks. When a person has a stroke and cannot speak, we know that the stroke occurred in the speech area of the brain and destroyed cells that are necessary for the person to express themselves. A stroke may cause extensive damage, but often the damage is limited to only a single area of the brain. In many of the illnesses that cause dementia, damage occurs in multiple areas and thereby affects many aspects of mental function. While a stroke does all its damage at once, Alzheimer disease gradually does more and more damage. This means that many cognitive abilities are damaged but in an uneven fashion. As a result, the person is able to do some things but not others. For example, they may be able to remember things from long ago but not from yesterday.

People who have brain damage may do things that don't make sense to us

Our brains do thousands of tasks, and we are usually not aware of most of them. We assume that other people's brains, like ours, are working as they should—but with a person who has dementia we cannot make this assumption. When the person does something odd or inexplicable, it is usually because some part of their brain has failed to do its job. In addition to controlling memory and language, the brain enables us to move our various body parts, helps filter out the things we don't need to pay attention to, gives feedback on the things we do, enables us to recognize familiar objects, and coordinates all the activities it is carrying out. When brain damage is uneven, people do things that don't make sense to us.

•

John Barstow can remember that he was angry with his spouse, but he cannot remember his spouse's explanation for the offending behavior. In fact, he may not even remember what his spouse did that made him angry in the first place.

•

Researchers have found that our brain stores and processes memories of emotions differently from memories of fact. It is possible for the dementia to damage one without damaging the other as much. Old social skills and the ability to make customary social remarks are often retained longer than insight and judgment. Thus, a person may sound fine to others but in fact be unable to care responsibly for themselves.

If the brain interferes with a person's ability to perform any step in a task, the person will not be able to do the rest of the task

---

It may be that damaged nerve cells, like a loose light bulb, connect sometimes and fail other times. This may be why a person can do something one day and not another. Even when we do something that seems simple, the brain must carry out many tasks. *If the illness that causes dementia prevents the brain from performing any one of the steps in a task, the task will not get done.*

•

"I asked my sister to make us both a cup of tea, but she ignored me. Then half an hour later, she went to the kitchen and made herself a cup of tea."

•

Obviously, this sister was still able to do this task but was not able to understand or act on spoken language even though she heard the request.

Behavioral and psychiatric symptoms are often caused by damage to the brain and are not something the person can control or prevent. Behavior that upsets you is rarely deliberate and almost never intended to "get your goat." Because the brain itself is damaged, the person is severely limited in their ability to learn new things or understand explanations. It is futile to expect the person to remember or learn, and it is frustrating to both of you to try to teach them something they can no longer master. The person does not *want* to act like this and *is trying as hard as they can.*

•

Mrs. Robinson helped out in her older daughter's kitchen, but when she visited her younger daughter, she only sat and criticized. The younger daughter felt that Mrs. Robinson had always preferred the older sister and that her refusal to help was a less-than-subtle reminder of her preference. In fact, the mother had been familiar with the older sister's kitchen before she became forgetful, so she could function pretty well in that kitchen, but she could no longer learn new information, even things as simple as where the dishes were kept in her younger daughter's unfamiliar kitchen.

•

A person's feelings also affect their behavior. The person who has dementia may feel lost, worried, anxious, vulnerable, or helpless much of the time. They may also be aware that they fail at tasks and feel that they are making a fool of themselves. Imagine what the person must feel like if they want to say something nice to their caregiver but all that comes out are curse words. Think how frightening it must be if a familiar home and familiar people now seem strange and unfamiliar. If we can find ways to make a person who has dementia feel more secure and comfortable, behavioral symptoms may decline.

Other things also affect behavior. When people are not feeling well, they will be less able to think. In Chapter 6 we discuss how illness, pain, and medication can make a person's thinking—and behavior—worse.

When you speak to a person with dementia, they need to hear you: the first step in the processes of communication is *sensory input*. The ability to repeat immediately what is heard may be retained, but the next step, to remember and process what was said, at least temporarily, is often lost in people who have Alzheimer disease. If the person cannot temporarily recall what you said, they cannot respond. Often a person can understand or recall only part of what was said and will act on only that part. If you say, "The grandchildren are coming to dinner, so you must have a bath," the person may comprehend or retain only "have a bath" and act accordingly. If he retains nothing of what you said, he may be angry when you lead him to the bathroom, because he has forgotten that company is coming.

As well as retaining what was heard, the person must comprehend what the words mean and evaluate what was said. Many things may go wrong in this process and may result in a reply that seems inappropriate to you. The person will act on what they *think* they heard. But they can act on only what their ears heard, their brain registered, their mental dictionary understood, and their mind processed. If their brain scrambles the message, they will respond in a way that is appropriate to what they understood. If, in their confusion, they think you are a stranger or that they are a youngster and you are their mother, their response will be based on the faulty understanding of the situation. A person who was usually placid may respond calmly, a person who was usually irritable may respond with anger, but whatever the response, it will be appropriate to the message *received*, not necessarily the message you gave.

The final step in communication is the person's answer. Things can go wrong here too. What comes out may not be what the person who has dementia intended. It may sound like an intentional evasion, an insult, or a foolish answer, but it is usually the result of an impairment in the person's ability to express themselves.

The person you are caring for may be unhappy but is doing the best they can

---

There is much that we do not know about this process. Neuropsychologists study the mind and try to understand these complex cognitive processes. Often a neuropsychologist or speech-language therapist can figure out why particular people act as they do, and sometimes the therapist can devise a way around the impairment. Although there is still an enormous amount to learn about how this process works, when people who have dementia say or do things that don't make sense or that seem nasty or deliberate, it is almost certainly the brain damage at work. *The person you are caring for is also often miserable and is doing the best they can.* In the rest of this book we show you many ways you can help.

You may not be able to figure out what the person with dementia understood or intended. Because the brain is so complex, even the best experts are often at a loss. In addition, many families do not have access to a neuropsychologist or speech-language therapist. Do the best you can; regard problems as the result of the brain damage, not as something you caused or something the person who has dementia intended. Affection, reassurance, and calm are best, even when things make no sense.

Caregiving: Some General Suggestions

Be informed. The more you know about the nature of the diseases that cause dementia, the more effective you will be in devising strategies to manage behavioral symptoms. The behavioral symptoms you have to cope with will vary with the specific disease the person has, which is one reason it is important to have an accurate diagnosis.

Share your concerns with the person who has dementia. When people's impairments are mild or moderate, they can take part in managing the problem. You may be able to share your grief and worries with each other. Together you may be able to devise memory aids that will help the person remain independent. People whose impairments are mild may benefit from counseling that can help them accept and adjust to their limitations. If the person does not recognize the problem, accept their point of view. Arguing with them will not help.

Try to solve your most frustrating problems one at a time. Families tell us that the day-to-day problems often seem to be the most insurmountable. Getting your mother to take her bath or getting supper prepared, eaten, and cleaned up can become daily ordeals. *If you are at the end of your rope, single out one thing that you can change to make life easier, and work on that.* Sometimes changing small things makes a big difference.

Get enough rest. One of the dilemmas many families face is that caregivers may not get enough rest or may not have the opportunity to get away from their caregiving responsibilities. This can make caregivers less patient and less able to tolerate irritating behavioral symptoms. If things are getting out of hand, ask yourself if this is happening to you. If so, you may want to focus on finding ways to get more rest or more frequent breaks from your caregiving responsibilities. We recognize that this is difficult to arrange. We discuss it in Chapter 10.

If you are at the end of your rope, find one thing you can change to make life easier and work on that

---

Use common sense and imagination. They are your best tools. Adaptation is the key to success. If something cannot be done in a certain way, ask yourself if it must be done that way. For example, when people can eat successfully with their fingers but cannot appropriately use a fork and spoon, don't fight the problem. Instead, serve as many finger foods as possible. Accept change. If the person insists on sleeping with a hat on, this is not harmful. Go along with it. Cognitive losses are uneven: accept what does not seem logical.

Use common sense and try to maintain a sense of humor

Maintain a sense of humor. It will get you through many crises. The person who has dementia is still a person. They need and enjoy a good laugh too. You may both be able to laugh when something goes wrong. Sharing your experiences with other families will help you. Surprisingly, these families may have faced the same

dilemma and found the shared experience funny as well as sad.

Try to establish an environment that allows as much freedom as possible but also offers the structure that people who have dementia need. Establish a regular, predictable, simple routine for meals, medication, exercise, bedtime, and other activities. Do things the same way and at the same time each day. If you establish regular routines, the person may gradually learn what to expect. Change routines only when they aren't working. Keep the person's surroundings reliable and simple. Leave furniture in the same place. Put away clutter.

Avoid talking *about* the person who has dementia when they are nearby—and remind others to avoid this too

---

Remember to talk to the person directly. Speak calmly and gently. Make a point of telling them what you are doing and why. Let them have a part in deciding things as much as possible. Avoid talking *about* the person when they are nearby, and remind others to avoid this also.

Have an ID bracelet made for the person who has dementia and consider a wearable tracking device. Include the nature of the person's disease (for example, "memory impaired") and your phone number on the ID bracelet. This is one of the single most important things you can do. Many people who have dementia get lost or wander away at one time or another, and an ID bracelet and wearable tracking device can save you hours of frantic worry. You can order a MedicAlert bracelet online. You may be able to purchase a bracelet with medical information on it from your drugstore or local chapter of the Alzheimer's Association. Phone apps and GPS devices that help you find a lost person are also available. See "The Management of Wandering" in Chapter 7 for more information.

> **An ID bracelet or necklace and a wearable tracking device or phone with a locator app can provide peace of mind and help you avoid hours of worry**

Keep the person active but not upset. Families often ask if computer programs, reality orientation, or keeping active will slow or stop the course of the disease. They may ask if being idle hastens the course of the disease. Some people who have dementia become depressed, listless, or apathetic. Families often wonder whether encouraging such a person to do things will help them to function better.

Activity helps to maintain physical well-being and may help prevent other illnesses and infections. Being active helps the person with dementia continue to feel that they are involved in the family and that their life has meaning.

Almost all people who have illnesses that cause dementia cannot learn as well as before because brain tissue has been damaged or destroyed. It would be unrealistic to expect them to learn new, complex skills. However, some individuals can learn simple tasks or facts if

they are repeated often enough. Many people who feel lost in a new place eventually "learn" their way around.

At the same time, too much stimulation, activity, or pressure to learn may upset the person who has dementia, may upset you, and may accomplish nothing. The key to this is balance:

- Accept that lost skills are gone for good (the person who has lost the ability to cook will not learn to fix a meal), *but* know that repeatedly and gently giving information that is within the person's abilities will help them function more comfortably (the person going into a strange day care setting will benefit from frequent reminders of where they are).

- Know that even small amounts of excitement—visitors, laughter, changes—can upset the person who has dementia, *but* plan interesting, stimulating things within their capabilities (a walk, visiting one old friend).

> **Keep the person active and engaged but avoid activities they can no longer do**

- Look for ways to simplify activities so that the person can continue to be involved within the limits of their abilities (the person who can no longer fix a whole meal may still be able to peel the potatoes).

- Look for things the person is still able to do and focus on them. A person's intellectual abilities are not all lost at once. Both of you will benefit from carefully assessing what they can still do and making the best use of those abilities. For example:

•

Mrs. Baldwin often cannot remember the words for things she wants to say, but she can make her meaning clear with gestures. Her daughter helps her by saying, "Point to what you want."

•

- Consider having a trained person come to the home to visit the person who has dementia or trying a group program such as day care designed for people with dementia (see Chapter 10). Day care often offers the right level of stimulation for some people and gives you time off as well.

- Give priority to keeping the person who has dementia calm and comfortable. Chapter 16 discusses some of the things you may have heard about that will prevent or delay the progress of an illness that causes dementia. While you may want to try some of these suggestions, such as "memory enhancing" games, keep in mind that if an activity or program upsets the person, you should stop using it.

Memory Problems

People who have dementia forget things quickly. For the person with memory impairment, life may be like constantly coming into the middle of a movie: one has no idea what happened just before what is happening now. People with illnesses that cause dementia may forget what you just told them, may start to prepare a meal and then forget to turn the stove off, or may forget what time it is or where they are. This forgetfulness of recent events can be puzzling when the person seems to be able to clearly remember events long past. There are some specific suggestions for memory aids throughout this book. You may think of others that will help you.

Forgetful people may remember events from the remote past more clearly than recent events, or they may remember some things and not others. This has to do with the way the brain stores and receives information; *it is not something the person does deliberately.*

The success of memory aids depends on the severity of the dementia. People who have mild dementia may devise reminders for themselves, while a person who has more severe dementia will only become more frustrated by their inability to use memory aids. Written notes and reminders may help people who have mild dementia.

It is often helpful to post a simple list of the day's activities on a piece of paper or a whiteboard where the person can easily see it. A regular daily routine is much less confusing than a frequently changing schedule.

Leave familiar objects (pictures, magazines, television remote) in their usual place where the person can see them easily. A tidy, uncluttered house will be less confusing to a person with dementia, and misplaced items will be easier to find. Putting labels on things occasionally helps. Labeling drawers, for example with "Rachel's socks" or "Rachel's nightgowns," may help.

Remember, however, that with an illness that causes a progressive dementia, the person will eventually be unable to read or to make sense of what they read. They may be able to read the words but be unable to act on them. Some families then use pictures instead of written messages.

As the disease progresses, the person will be unable to remember what you tell them *even for a minute*. You will need to repeat yourself and remind and reassure them over and over.

Overreacting, or Catastrophic Reactions

Even though Miss Ramirez had told her sister over and over that today was the day to visit the doctor, her sister would not get into the car until she was dragged in, screaming, by two neighbors. All the way to the doctor's office, she shouted for help, and when she got there she tried to run away.

•

Mr. Lewis suddenly burst into tears as he tried to tie his shoelaces. He threw the shoes in the wastebasket and locked himself, sobbing, in the bathroom.

•

Mrs. Coleman described several incidents similar to this one, in which her husband had mislaid his glasses.

"You threw out my glasses," he told her.

"I didn't touch your glasses," she answered.

"That's what you always say," he responded. "How do you explain that they are gone?"

"You do this to me every time you lose your glasses."

"I did not lose them. You threw them out."

Reflecting back, Mrs. Coleman knew that her husband had changed. In the past he would have merely asked her if she knew where his glasses were instead of accusing her and starting an argument.

•

People with brain diseases often become excessively upset and experience rapidly changing moods. Strange situations, confusion, groups of people, noises, being asked several questions at once, or being asked to do a task that is difficult for them can trigger these reactions. The person may weep, blush, or become agitated, angry, or stubborn. They may strike out at those trying to help them. They may cover their distress by denying what they are doing or by accusing other people of things.

Emotional overreaction is common when a situation overwhelms the limited thinking capacity of a person who has dementia. Many of us do this when we are bombarded with more things at one time than we can handle. People who have dementia have the same reaction to simpler, everyday experiences. For example:

•

Every evening, Mrs. Hamilton gets upset and refuses to take a bath. When her daughter insists, she argues and shouts. This makes the rest of the family tense. The whole routine is dreaded by everyone.

•

Taking a bath means that Mrs. Hamilton must think about several things at once: undressing, unbuttoning, finding the bathroom, turning on faucets, and climbing in the tub. At the same time, she feels insecure without clothes on and feels she has lost her privacy and independence. This is overwhelming for a person who cannot remember doing these tasks before, who can't remember how to do all these tasks, and whose mind cannot process all these activities at once. One way to react is to refuse to take a bath.

We use the term *catastrophic reaction* to describe this behavior. (The word *catastrophic* is used in a special sense; it does not mean that these situations are necessarily very dramatic or violent, only that the person *acts as if* a catastrophe has happened.) *Often a catastrophic reaction does not look like behavior caused by an illness that causes dementia. The behavior may look as if the person is merely being obstinate, critical, or overemotional.* It may seem inappropriate to get so upset over such a little thing.

Catastrophic reactions are upsetting and exhausting for you and for the person who has dementia. They are especially upsetting when it seems as if the person you are trying to help is being stubborn or critical. The person may get so upset that they refuse necessary care. Learning how to avoid or lessen catastrophic reactions is a major key to easier management of them.

Sometimes catastrophic reactions and forgetfulness are the first behaviors family members see when they begin to realize that something is wrong. The person with a mild impairment may benefit by being reassured that their panic is not unusual and that you understand their fear.

The things that can help prevent or reduce catastrophic reactions depend on you, on the individual who has dementia, and on the extent of their limitations. You will gradually learn how to avoid or limit these reactions. *First, you must fully accept that these behaviors are not just stubbornness or nastiness but a response that the person who has dementia cannot help.* The person is not just denying reality or trying to manipulate you. Though it seems strange, you may have more control over the person's reaction than they do.

The best way to manage catastrophic reactions is to stop them before they happen. The things that trigger these outbursts vary from one person to another and from one time to another, but as you learn what upsets your family member, you will be able to reduce the severity and frequency of outbursts. Some of the common triggers of catastrophic reactions are listed here:

- needing to think about several things at once (for example, all the tasks involved in taking a bath)

- trying to do something that they can no longer manage

- being cared for by someone who is rushed or upset

- not wanting to appear inadequate or unable to do things (for example, if the doctor asks a lot of questions that the person cannot answer)

- being hurried (when the person is thinking and moving more slowly than they used to)

- not understanding what they were asked to do

- not understanding what they saw or heard

- being tired (none of us are at our best when we are tired)

- not feeling well

- not being able to make themselves understood (see also the following section)

- feeling frustrated

- being treated like a child

- feeling sick and not knowing why

Anything that helps remind the person who has dementia about what is going on, such as following familiar routines, leaving things in familiar places, and having written instructions (for people who can manage them), can help to reduce catastrophic reactions. Because catastrophic reactions are brought on by having to think of several things at once, simplify what the person has to think about. Take things one step at a time, and give instructions or information step by step. For example, when you help a person bathe, tell them one thing at a time. Say, "I'm going to unbutton your shirt" and then reassure them, "It's all right." Say, "Now I'm going to slip your shirt off. That's

fine. Now take a step up into the tub. I will hold your arm."

Give the person who has dementia time to respond. They may react slowly and become upset if you rush them. Wait for them. If a person is having frequent catastrophic reactions, try to reduce the confusion around them. This might mean having fewer people in the room, having less noise, turning off the television, or reducing clutter in the room. The key is to simplify, to reduce the number of signals the impaired, disoriented brain must sort out.

If a person is having frequent catastrophic reactions, try to reduce the confusion around them

---

Find things the person who has dementia can realistically do. If strange places upset them, you may not want to take them on a trip. If they get tired or upset quickly, plan shorter visits with friends.

Plan demanding tasks for the person's best time of day. Avoid asking them to do things when they are tired. Know what the person's limits are and try not to push the person beyond them.

•

Mr. Lewis's family recognized that tying shoelaces had become too difficult for him but that he needed to remain as independent as possible. Buying him slip-on shoes solved the problem.

•

Mrs. Coleman's husband often lost things because he forgot where he put them. She found it helpful to ignore his accusations and help him find his glasses. Knowing that accusing her was his way of reacting to his forgetfulness made it easier for her to accept the insult.

•

Do the parts of a task yourself that the person who has dementia finds difficult. Families often worry that they are doing too much for a person and might make them more dependent. A good rule is to let people do activities themselves until they show the *first signs* of frustration, then assist them *before* they become more upset. Urging them on will usually only upset them more.

If a person seems more irritable than usual, check carefully for signs of illness or pain. *Even minor illness or discomfort can make the person's thinking worse.* Reactions to medication sometimes cause these outbursts. Have the person's medications been changed in the past month?

Reconsider your approach. Are you unintentionally rushing the person? Did you misunderstand them? Did you ignore their protests? Are your behavior and voice communicating your own frustration to them? Although it's easy to treat a person who is so dependent like a child, this may make them angry and trigger an outburst.

Reduce the number of tasks the person must do or think about at one time

Often multiple small stressors build up for the person who has dementia. Just trying to make sense of things, being tired, noise from the television, a delay in having lunch, feeling rushed—all may add up so that when you suggest a bath, the person is already so stressed that they blow up. The person may be so stressed that they are on the edge of an outburst much of the time. Reducing the overall stress level may make a necessary task like bathing easier.

When you are interacting with the person, watch for signs of increasing stress, such as irritability, stubbornness, flushing, and refusing to do things. If you notice any of these, stop what you are doing and let the person calm down.

Medications, pain, and newly developed illnesses are common causes of a sudden decline

When the person does become upset or resistant, remain calm and remove them from the situation in a quiet, unhurried way. Often the emotional storm will be over as quickly as it began, and the person will be relieved that the upset is over. Their short memory may work to your advantage: they may quickly forget the trouble.

As a person who has dementia becomes upset, their ability to think and reason temporarily declines even more. It is useless to argue with them, explain things to them, or even ask them to complete a task when they are in the grip of a catastrophic reaction. Arguing, explaining, or restraining them may make things worse. Help the person calm down and relax so that they can think as well as possible. Take them away from what upset them, if possible.

You may lose your temper with a person who is having catastrophic reactions or is unable to do what seems like a simple task. This usually will make the person's behavior worse. Losing your temper occasionally is not a calamity; take a deep breath and try to approach the problem calmly. The person will probably forget your anger much more quickly than you will.

> Take things one step at a time. Move slowly and quietly. Remember that the person is *not* being obstinate or doing this intentionally.

Try not to express your frustration or anger to the person who has dementia. Your frustration will further upset them when they cannot understand your reaction. Speak calmly. Take things one step at a time. Move slowly and quietly. Remember that the person is *not* being obstinate or doing this intentionally.

Gently holding a person's hand or patting them may help calm them, but the person may feel that you are restraining them and become more upset. Physically restraining a person often adds to their panic. Restrain a person only if it is absolutely essential for safety and if nothing else works.

If catastrophic reactions are happening often, keeping a log may help you identify their triggers. After the outburst is over, write down what happened, when it happened, who was around, and what happened just before the outburst started. Look for a pattern. Are there events, times, or people that might be triggering upsets? If so, can you avoid them?

These overreactions are distressing to the person who has dementia as well as to you. After they have calmed down, reassure them. Tell them that you recognize their distress and that you still care for them.

If you find that catastrophic reactions are occurring frequently and that you are responding with anger and frustration, this is a warning that you are overtired and overwhelmed. You are caught in a vicious circle that is bad for both you and the person who has dementia. You must have time away from the person. Read Chapter 10, "Getting Outside Help," and make the effort to take some time off for yourself even if you feel too tired and overwhelmed to do so.

You may feel that none of these suggestions will work, that you are caught in an endless battle. The suggestions we offer may not work, but if you are feeling that nothing will help you, this may be an indication of your own depression (see page 222). In fact, things can be found that will reduce catastrophic reactions in most people who have dementia.

> After the outburst is over, think about prior upsets and look for a pattern

Identifying triggers and reducing stressors can be challenging. Brainstorming with other family members in a support group is particularly helpful (see pages 239–41).

Combativeness

Mrs. Frank was having her hair done. The beautician was working on the back of her head, and Mrs. Frank kept trying to turn around. When this happened, the beautician would turn Mrs. Frank's head back. Then Mrs. Frank began batting at the beautician's hands. She looked as if she were about to cry. Finally, Mrs. Frank turned around in the chair and hit the beautician.

Mr. Williams stood close to a group of nurses who were talking. He bounced up and down on his toes. The nurses ignored him even though he bounced faster and faster. When he began to shout, one of the nurses took his arm to lead him away. He pulled away from her but she held on. When she did not let go, he struck her.

When an individual who has dementia hits (or bites, pinches, or kicks) another person, it is upsetting for everyone. Sometimes this happens frequently and the family caregiver or nursing home staff may feel that they cannot continue to provide care.

Combativeness is almost always an extreme catastrophic reaction. It often can be prevented by being alert to the person's signals that their stress level is rising. Perhaps if the beautician had continually talked to Mrs. Frank about what she was doing and showed her in a mirror how her hair was coming along, Mrs. Frank would have understood what was going on and would have been less upset. Turning and batting at the hairdresser were warnings that she was becoming distressed.

> **When people become agitated, stop whatever is upsetting them and let them relax**

Perhaps Mr. Williams wanted to join the conversation. If the nurses kept a log of his outbursts, they might observe that bouncing on his toes was a sign of his rising agitation. If the nurses had included him in their conversation or suggested something else he might enjoy doing, he might not have gotten upset. Physically holding or pulling someone is often perceived by the person as an attack and leads to an angry response.

When a person becomes agitated, immediately stop whatever is upsetting them and let them relax. Do not continue to push them. Reread the material on catastrophic reactions in this section and in other books. Look for ideas for preventing outbursts or stopping them when they first begin. As a last resort, small amounts of medication may be necessary to help people who are upset much of the time stay calm; however, medication is not a substitute for changing the things going on around the person or altering how caregivers respond to the person. See "Medications" in Chapter 6.

Problems with Speech and Communication

You may have problems understanding or communicating verbally with the person who has dementia. There are two kinds of communication problems: the problems people who have dementia have in expressing themselves to others, and the problems they have in understanding what people say to them. They may understand more than they can express or may express more than they can understand. Do not make assumptions about what a person understands.

Problems People Who Have Dementia Experience in Making Themselves Understood

The nature of communication problems and whether or not they will get worse depend on the specific disease. Do not assume that things will get worse.

Some people have only occasional difficulty finding words. They may have trouble remembering the names of familiar objects or people. They may substitute a word that sounds similar, such as saying "tee" for "tie" or "wrong" for "ring." They may substitute a word with a related meaning, such as saying "wedding" for "ring" or "music thing" for "piano." They may describe the object they cannot name, such as "it's a thing that goes around" for "ring" or "it's to dress up" for "necktie." Such problems usually do not interfere with your ability to understand what the person means. Some people have difficulty communicating their thoughts.

Mr. Zuckerman was trying to say that he had never had a neurological examination before. He said, "I really have not, not really, ever have been done, I have never ..."

With some language problems, the person cannot communicate the whole thought, but they can express a few of the words in the thought.

Mr. Mason wanted to say that he was worried about missing his ride home. He could say only, "Bus, home."

Sometimes people are able to ramble on quite fluently, and it seems as if they are talking a lot. They will often string together commonly used phrases, so what they say at first seems to make sense, but on reflection listeners may not be sure they understood the thought being expressed.

Mrs. Simmons said, "If I tell you something, I might stop in the middle and ... I'll be real sure about what I've done, ... said, ... sometimes I stop right in the middle and I can't get on with ... from ... that. In past records ... I can be so much more sure of the ... After I get my bearing again I can just go on as if nothing happened. We thought it was high time to start remembering. I just love to ... have to ... talk."

In these examples, it is possible to understand what the person is saying if we know the context.

When the limitations in ability to communicate frustrate the person and frustrate you, they can lead to repeated catastrophic reactions. For example, the person with an impairment may burst into tears or stomp out of the room when no one understands them.

Sometimes a person is able to conceal language problems. When a doctor asks a person if they know the word for a wristwatch (a common question used to evaluate language problems), the person may say, "Of course I do. Why do you ask?" or "I don't want to talk about it. Why are you bothering me?" when they cannot think of the word.

Some people begin to use curse words, even if they have never used such language before. This disturbing behavior appears to be a strange quirk of diseases that take away important language skills. It is commonly seen after a stroke that affects the language area of the brain. It must be like opening a "mental dictionary" to say something and having only curse words come out. One person who was asked why he cursed the day care staff said, "These are the only words I have." This behavior is rarely deliberate and sometimes upsets the person who curses as much as it does you.

With severe language problems, people may remember only a few key words, such as "No," which they may use whether or not they mean it. Eventually the person may be unable to speak. They may repeat a phrase, cry out intermittently, or mumble unintelligible phrases. In some language problems there seems to be no meaning in the jumbled words the person produces. Family members and caregivers often grieve when this happens and they can no longer communicate verbally with a loved one. We sense that language is the most human of mental skills. In some families the person with dementia continues to be a friend and companion—although a forgetful one—for a long time, but when they are unable to communicate anymore, the family feels they have lost that companionship. You may worry that the person will be sick or in pain and be unable to tell you.

How you help the person communicate depends on the kind of difficulty they are having. If they have been diagnosed as having had a stroke that interferes with language function, they should be seen by a stroke rehabilitation team as soon as possible after the stroke is diagnosed. Much can be done to rehabilitate people who have had strokes.

If the person is having difficulty finding the right word, it is usually less frustrating for them to have you supply the word for them than it is to let them search and struggle for the word. When a person uses the wrong word and you know what they mean, it may be helpful to supply the correct word. However, if doing so upsets them, it is better to ignore it. When you don't know what they mean, ask them to describe it or point to it. For example, the nurse did not know what Mrs. Kealey meant when she said, "I like your wrong." If the nurse had said, "What?" Mrs. Kealey might have become frustrated in trying to express herself. Instead, the nurse asked, "Describe a wrong." Mrs. Kealey said, "It's a thing that goes around." "Point to it," said the nurse. Mrs. Kealey did and the nurse responded, "Oh, yes, my ring." If the person gets lost in the middle of what they are saying, repeat their first few words—this may help get them started again.

When a person is having trouble expressing an idea, you may be able to guess what they are trying to say. *Ask* if you are guessing correctly. You might guess wrong, and if you act on an erroneous guess you will add to the person's frustration. Say, "Are you worried about catching the bus home?" or "Are you saying you have never had an examination like this before?"

People who have dementia communicate better when they are relaxed. Try to appear relaxed yourself (even if you have to pretend) and create a calm environment. Never rush the person who is trying to make themselves understood.

When a person cannot communicate verbally, establish a routine of regularly checking their comfort

---

Even when you cannot communicate with the person in the usual way, you can often guess what a person is trying to tell you. Remember that their feeling is usually accurate, although it may be exaggerated or not appropriate to the situation, but their explanation of why they feel a certain way may be confused. If Mr. Mason says, "Bus, home," and you say, "You aren't going on the bus," you will not have responded to his feelings. If you correctly guess that he is worried about going home, you can reassure him by saying, "Your daughter is coming for you at 3:00."

If a person can still say a few words or shake or nod their head, you will need to ask them simplified questions about their needs. Say, "Do you hurt?" or "Does this hurt?" Point to a body part rather than name it.

When a person cannot communicate, you must establish a regular routine of checking their comfort. Make sure that clothing is comfortable, that the room is warm, that there are no rashes or sores on their skin, that they are taken to the toilet on a regular schedule, and that they are not hungry or sleepy.

When a person repeats the same thing over and over, try distracting them. Change the subject, ask them to sing a familiar song, or talk about the feelings behind the statement. For example, if a person is searching for their mother, try saying "You must miss your mother" or "Tell me what your mother was like."

Problems People Who Have Dementia Experience in Understanding Others

Often people who have dementia have difficulty comprehending what you and others tell them. This is a problem that families sometimes misinterpret as uncooperative behavior. For example, you may say, "Mother, I am going to the grocery store. I will be back in half an hour. Do you understand?" Your mother may say, "Oh yes, I understand," when in fact she does not understand at all and will get upset as soon as you are out of sight.

People who have dementia also quickly forget what they did understand. When you give them a careful explanation, they may forget the first part of the explanation before you get to the rest of it.

People who have dementia can have trouble understanding written information even when they can still read the letters or words. For example, to determine exactly what a person can still comprehend, we may hand them a newspaper and have them read the headline, which they may be able to do correctly. Then when we hand them the written instructions "Close your eyes," they do not close their eyes although they correctly read the words aloud. This indicates that they cannot understand what they are reading.

•

Jan told her mother that lunch was in the refrigerator. She left a note on the refrigerator door to remind her mother. Her mother could read the note aloud but could not understand what it said, so she didn't eat her lunch. Instead she complained that she was hungry.

•

This can be infuriating until you consider that reading and understanding are two different skills, one of which may be lost without the loss of the other. It is not safe to assume that a person can understand and act on messages they can hear or read. You will need to observe them to know whether they can act on them. If they do not act on instructions, assume they have a problem in understanding language.

The person who can understand what they are told in person may not be able to comprehend what they are told over the phone. When a person who has dementia does not understand what you told them, the problem is not inattentiveness or willfulness, but an inability of the malfunctioning brain to make sense of the words it receives.

It is not safe to assume that a person can understand and act on messages that they repeat or read aloud

---

There are several ways to improve your verbal communication with a person who has dementia:

- Make sure the person does hear you. Hearing acuity declines in later life, and many older people have a hearing deficit.

- Lower the tone (pitch) of your voice. A raised pitch is a nonverbal signal that one is upset. A lower pitch is also easier for a hearing-impaired person to hear.

- Eliminate distracting noises and activities. The inability to tune out extraneous stimuli can make a person unable to understand you if other noises or distractions are present.

- Use short words and short, simple sentences. Avoid complex sentences. Instead of saying, "I think I'll take the car to the garage tonight instead of in the morning because in the morning I will get caught in traffic," just say, "Taking the car to the garage now."

- Ask only *one* simple question at a time. Avoid questions like "Do you want an apple or pie for dessert, or do you want to have dessert later?" Complex choices may overload the person's decision-making ability.

- Ask the person to do one task at a time, not several. They may not be able to remember several tasks or may be unable to make sense of your request. Most of the things we ask a person to do—take a bath, get ready for bed, put on a coat so we can go to the store—involve several tasks. The person who has dementia may not be able to sort out these tasks. We help them by breaking down each task into individual steps and asking them to do one step at a time.

- Speak slowly, and wait for the person with dementia to respond. The person's response may be much slower than what seems natural to us. Wait.

You can also improve communication with the person and your understanding of their needs by using the nonverbal aspects of communication. We communicate through both what we say and the way we move our faces, eyes, hands, and bodies. Everyone uses this nonverbal system of communication without thinking about it. For example, we say, "He looks mad," "You can tell by the way they look at each other that they are in love," "You can tell by the way she walks who's boss," "I know you aren't listening to me," and so on. These are all things we are communicating without words. People who have dementia can remain sensitive to these nonverbal messages when they cannot understand language well, and they often remain able to express themselves nonverbally.

For example, if you are tired, you may send nonverbal messages that upset the person. Then they may get agitated, which will upset you. Your hands, face, and eyes will reveal your distress, which further agitates the person who has dementia. If you are unaware of the significance of body language, you may wonder what happened to upset them. In fact, we all do this all the time. For example, "No, I am not upset," you tell a spouse. "But I know you are," they reply. They can tell by the set of your shoulders that you are upset.

If you are living with a person who has dementia, you have already learned to identify many of the nonverbal clues that they send to make their needs known. Here are some additional ways to communicate nonverbally:

- *Remain pleasant, calm, and supportive.* Even if you feel upset, your body language will help to keep the person calm.

- *Express affection, if you know this helps.* Smile, take the person's hand, put an arm around their waist, or show affection in some other physical way.

- *Look directly at them.* Look to see if they are paying attention to you. If they use body language to signal that they are not paying attention, try again in a few minutes.

- *Use other signals besides words.* Point, touch, hand the person things. Demonstrate an action or describe it with your hands (for example, brushing teeth). Sometimes if you get a person started, they will be able to continue the task.

- *Avoid assuming complex reasons for the person's behavior.* Because the person's brain can no longer process information properly, they experience the world differently from the way you do. Because nonverbal communication depends on a whole different set of skills than verbal communication, you may be better able to understand the person by considering what it *feels* like they are saying rather than what you *think* they are saying, through either actions or words.

Even when a person is unable to communicate, they still need and enjoy affection. Holding hands, hugging, or just sitting companionably together is an important way to continue to communicate. The physical care that you give a person who has a severe dementia communicates to them your concern and that they are protected.

Loss of Coordination

Because illnesses that cause dementia affect many parts of the brain, the person who has dementia may lose the ability to make their hands and fingers do certain familiar tasks. They may understand what they want to do, and although their hands and fingers are not stiff or weak, the message just does not get through from the brain to the fingers. Doctors use the word *apraxia* to describe this failure of the brain to communicate with muscles. An early sign of apraxia is a change in a person's handwriting. Another, later indication is a change in the way a person walks. Apraxias may progress gradually or change abruptly depending on the disease. For example, at first a person may seem only slightly unsteady when walking but later will gradually develop a slow, shuffling gait.

It can be difficult for a person not trained to evaluate illnesses that cause dementia to separate problems of memory (can the person remember what they are supposed to do?) from problems of apraxia (can the person make their muscles do what they are supposed to do?). Both problems occur when the brain is damaged by disease. It is not always necessary to distinguish between them in order to help the person manage as independently as possible.

When apraxia begins to affect walking, the person may be slightly unsteady. You must watch for this and provide either a handrail or someone to hold on to when the person is using stairs and stepping up onto or down off a curb. If you have the person hold on to you, be sure your own footing is secure.

Losses of coordination and manual skills may lead to problems in daily living such as bathing, managing buttons or zippers, dressing, pouring a glass of water, and eating. Using a phone requires good coordination, and a person who does not appear to have any motor impairment may in fact be unable to use a phone to call for help.

Some of the things a person has difficulty with may have to be given up. Others can be modified so that the person who has dementia can remain partially independent. When you modify a task, the key is to simplify, rather than change, the task. Because of their intellectual impairment, people who have dementia may be unable to learn even a simpler *new* task. Consider the nature of each task. Ask yourself if it can be done in a simpler way. For example, shoes that slip on are easier to put on than shoes with laces. It is easier to drink soup out of a mug than to spoon it from a bowl. Finger foods are more easily managed than foods that must be cut with a knife and fork. Can the person do part of the task if you do the difficult part? You may already have discovered that the person can dress themselves if you help with buttons or snaps.

A person may feel tense, embarrassed, or worried about their clumsiness. They may try to conceal their increasing disability by refusing to participate in activities. For example:

·

Mrs. Fisher had always enjoyed knitting. When she abruptly gave up this hobby, her daughter could not understand what had happened. Mrs. Fisher said only that she no longer liked to knit. In fact, her increasing apraxia was making knitting impossible, and she was ashamed of her awkwardness.

·

A relaxed atmosphere often helps make the person's clumsiness less apparent. It is not unusual for a person to have more difficulty with a task when they are feeling tense.

Sometimes a person can do something one time and not another time. This may be a characteristic of the brain impairment, not laziness. Being hurried, being watched, being upset, or being tired can affect the person's ability to do things—just as it does for anyone. Having a brain disease makes these natural fluctuations more dramatic. Sometimes people can do one task with no problem, such as zipping up pants, but be unable to do another similar task, such as zipping up a jacket. It may seem that the person is being difficult, but the reason may be that one task is impossible because it is different in some way.

Sometimes a person can do a task if you break it down into a series of smaller tasks and take one step at a time. For example, brushing your teeth involves picking up the toothbrush, putting toothpaste on it, putting the toothbrush in your mouth, brushing, rinsing, and so on. Gently remind the person of each step. It may help to demonstrate. You may have to repeat each step several times. Sometimes it helps to put the familiar necessary tool, such as a spoon or comb, into the person's hand and gently start their arm moving in the right direction. Beginning the motion seems to help the brain remember the task.

An occupational therapist is trained to assess what motor skills the person has retained and how they may make the best use of them. If you can obtain an occupational therapy evaluation, this information can help you give the person who has dementia the help they need without taking away their independence.

In the later stages of some of the diseases that cause dementia, extensive loss of muscle control occurs, and the person may bump into things and fall down. We discuss this in Chapter 5.

People who have dementia may have other physical conditions that also interfere with their ability to do daily tasks. Part of the problem may be in the muscles or joints and another part of the problem in the impaired brain. Such complicating conditions include tremors (shaking), muscle weakness, joint or bone diseases such as arthritis, and stiffness caused by medication or by Parkinson disease.

Some people have tremors. These are shaking movements of the hands or body. These can make many activities difficult for a person, but an occupational therapist or physical therapist may be able to show you how to minimize the effects of tremors. Medications may help.

Some people with neurological conditions, especially Parkinson disease, have difficulty starting a movement or get "stuck" in the middle of a movement. This can be frustrating for both of you. If this is a problem, here are some helpful hints:

- If the person becomes "glued to the floor" while walking, tell them to walk toward a goal or to look at a spot or a line on the floor a few feet in front of them. This may help them get going again.

- It may be easier to get out of a chair that has armrests. Also, try raising the sitting person's center of gravity by raising the chair seat two to four inches. A firm seat is needed. Use a firm pillow or a higher chair such as a dining room chair or a director's chair. Avoid low chairs with soft cushions. Instruct the person to move forward to the edge of the chair and spread their feet about one foot apart to give a wider base to stand on. Ask the person to put their hands on the armrests and then to rock back and forth to gain momentum. On the count of three, have them get up quickly. Have them take time to gain their balance before beginning to walk.

- Sitting down in a chair may be easier to do when the person puts both hands on the armrests, bends forward as far as possible, and sits down slowly.

Muscle weakness or stiffness may occur when a person does not move around much. Remaining active is important for memory-impaired people.

Occasionally, a person who is taking one of the major tranquilizers or neuroleptic drugs will become stiff and rigid or may become restless. These may be side effects of the medication. They can be very uncomfortable. Notify your doctor. If the medication is necessary, the dosage can be changed or a different medication can be prescribed to overcome this side effect.

Arthritic joints can be painful to move. If the person resists or fights when you help them dress, consider that you may be hurting them when you move their limbs. A physical therapy consultation can help you with this problem.

There are many techniques and devices to help people with physical limitations remain independent. When you consider these techniques or devices, remember that most of them require the ability to learn to do something a new way or to learn to use a new gadget. People who have dementia may not be able to learn the new skills needed.

Loss of Sense of Time

A person who has dementia loses the uncanny ability normal individuals have for judging the passage of time. They may repeatedly ask you what time it is, feel that you have left them for hours when you are out of sight for only a few minutes, or want to leave a place as soon as they have arrived. It is not hard to understand this behavior when you consider that, to know how much time has passed, one must be able to remember what one has done in the immediate past. The person who forgets quickly has no way to measure the passage of time.

In addition to this defect of memory, it appears that diseases that cause dementia can affect the internal clock that keeps us on a reasonably regular schedule of sleeping, waking, and eating. It will be helpful to you to recognize that this behavior is not deliberate (although it can be irritating). It is the result of the loss of brain function.

The ability to read a clock may be lost early in the course of the disease. Even when a person can look at the clock and say, "It is 3:15," they may be unable to make sense of this information.

Not being able to keep track of time can worry the forgetful person. Many of us, throughout our lives, are dependent on a regular time schedule. Not knowing the time can make people worry that they will be late, be forgotten, miss the bus, overstay their welcome, miss lunch, or miss their ride home. The person who has dementia may not know just what they are worried about, but a general feeling of anxiety may make them repeatedly ask you what time it is. And, of course, as soon as you answer them, they will forget the whole conversation and ask again.

> **The person who forgets quickly has no way to measure the passage of time**

Sometimes a person feels that you have deserted them when you have been gone only briefly. This is because they have no sense of how long ago you left. Setting a timer or an old-fashioned hourglass or writing a note—"I am in the backyard gardening and will be in at 3:00 p.m."—might help the person wait more patiently for your return. Be sure to select a cue (timer, note) that the person can still comprehend. Perhaps you can think of other ways to reduce this behavior. For example:

When the Jenkinses went to dinner at their son's house, Mr. Jenkins would almost immediately put his hat and coat on and insist that it was time to go home. When he could be persuaded to stay for the meal, he insisted on leaving immediately afterward. His son thought he was just being rude.

•

Things went more smoothly when the family understood that this was because the unfamiliar house, the added confusion, and Mr. Jenkins's lost sense of time upset him. The family thought back over Mr. Jenkins's life and hit upon an old social habit that helped them. In earlier years he had enjoyed watching the football game after Sunday dinner. Now his son turned on the television as soon as Mr. Jenkins finished eating. Because this was an old habit, Mr. Jenkins would stay for about an hour, giving his wife time to visit, before he got restless for home.

Symptoms That Are Better Sometimes and Worse at Other Times

F amilies often observe that the person can do something one time but not another time.

•

"In the morning my mother does not need as much help as she does in the evening."

•

"My wife can use the bathroom alone at home, but she insists she needs help at our daughter's house."

•

"My husband does not get as angry and upset at day care as he does at home. Is this because he is angry with me?"

•

"Bill said a whole sentence yesterday, but today I can't understand a thing he says. Was he trying harder yesterday?"

•

Fluctuations in ability are common in people with diseases that cause dementia. While everyone has fluctua-tions in ability, they are more noticeable in people with dementia. People who have dementia have good days and bad days; some are better in the morning, when they are rested; some have more problems in less familiar settings; some do better when they feel more relaxed. Some fluctuations have no explanation. Whatever the likely reason, such fluc-tuations are normal and do not signal a change in the course of the disease.

People who have dementia are more vulnerable than others to minor changes in health (see Chapter 6). An abrupt change in the ability to do some-thing or in the overall level of function may indicate a medication reaction or a new illness. If you suspect this kind of change, it is important to contact the person's physician.

The brain damage itself accounts for some fluctuation. It is possible that damaged nerve cells that fail most of the time do work occasionally. It is also possible that less damaged or undamaged areas can intermittently take over and temporarily "fix" a defective system.

Fluctuations in ability are normal and do not signal a change in the course of the disease

---

Unrecognized changes in the environment can also lead to fluctuations in the person's ability to function. Carefully examining whether the environment has changed will allow you to rearrange things to make the person more comfortable.

All these causes of variation in ability are beyond the person's deliberate control. People who have dementia are usually trying as hard as they can. You can help them the most by learning which things in their environment bring out their best and which things cause more disability.

CHAPTER 4

Problems in Independent Living

Mild Cognitive Impairment

Because most diseases that cause dementia start imperceptibly and progress gradually, and because early identification will be important when effective treatments are available, researchers have increasingly focused on identifying dementia at its very beginnings. This has proved to be a challenging task because the brain changes in Alzheimer disease begin ten to twenty years before recognizable symptoms can be identified and the subtle changes that occur with normal aging are similar to the beginning symptoms of dementia. These challenges are being intensively studied, and earlier detection, even detection at the very beginnings of the brain changes, might be possible in the future.

The difficulty of the task at present is illustrated by the lack of consensus on how to define the earliest symptoms. Doctors use the term *mild cognitive impairment* (MCI) to identify people who have the earliest detectable symptoms (see Chapter 17, pages 295–96). About half of people with a diagnosis of MCI will develop dementia over the next five years, but half will not.

When a diagnosis of MCI has been made, the uncertainty of the future is a challenge. For this reason, we suggest that people with MCI stay as active and busy as possible. Follow-up with the doctor or clinic that made the diagnosis is essential to determine whether the symptoms have progressed, stayed the same, or improved.

> The uncertainty of the future is a challenge when a diagnosis of mild cognitive impairment has been made

Once a person has received a diagnosis of MCI, make sure they have prepared a will and an advance directive (see Chapter 14). Discuss preferences for future care in case the symptoms do progress. Most individuals with MCI are aware of their difficulties. Many find it beneficial to express their frustrations, but continued focus on their memory problems can make it even harder for them to remember. Encouraging the use of a memory pad, as well as avoiding situations in which pressure to remember is high, can help the person function better. Encourage the use of "to do" lists and reminder notes. Keeping the person's living area neat helps to avoid losing things. Routines help some people. The Alzheimer's Association offers support groups for people with MCI and provides social networking site chat rooms for people with MCI.

Make sure that medical problems are optimally treated and that medications that can impair memory are elim-inated or minimized. Reduce the risk of forgetting medications or taking a dose twice by keeping medications in a pill container that has a compartment for each day of the week. Depression and anxiety, if present, should be treated.

The key to living with MCI is the same as living with any of the other health problems of later life: do not panic, because the condition may not worsen. Continue to enjoy life.

Managing the Early Stages of Dementia

As people begin to develop a disease that causes dementia, they may begin to have difficulty managing in-dependently. You may suspect that the person is mismanaging their money, worry that they should not be driving, or wonder if they should be living alone. Surprisingly, about 20 percent of people with dementia are living alone.

People who have early stage de-mentia often appear to be managing well, and they may insist that they are fine and that you are interfering. It can be difficult to know when you should take over and how much you should take over. It can also be painful to take away the outward symbols of a person's independence, especially if the person adamantly refuses to move, to stop driving, or to relinquish their financial responsibilities.

One reason these changes are so difficult is that they reflect a loss of in-dependence and responsibility. This is often upsetting not only to the person with early symptoms but also to family members and friends. (We discuss these role changes in Chapter 11.) Making necessary changes may become easier when people understand the feelings involved.

The first step in deciding whether the time has come to make changes in a person's independence is to get an evaluation. This will tell you what the person is still able to do and what they are no longer able to do. It can also give you the authority to insist on necessary changes. When a professional eval-uation is not available, you and your family must analyze each task as thor-oughly and objectively as possible and decide whether the person can still do each specific task *completely, safely,* and *without becoming upset.*

The illnesses that cause dementia bring about many kinds of losses. Among them are loss of independence, skills, control over one's daily activities, and the ability to do those things that make one feel useful or important. The diseases that cause dementia limit the possibilities the future can hold. While others can look forward to things getting better, the person who is developing dementia must gradually realize that their future is limited. Perhaps the most terrible loss of all is the loss of memory. Losing one's memories means losing one's day-to-day connections with others and with the past. The distant past may seem like the present. Without a memory of today or an understanding that the past is past, the future ceases to have meaning.

> **One reason changes are so difficult for people with dementia is that the changes represent a loss of independence and responsibility**

As losses accumulate in a person's life, it is natural for them to cling even more tightly to the things that remain. Understandably, they might respond to such changes with resistance, denial, or anger. The person's need for familiar surroundings and the determination of most people not to be a burden to anyone make it understandable that a person who has dementia will not want to give up these things. Accepting the necessity to do so means facing the extent and finality of an illness, something that many people find hard to do.

In addition, the person who has dementia might be unable to make complete sense of what is going on. Even early in the disease, they may completely forget recent events. Without a recollection of leaving the stove on or of having an auto accident, they may reasonably insist that they can take care of themselves or that they are still a good driver. They are not "denying" the reality of the situation—they just cannot remember the mistakes that are evidence of their impairment. If they are not able to assess their own limitations, it may seem to them as if things are being unfairly taken away from them and that their family is "taking over." By recognizing how the person may feel, you will be able to find ways to help them make the necessary changes and still feel that they are in control of their life.

When a Person Must Give Up a Job

The time when a person must give up their job depends on the kind of job they have and whether they must drive as part of their job. Sometimes an employer will tell you or the person directly that they must retire. Some employers will be willing to retain a person in a job that is much less demanding.

Sometimes the family must make this decision. You may realize that this time has come.

If the person must give up their job, there are two areas that you must consider: the emotional and psychological adjustments involved in such a major change, and the financial changes that will be involved. For most people, their job is a key part of how they define who they are. This is one reason a person who has dementia may resist giving up their job or may insist that nothing is wrong. Adjustment to retirement may be painful and distressing. A counselor or social worker can be invaluable in helping a person who is having difficulty.

It is important that you consider the financial future of the person who has dementia. (This is discussed in Chapter 14.) Retirement can create special problems. Individuals who are forced to retire early because of an illness that causes dementia should be entitled to the same retirement and disability benefits as a person with any other disabling *disease*. In some cases, benefits have been denied on the erroneous grounds that declining job performance is not a disease. Such a decision can substantially reduce income. If this happens, it is important to establish that dementia is the cause of the declining performance. If this approach is unsuccessful, you may want to obtain legal counsel.

Federal law (the Social Security Disability Act) provides assistance to people who become disabled before age 65, either as Social Security Disability Income (SSDI) or Supplemental Security Income (SSI). To receive SSDI, the disabled person must have worked twenty out of the past forty calendar quarters and no longer be able to do gainful work because of a medically determinable physical or mental illness that will result in death or that has lasted for at least twelve months. The amount of the financial benefit is based on the person's earnings at the time they stop working. Thus, a person who is developing symptoms of dementia and tries a lower-paying job before applying for SSDI may receive a lower payment than a person who applies for SSDI directly after stopping their original job. People who have dementia often have no difficulty obtaining benefits, but some claims are still being denied. Preparing for and applying for SSDI is especially important for anyone who must retire early and for people who have frontotemporal dementia (because their impairments are often not obvious to others).

Many people are denied disability on their initial application and give up. But persistence through the appeals process often results in reversal of the initial decision. A diagnosis of early onset dementia should automatically qualify the person for expedited review of a claim for SSDI or SSI.

When a Person Can No Longer Manage Money

The person who has dementia may lose the ability to make change, become irresponsible with their money, or be unable to balance their checkbook or pay their bills. Occasionally, when a person can no longer manage their money, they will accuse others of stealing from them.

Said Mr. Fried, "My wife has kept the books for the family business for years. I knew something was wrong when my accountant came to me and told me the books were a terrible mess."

Mr. Rogers said, "My wife was giving money to the neighbors, hiding it in the wastebasket, and losing her purse. So I took her purse—and her money—away from her. Then she was always saying I stole her money."

Money often represents independence, so it is not surprising that people with dementia are often reluctant to give up control of their finances

Because money often represents independence, some people are psychologically unwilling to give up control of their finances. Sometimes you can take over the household accounts by simply correcting the efforts of the person affected by dementia after she has done her work. If you have to take a debit or credit card away against a person's wishes, it may help to write a memo such as "My son Alex now takes care of my banking" and put the note where the person can refer to it to refresh their memory.

It can be upsetting when a person accuses others of stealing, but this is easier to understand when you think about human nature. We have been taught all our lives to be careful with money, and when money disappears, most of us wonder if it was stolen. As a person's brain becomes less able to remember what is really happening, it is not surprising that they become anxious and suspicious that their money is being stolen. Avoid getting into arguments about it. That may upset the person more.

Some families find that giving the forgetful person a small amount of spending money (perhaps small change or several one-dollar bills) helps. If the money is lost or given away, it is only a minimal amount. Since many people feel secure if they have a little bit of cash on hand, this is one way to avoid conflicts about money. One peculiarity of the diseases that cause dementia is that a person can lose the ability to make change before they lose the knowledge that they need money.

Mrs. Hutchinson has always been fiercely independent about her money, so Mr. Hutchinson gave her a purse with some change in it. He put her name and address in the purse in case she lost it. She insisted on paying her hairdresser by check long after her husband had arranged to pay the bill by debit. So Mr. Hutchinson gave her some checks stamped VOID by the bank. Each week she gives one to the hairdresser. Mr. Hutchinson privately arranged with the hairdresser that these would be accepted and that he would continue to pay ahead of time by debit.

This may seem extreme. It may also seem unfair to dupe one's wife this way. In reality, it allows her to continue to feel independent, and it allows her tired and burdened husband to manage the finances and keep the peace.

Money matters can cause serious problems, especially when the person who has dementia is suspicious or when other members of the family disagree on how to handle the issues. (It may be helpful here to read "Suspiciousness" in Chapter 8 and "Coping with Role Changes and Family Conflict" in Chapter 11.) Your ingenuity can be a great help to you in making money matters less distressing.

When a Person Can No Longer Drive Safely

The time may come when you realize that your family member can no longer drive safely. While some people will recognize their limits, many are unwilling to give up driving. As a group, people who have dementia and continue to drive are much more likely to have accidents than other people their age.

For most experienced drivers, driving is a skill so well learned that it is partly "automatic." A person can go back and forth to work every day with their mind on other things—perhaps answering calls or listening to music. It does not take much concentration to drive, but when the traffic pattern suddenly changes, we rely on our mind to immediately focus on the road and respond swiftly. Because driving is a well-learned skill, a person who has dementia can still *appear* to be driving well when they are not really a safe driver. Driving requires a highly complex interaction of eyes, brain, and muscles and the ability to solve complicated problems quickly. A person who is still apparently driving safely may have lost the ability to respond appropriately to an unexpected problem on the road. They may be relying entirely on the automatic aspects of driving and be unable to shift quickly from a habitual response to a different response when the situation demands it.

Often people make the decision themselves to stop driving when they feel that they "aren't as sharp as they used to be." But if your family member does not, you have a responsibility to them and to others to carefully determine whether or not their driving is dangerous, and to intervene when it is. This may be one of the first situations in which you take a decision out of the hands of the person who has dementia. You may feel hesitant to do this, but you will probably be relieved once you have stopped a forgetful person from driving. Do not push someone who hesitates to drive to continue to drive.

There is some controversy over whether a person who has dementia can continue to drive in the early phases of the illness. No test score can determine this, but a trained occupational therapist can evaluate driving skills. To decide whether the time has come for the person to stop driving, look at the skills that are needed to drive safely and evaluate whether the person still has these skills—both in the car and in other situations:

- *Good vision.* A person must have good vision, or vision corrected with glasses, and be able to see clearly *both* in front and out of the corners of their eyes (peripheral vision) so that they see things coming toward them from the sides.

- *Good perception.* The brain merges the sensory information it receives in a way that makes it understandable. For example, it integrates all the visual information it receives while a person is driving so that it can quickly identify something out of the ordinary, such as a young child standing on a curb—this should alert the driver that the child may dart out into the street. Diseases that cause dementia impair the brain's ability to put information together in the correct way and therefore can affect a basic aspect of driving ability.

- *Good hearing.* A person must be able to hear well, or have their hearing corrected with hearing aids, so that they are alert to the sounds of approaching cars, horns, and so forth.

- *Quick reaction time.* A driver must be able to react quickly—to turn, to brake, and to avoid accidents. Older people's reaction time, when it is formally tested, is slightly slower than that of young people, but in older people who are healthy it does not slow enough to interfere with driving. However, if you see that a person seems slowed down or reacts slowly or inappropriately to sudden changes around the house, this should alert you to the possibility of the same limitations when they are driving.

- *Ability to make decisions.* A driver must be able to make *appropriate* decisions rapidly and *calmly*. The ability to make a correct decision when a child darts in front of the car, a driver honks, and a truck is approaching all at once necessitates being able to solve complicated, unfamiliar problems quickly and without panicking. People who have dementia often rely on habitual responses, and the habitual response may not be the correct one in a given driving situation. Some people also become confused and upset when several things happen at once. You will see these problems, if they are occurring, around the house as well as in the car.

- *Good coordination.* Eyes, hands, and feet must all work together well to handle a car safely. If a person is getting clumsy, or if their way of walking has changed, it should alert you that they may also have trouble getting their foot on the brake.

- *Alertness to what is going on around one.* A driver must be alert to all that is going on without becoming upset or confused. If a person is "missing things" that happen around them, they may no longer be a safe driver.

Sometimes driving behaviors alert you to problems. Forgetful people may get lost on routes that would not have confused them previously. Being lost can distract the driver and further interfere with their ability to react quickly. Sometimes driving too slowly is a clue that the driver is uncertain of their skills—but this does not mean that every cautious driver is an impaired driver. Drivers who have dementia may hit the accelerator when they mean to hit the brake.

People who have dementia may become angry or aggressive when they drive, or they may inappropriately believe that other drivers are "out to get them." This is dangerous. Occasionally a person who has dementia is also drinking too much. Even small amounts of alcohol impair the driving ability of people who have dementia. If this dangerous combination affects your family member, you must intervene.

The "grandchild test" is one way to decide whether a person should still be driving. If you would not let a person drive your child or grandchild, then that person should not be driving.

Some people voluntarily give up driving. Others require the involvement of the Department of Motor Vehicles.

If you are concerned about the driving ability of a person who has dementia, you should first approach the problem by discussing it frankly with them. Even though a person is cognitively impaired, they are still able to participate in decisions that involve them. How you initiate such a discussion may affect their response. People with brain impairments are sometimes less able to tolerate criticism than they were before, so you will want to use tact in such a discussion. If you say, "Your driving is terrible. You're getting lost, and you're just not safe," the person may feel they have to defend themselves and argue

with you. Instead, by gently saying, "You are getting absentminded about stop lights," you may be able to give them an easy way out. Giving up driving means admitting one's increasing limitations. Look for ways to help the person save face and maintain their self-image at the same time that you react to the need for safety. Try offering alternatives: "I'll drive today and you can look at the scenery." As a last resort some families have sold the car and told the person who has dementia that it could not be repaired.

Sometimes families are pleasantly surprised.

•

Mr. Solomon was a strong-minded, independent man. The family knew that his driving skills were poor but felt it would break his heart to lose his independence. They also anticipated a terrible fight over driving. However, a neighbor notified the Department of Motor Vehicles. When Mr. Solomon came home from his driving test, he tossed his license on the table and said he could no longer drive. After that, he never, despite the family's fears, seemed upset or inconvenienced. The Department of Motor Vehicles probably made this easier by telling him this was a routine check of people his age.

•

Sometimes a person will absolutely refuse to give up driving despite your tact. It may help to enlist the support of the doctor or family lawyer. Some physicians will write an order on a prescription pad that says, "Do not drive." Families report that having the physician be the "bad guy" takes pressure off the caregiver. Often a person will cooperate with the instructions of an authority when they may regard your advice as nagging. As a last resort, you may have to take away the car keys or have a mechanic disable the starting mechanism.

States vary in their policies regarding driver's licenses. Some states require that physicians report drivers who have dementia. In most states the Department of Motor Vehicles will issue any nondriver an ID card that can be used to board airplanes and the like. They may also investigate a complaint from any citizen, even if it is anonymous, and will sometimes suspend a license if they receive a written opinion from a physician that the person's health makes them an unsafe driver.

Some states issue limited licenses that allow a person to drive only under certain circumstances, such as only in daylight. Call the state police or the Department of Motor Vehicles to find out the policy in your area. If a person has been told by a physician not to drive, the caregiver may be found negligent if the person drives and has an accident. If someone is injured or killed in the accident, it could bankrupt the family. One wife who did not drive sold the car and put the money aside in a safe place. Every week she added the amount they used to spend on gas, maintenance, and car insurance. She said it was easier to spend money on taxis knowing they used to spend it on the car.

When a Person Can No Longer Live Alone

When a person has lived alone but can no longer do so, the move to live with someone else can be difficult for everyone. Some people welcome the sense of security that living with others provides. Others vigorously resist giving up their independence.

Often people who have dementia go through a series of stages from complete independence to living with someone. If a gradual transition from independence is possible, it may be easier for the person to adjust and it may postpone the time when they must live with someone. For example, at first the help of the neighbors or a Meals on Wheels program may be adequate; later, a family member or a paid helper may spend part of the day with the person. A few people may need someone to come in only to give medications or help with a meal.

When You Suspect That Someone Living Alone Is Developing Dementia
You need to be alert to the possibility that the person's ability to function alone may change suddenly: some minor stress or even a mild cold can make a person with dementia worse. Sometimes you will not notice the gradual, insidious decline until something happens. Families often wait too long before taking action.

When things do go wrong, the person may react by trying to "cover up." Some people who have dementia do not realize they have problems;

others may blame the family or withdraw. Close family members may also deny that there are problems. Therefore, it can be difficult to know for sure what is going on. Here are some questions to consider when deciding whether a person who is living alone is in need of help.

Changes in Personality or Habits

Is the person uncharacteristically withdrawn, apathetic (lacking interest or concern), negative, pessimistic, suspicious, or fearful of crime?

Do they insist that everything is fine, or not admit that there are problems when you know there have been?

Is the person able to manage their own personal care and grooming? Are they wearing dirty clothes, forgetting (or refusing) to bathe or brush their teeth, or in other ways neglecting themselves?

Have they become isolated? Do they say they are going out when they do not?

Phone Calls

Have their conversations become increasingly vague? (Details require more memory.)

Do conversations ramble, or does the person seem to forget what they were saying? Do they repeat themselves?

Does the person more often become "edgy" when talking on the phone? Are they less tolerant of frustration?

Are you receiving fewer phone calls from them, too many calls, or calls late at night?

Do they repeat the same story in each conversation as if it were new?

Emailing and Writing

Has the person stopped emailing, using Facebook, writing letters, or sending cards, or are their writings uncharacteristically rambling? Has their handwriting changed? Is it now hard to understand what they are trying to get across?

Meals and Medications

Is the person eating their meals and taking their medications correctly? A person who has dementia may not eat, or may eat only sweets even when you have provided a hot meal. The person may take too much medicine or forget their medicine. This can jeopardize their physical health and make their thinking impairments worse. If the person is safe in other ways, they may be able to live alone if someone else helps daily with food and medicine, but it has been our experience that people who forget to eat properly are experiencing sufficient cognitive impairment that they very likely cannot safely live alone.

Is the person forgetting to turn off the stove or burning the food? People who appear to be managing well often forget to turn off the stove. Have they stopped cooking? Are pots burned? Is the person using candles or matches? It can be hard to believe that a person is really a danger to themselves when they look so well, but fire is a real and serious hazard. Cases of severe or even fatal accidental burns are not uncommon. If you suspect that the person is forgetting to turn off the stove, you must intervene.

Other Problems

Has the person wandered away from home even once? If so, there is a real chance they could get lost or be robbed or assaulted. Are they wandering around outside at night? Such behavior is dangerous. Have friends or neighbors called you with concerns about the person's behavior or safety? Have they failed to keep appointments or not come to family events? Have they given you confusing reports of a mishap, such as a car accident? Did they retire from work early or abruptly?

If you suspect that the person is forgetting something dangerous like turning off the stove, you must take action, for everyone's safety

---

Is the person keeping the house tidy, reasonably clean, and free of hazards? The person may spill water in the kitchen or bathroom and forget to clean it up, creating a fall hazard for themselves. Sometimes people forget to wash the dishes or forget to flush the toilet or in other ways create unsanitary conditions. If the house is badly cluttered, they can trip and fall. A person who has dementia may pile up newspapers and rags, which become a fire hazard. Does the house smell of urine? These are signs that the person is unable to manage alone or is ill.

Is the person keeping warm enough or cool enough? They may keep the house too cold or dress improperly for cold weather. Their body temperature can drop dangerously low in such circumstances. In hot weather they may dress too warmly or may be afraid to open the house for adequate ventilation. This can lead to heat stroke.

Is the person acting in response to "paranoid" ideas or unrealistic suspiciousness? Such behavior can get them in trouble in the community. Sometimes people call the police because of their fears and make their neighbors angry. Sometimes, too, people who are elderly or who have dementia become the targets of malicious teenagers or adults. Such problems can occur in any neighborhood.

Is the person showing good judgment? Do they have new "friends" of questionable character? Are they donating money to questionable causes? Are they sending money to every charity that sends them an appeal in the mail, even if they are uninterested in its work? Do they repeatedly send money to the same charity because they have forgotten that they had already donated? Some people who have dementia show poor judgment about whom they let in the house and can be robbed by the people they invite in, or they may give away money or do other inappropriate things.

Who is paying the bills? Often the first indication family members have that something is wrong is when the heat or water is shut off because the bill has not been paid or because the person will not let the meter reader in. The person may stop managing their finances or change their spending habits. Has the person skipped filing income taxes when they were always careful about such matters?

Such clues indicate that *something* may be wrong—but not necessarily that the person has an illness that causes dementia. Once you are aware that there may be a problem, it is essential to get a complete assessment for the person. These changes can indicate many other treatable conditions.

What You Can Do

Contact the Alzheimer's Association chapter in your community. Most chapters have had experience helping families who live at a distance and can give you valuable information. Talk to other family members and the person's friends, neighbors, and clergyperson to get as complete a story as possible. If the person lives in an apartment, talk to the landlord or doorkeeper. If they live in a rural area, talk to their mail carrier or the manager of a store they frequent. They may be aware of problems. Give these people your phone number and ask them to alert you if they notice something you should know about.

Visit in person to assess the situation and to arrange for a diagnosis. Talk to the Alzheimer's Association, the office on aging, or a family social agency in your relative's town. They will be able to tell you about local resources.

Sometimes a person can continue to live independently for a while if you arrange for supervision. Perhaps the person's physician can give you an idea of how able they are to continue functioning alone. In major cities there are geriatric case managers who will, for a fee, function as a stand-in relative, taking a person for appointments, helping with the finances, and keeping an eye on things. You should check the credentials of anyone who offers to provide these services. Ask for references. Contact the references and inquire about the applicant's honesty and reliability, how long they have known the applicant, and what the applicant did for them. Find

out whether any state agency regulates this service, and check to see if any complaints have been registered against the applicant. Tell your relative who is showing symptoms of confusion that you are concerned about them and will be checking on them frequently.

Moving to a New Residence

If you believe that your relative can no longer live alone, you must make other arrangements for them. You might consider full-time help, or you may arrange for the person to move into someone else's home, an assisted living facility, a nursing home, or a retirement community. (These facilities are described in detail in Chapter 15.)

•

Mr. Sawyer reports, "Mother simply cannot live alone anymore. We hired a housekeeper and Mother fired her—and when I called the agency, they said they could not send anyone else. So we talked with Mother and told her we wanted her to come live with us. But she absolutely refused. She says nothing is wrong with her, that I am trying to steal her money. She won't admit she isn't eating. She says she changed her clothes, and we know she hasn't. I don't know what to do."

•

If a person who is confused refuses to give up their independence and move into a safer setting, your understanding of what they might be thinking and feeling may help make the move easier. A transition from independent living to living with someone else may mean giving up their independence and admitting impairment. Moving means more losses. It means giving up a familiar place and often many familiar possessions. That place and those possessions are the tangible symbols of the person's past and serve as reminders when their memories fail.

If you believe that your relative can no longer live alone, you should make other arrangements for them

The person who is developing dementia is dependent on a familiar setting to provide them with cues that enable them to function independently. Learning one's way around a new place is difficult and sometimes impossible. They feel dependent on familiar surroundings to survive. The person who has dementia may forget the plans that have been discussed or may be unable to understand them. You may reassure your mother that she is coming to live in your house—which is very familiar to her—but all her damaged mind can perceive is that a lot of things are going to be lost. She may not understand the need for a move because she does not remember the problems she is having.

As you make plans for the person to live with someone, there are several things to consider.

1. *Take into careful consideration the changes that this move will mean in their life and yours. Plan, before the move, for financial resources and emotional outlets and supports for yourself.* If the person is to move in with you, what effect will this have on their income? A state may reduce public assistance benefits to people who begin living with someone. You will also want to review such things

as whether you can claim the person as a dependent on your income tax return.

If the person is coming to live with you, how does the rest of the family feel about it? If there are children or teenagers in your family, will their activities upset the person, or will the person's "odd" behavior upset them? How does your spouse feel about this? Is your marriage already under stress? Having a person who has dementia in the home creates burdens and stresses under the best of circumstances. If the person who has dementia and their spouse are both moving in, you must also consider how their spouse will interact in the household. All of the people affected need to be involved in the decision and need the opportunity to express their concerns.

If you have had a long-standing poor relationship with the person who now has dementia, that poor relationship can make things more difficult for you

Assuming the care of a forgetful person may mean changes in other areas of your life: leisure time (you may not be able to go out because there is no one to stay with the person), peace and quiet (you may not be able to read the news or talk to your spouse because the person is pacing the floor), money (you may have increased medical bills or bills for remodeling the bathroom), rest (the person who has dementia may be awake at night and wander about the house), and visitors (people may stop visiting if the person's behavior is embarrassing). These are among the things that make life meaningful and help to reduce your stress. It is important to plan ways for you and your family to relax and get away from the problems of caring for a person who has dementia. Remember also that other problems are not going to go away: you may still worry about your children, come home exhausted from your job, or have the car break down.

> **If people who have dementia move before their illness becomes severe, they have a better chance of adapting to their new environment**

Is the person you are bringing into your home someone you can live with? If you never could get along with your parent or sibling, and if their illness has made their behavior worse instead of better, having them move in with you may be disastrous. If you have had a long-standing poor relationship with the person who now has dementia, that poor relationship is a reality that can make things more difficult for you.

2. *Involve the person as much as possible in plans for the move, even if they refuse to move.* The individual who has dementia is still a person, and their participation in plans and decisions that involve them is important unless they are too severely impaired to comprehend what is happening. People who have been hoodwinked into a move may become even angrier and more suspicious, and their adjustment to the new setting may be extremely difficult. Certainly, the extent and nature of the

person's participation depend on the extent of their illness and their attitude toward the move.

Keep in mind that there is a key difference between making the decision, which you may have to do, and participating in the planning, which the person who has dementia can be encouraged to do. Perhaps Mr. Sawyer's story above will continue this way:

•

"After we talked it over with Mother, she still absolutely refused to consider a move. So I went ahead with the arrangements. I told Mother gently that she had to move because she was getting forgetful.

"I knew too many decisions at once would upset her, so we would just ask her a few things at a time: 'Mother, would you like to take all your pictures with you?' 'Mother, let's take your own bed and your lovely bedspread for your new bedroom.'

"Of course, we made a lot of decisions without her—about the stove and the washer, and the junk in the attic. And of course she kept saying she wasn't going and that I was robbing her. Still, I think some of it sank in, that she was 'helping' us get ready to move. Sometimes she would pick up a vase and say, 'I want Carol to have this.' We tried to comply with her wishes. Then after the move, we could honestly tell her that the vase was not stolen: she had given it to Carol."

•

When a person is too impaired to understand what is happening around them, it may be better to make the move without the added stress of trying to involve them in it.

3. *Be prepared for a period of adjustment.* Changes are frequently upsetting to

people who have dementia. No matter how carefully and lovingly you plan the move, this is a major change, and the person may be upset for a while. It is easy to understand that it takes time to get over the losses a move involves. A person who has dementia also needs extra time to learn their way around a new place.

When people who have dementia move before their illness becomes severe, they are often better able to adjust to their new environment. They have greater ability to learn new things and to adapt. Waiting until someone is "too far gone to object" may mean that they will not be able to learn their way around or recognize that they are in a new setting.

Reassure yourself that after an adjustment period most people settle into their new surroundings. Signs on doors occasionally help people find their way around an unfamiliar home. Try to postpone other activities and changes until after everyone has adjusted to the move.

Reassure yourself that, after an adjustment period, most people settle into their new surroundings

---

Occasionally a person who has dementia never really adjusts to moving. Don't blame yourself. You did the best you could and acted for their well-being. You may have to accept their inability to adjust as being the result of their illness.

CHAPTER 5

Problems Arising in Daily Care

Hazards to Watch For

People who have dementia may not be able to take responsibility for their own safety. They are no longer able to evaluate consequences the way the rest of us do, and because they forget so quickly, they are at high risk of having a serious accident. They may attempt to do familiar tasks without realizing that they can no longer manage them. For example, the disease may affect those portions of the brain that coordinate how to do simple things, such as using the microwave or slicing meat. This inability to do manual tasks is often unrecognized and can lead to serious mishaps. Because the person also cannot learn, minor changes in routine can lead to dangerous situations. And because a person seems to be managing well, you may not realize they have lost the judgment they need to avoid accidents. Families often need to take responsibility for the safety of people who have dementia even when they are only mildly impaired.

Accidents are most likely to occur when people are cross or tired, when everyone is hurrying, when there is an argument, or when someone in the household is sick. At these times you are less alert to the possibility of an accident, and the person who has dementia may misunderstand or overreact to even the slightest mishap by having a catastrophic reaction.

Do what you can to reduce confusion or tension when it arises. This is difficult when you are struggling with the care of a person who has dementia. If you are rushing with them to keep an appointment or finish a job and they are beginning to get upset, *stop*, even if it means being late or not getting something done. Catch your breath, rest a minute, and let the person calm down.

Be aware that even minor mishaps can be warning signs of impending accidents: you banged your shin on the edge of the bed or dropped and broke a cup, and the person who has dementia became upset. This is the time to create a change of pace, before a serious accident occurs. Alert others in the household to the relationship between increased tension and the greater likelihood of accidents. At such times, every-one can keep a closer eye on the person who has dementia.

Be sure you know the limits of the person's abilities. Do not take their word that they can heat their own supper or get into the bathtub alone. An occupational therapist can give you an excellent picture of what the person can do safely. If you do not have this resource, observe the person closely as they do various tasks.

Have an emergency plan ready in case something bad does happen. Whom will you call if someone—including you—is hurt? If there is a fire, how will you get the person who has dementia and is upset to leave? Remember that they may misinterpret what is happening and resist your efforts to help.

> ### Making the environment safer is one of the best ways to lower the risk of accidents

Change the environment to make it safer. This is one of the most important ways to avoid accidents. Hospitals and other institutions have safety experts who regularly inspect for hazards. You can, and should, do the same thing.

Select a time when the person who has dementia is not with you, and carefully consider the person's home, yard, neighborhood, and car, looking for things they could misuse or misinterpret that might cause an accident. Consider that the person may easily become confused by clutter, may try to do things that are no longer safe (like using the stove), and may gradually become clumsy enough to trip over

things like low furniture or loose throw rugs. Consider the person's level of impairment now, but also plan ahead for increasing impairment. The person can decline without your realizing their increased risk. As the illness progresses, repeat your survey. The National Institute on Aging has helpful resources to advise you.

Make key changes right away, and write out a list of other things that you will want to change over time or that you will want to ask others to help you with. Think of yourself also. What can you do to save yourself steps, keep yourself from falling, and prevent fires? You may find making changes difficult. It means facing the reality that the person who has dementia is changing. It may also mean doing things differently from the way you have always done them.

In the House

Put away dangerous items such as medications, kitchen knives, matches, power tools, and electric gadgets like hair dryers that, if misused, could start a fire or hurt the person who is impaired. Safely lock away insecticides, gasoline, paint, solvents, cleaning supplies, soap pods, and the like—or, better yet, get rid of them. People with even a mild impairment may use them inappropriately. For things you need ready access to, look in the hardware store for childproof locks for drawers and cabinets. There are several kinds, and they are easy to install. You will want more than one locked or childproof cabinet in which to store things. Be sure your smoke detectors work and that the batteries are fresh.

Simplify, simplify, simplify. Clutter means the person who has dementia must try to think through more things, and this leads to accidents. Get rid of clutter, especially on stairs, in the kitchen, and in the bathroom. Think about where the person walks. Remove clutter that they must walk around. Put away low furniture and throw rugs that they could trip over. Remove any extension cords that the person could trip on. A neat house with less clutter also makes it easier for you to find things that the person with an impairment misplaces or hides.

Simplify, simplify, simplify

As people grow older, their eyes need more light, but often people become accustomed to low light in their homes. Increasing the light in the home and adding night-lights will reduce accidents and help the person who has dementia to function as well as possible. You can increase light by leaving the drapes open in the daytime and by using higher lumen bulbs in lamps. Turn lamps on during the daytime in dimly lit rooms. Newer light bulbs are more economical because they use less electricity. The added light helps reduce the person's confusion and can prevent them from stumbling over things.

The bathroom is usually the most dangerous room in the house. Hazards include falls, poisons, cuts, and burns. Lock up medications and put other items like shampoo—substances that the person might eat or drink—in a cabinet with a childproof lock. Replace glass cups with plastic ones that won't break.

Lower the temperature on the water heater to prevent scalds. Make hot radiators inaccessible.

People who have dementia may try to cook or "just heat up something," especially at night when you are sleeping. They may put an empty pan on a hot burner. *This is a serious fire hazard.* They may also hide things under the stove burners, which can start a fire. You can take several steps to decrease these risks. Begin by taking the knobs off the stove when you are not using it. You can also have someone install timers on the stove and other appliances, such as the microwave, that will turn them off after a certain period of time. You can have a switch installed on the stove or any other electrical appliance so that you can turn it off when you are not using it. It is wise to put this switch out of sight in a cabinet where the person who has dementia will not find it.

Don't keep medications out in the open. Get in the habit of storing them away where you are sure the person who has dementia cannot get to them. If they take medication and then forget that they took it, see the bottle, and take it again, they could become seriously ill from an overdose.

Look at the areas the person walks through. In Chapter 7 on page 132 we discuss ways to lock doors. Secure any doors you do not want the person to enter. Put clear signs on doors or cabinets that help the person find what they want or where they are going. Use nonskid rugs. Remove furniture from the hallways. Look for things the person could trip over.

Can the person lock themselves in a room so that you cannot get in? Remove the lock, take the tumblers out, and replace the knob or securely tape the latch open.

Stairs are dangerous. Dementia causes people to become unstable and to pay less attention to steps. They can easily get "turned around" and fall down the steps, especially at night. Check the handrails on stairs: be sure they are sturdy. They should be anchored into the wall stud and not into drywall or plaster. They will not hold a person's weight if they are not securely fastened.

If at all possible, set up the person's bedroom on the ground floor early in the person's illness so that they do not have to go up and down steps. Put gates at both the top and the bottom of stairs or block them off. Be sure the person cannot climb over the gates and tumble down the flight of stairs.

Most people who have dementia will at some point in their illness walk into areas that are unsafe or wander away. Begin beforehand to make the person's home secure. We talk about wandering in Chapter 7.

A person who has dementia can easily lean too far out of a window or over a balcony rail and fall—a particular danger in a high-rise building. Install security locks on windows and balcony doors. Be aware that people can climb over railings. When people have a catastrophic reaction and feel panicky, they may be so confused that they will climb over a balcony or fence or out a window to escape what they perceive to be a danger. Prepare for this in advance so that you never have to struggle to hold them back.

At the same time that you look for ways to make the home safe, look for ways to make it comfortable for the person who has dementia. Easily understood signs occasionally help people remain independent. Use stable chairs that are easy to get in and out of (see page 41). Place a comfortable chair near the area where you often are, such as close to the kitchen, so that the person can watch you. Set up a comfortable, safe seating area in the yard with a chair by the window so you can keep an eye on the person.

At the same time that you look for ways to make the home safe, look for ways to make it more comfortable

---

Reduce the clutter in the person's bedroom, but make the bedroom welcoming and leave some drawers that the person can rummage through. You may want to lower the bed so that if the person falls, they will be less likely to be injured. Bed rails are available from medical supply stores and drugstores, but they are dangerous because people with dementia often try to climb over them and put themselves at risk of falling.

If you live in an apartment or condominium building that has a doorkeeper or security staff, let these people know that this member of your family is forgetful and may have trouble finding their apartment. They may be willing to alert you if the person tends to wander away.

Outdoors

Both adults and children can easily fall or put a hand through the glass in a storm door. Consider covering storm doors with a protective grillwork. Sliding glass patio doors should be well marked with stick-on decals.

Porches and decks without walls or railings are major fall hazards. Be sure rails are sturdy. If there are steps, attach outdoor nonskid tape to the edges, and install a banister.

Be sure that garages, hobby or tool areas, and outdoor sheds are inaccessible. These areas are dangerous. One man who had a mild dementia was repairing the toaster, but he left it plugged in while he worked on it. Such mistakes are common and serious.

Check for uneven ground, cracked pavement, holes in the lawn, fallen branches, thorny bushes, or molehills that the person can trip over. Take down the clothesline so the person will not run into it.

If you have an outdoor grill, never leave it unattended while the coals are hot. Make sure the coals are cold. If you have a gas grill, be sure the person who has dementia cannot operate it.

Check yard furniture to be sure it is stable, will not tip or collapse, and has no splinters or chipped paint.

Lock up garden tools. Fence in or dispose of poisonous flowers.

Lawn mowers are dangerous. The person who is impaired may try to unjam a lawn mower while the blades are turning. Occasionally a person who can no longer safely drive a car will drive away on a riding mower. Push and riding mowers are especially risky on hilly terrain, because they can turn over.

A fence may help to keep a person who wanders from leaving the yard, but all fences can be climbed, and the person may fall trying to get out. A taller fence is safer than a short one. However, you will still need to watch a person who tends to wander.

Swimming pools are very dangerous. Be sure that your or your neighbor's pool is securely fenced and locked so that the person who has dementia cannot get to it. You may have to explain carefully the nature of the person's impairment to the owner of the pool, making certain that the person is not ever assumed to be competent around a pool. Even if they have always been good swimmers, people who have dementia may lose their judgment or ability to handle themselves in the water.

Ice and snow are serious hazards for both of you. The person who has dementia is not able to pay attention to stepping carefully, and even if you remind them, their shuffling gait makes things worse. You may also be off-balance as you try to help them or distracted as you pay attention to them. Falls have serious consequences for the person who does not understand an injury, and if you are hurt, you will be unable to be a caregiver. Have someone keep your steps and walkway shoveled and salted. Do not take the person out in icy weather except in an emergency, and then only with help. Kitty litter is a good substitute for salt and does not damage lawns.

Riding in the Car

Problems with driving are discussed in Chapter 4. Never leave a person who has dementia alone in a car. They may wander away, fiddle with the ignition, become frightened by not being able to lower the window, be harassed by strangers, or run the battery down by keeping the lights on. Some automatic windows are dangerous for people who have dementia and for children, who may close the window on their head or arm. Engage the automatic window locks so that only the driver can control them.

Occasionally a person will open the car door and attempt to get out while the car is moving. Locking the doors may help. Most cars have child safety locks on the rear doors. This will keep a person from getting out of the backseat until the driver unlocks the doors. If getting out of a moving car is a potential problem, you may need a third person to drive while you keep the person who has dementia calm.

> Never leave a person who has dementia alone in a car

A swivel cushion for cars raises the car seat slightly and makes it easier for the person to get into the car without having to slide in and out. Another useful product is a support handle (HandyBar is a popular brand) that locks into the striker on the vehicle door frame and saves you from having to lift the person in and out of the car.

Highways and Parking Lots

Highways are dangerous. If you think the person who has dementia may be walking along a highway, notify the police immediately. You should not be concerned that you are bothering the police unnecessarily. Notifying the police when it turns out to be unnec-essary is much better than not alerting them and having a tragedy occur.

People driving in parking lots often assume that pedestrians will get out of their way. People who have dementia may not anticipate cars coming or may move slowly. Be especially alert to en-trances into enclosed garages. These often put the pedestrian directly in the path of cars.

Smoking

If the person smokes, the time will come when they lay down a lighted cigarette and forget it. *This is a serious hazard.* If allowing the person to smoke poses a hazard, you must intervene. Try to discourage smoking. Talk with the person's doctor to see whether it might be possible to get a medication that decreases the craving to smoke. Many families have been able to take ciga-rettes completely away from a person who has dementia. This may be diffi-cult for a few days or weeks, but it is much easier in the long run. However, some people forget they ever smoked and thus do not complain when you take their cigarettes away. Other fam-ilies allow the person to smoke only under their supervision. All smoking materials and kitchen or fireplace matches must be kept out of reach of the forgetful person. The person who has cigarettes but not matches may use the stove to light their cigarette and may leave the stove on. (See the sug-gestions for disabling the stove given earlier in this chapter.)

Hunting

The use of firearms requires complex mental skills that are usually lost early in dementia. Firearms must be put in a safe place under lock and key. If necessary, ask your doctor or clergyperson to explain to the person's hunting buddies that hunting is now too dangerous for them. Ask the local police or sheriff's department if they can help dispose of a firearm if you do not know how to do so. If you have pistols or rifles in the house, make sure they are under lock and key and that the person with dementia cannot access the key.

Nutrition and Mealtimes

Good nutrition is important to both you and the person who has dementia. If you are not eating well, you will be more tense and more easily upset. It is not known to what extent a proper diet affects the progress of dementia, but we do know that forgetful people often fail to eat properly and can develop nutritional deficiencies. Poor nutrition leads to numerous dental and health problems, which can add to behavioral symptoms.

Talk to your doctor about a diet that is healthy for both of you. Studies indicate that a diet that is good for the heart is also good for the brain—ask your doctor if they recommend a heart-healthy diet. The National Institute on Aging has current information on these findings. If the person is at risk for strokes, your physician may add supplements or medications to reduce this risk. If your doctor has recommended a special diet for managing other diseases like diabetes or heart disease, it is important that you find out what food you should serve in order to maintain a balanced diet.

Ask your doctor to refer you to a nutritionist who can help you plan meals that are good for both of you, that the person will eat, and that you can easily prepare.

If the person who has dementia is active, wandering, or pacing and has difficulty sitting still long enough to eat, try preparing sandwiches. Cut them into quarters and give them one piece at a time to eat as they walk.

Meal Preparation

When you must prepare meals in addition to all your other responsibilities, you may find yourself taking shortcuts such as fixing just a cup of coffee and toast for yourself and the person who has dementia. If preparing meals is a job you had to take on for the first time when your family member became ill, you may not know how to serve good nutritious meals quickly and easily and you may not want to learn to cook. There are several alternatives. We suggest you plan a variety of ways to get good meals with a minimum of effort.

Already cooked food is available in many supermarkets. Partially prepared meals that are delivered on a regular basis are available from many companies. They can be found by searching online for "meal delivery services." Some companies make meals that require reheating in an oven or microwave. Others send ingredients that require some meal preparation and cooking. Choose a service that meets your needs. Don't put pressure on yourself to do more than you have the time or inclination to do.

There are Eating Together programs for people over 60 and Meals on Wheels programs in most areas. Both services provide one hot, nutritious meal a day. You can find out what meal services are available through a social worker or the local office on aging. Meals on Wheels programs bring a meal to your home. Eating Together programs, offered at senior centers and funded under the Older Americans Act, provide lunch and often a recreational program in the company of other retired people at a community center. Transportation is often provided.

Many restaurants provide takeout meals. This helps when a person can no longer eat in public.

Numerous inexpensive cookbooks on the market explain the basic steps in easy meal preparation. Some are available in large print. Friends who enjoy cooking can show you how to prepare quick, easy meals. The nutrition educator in your county extension office or a public health nurse can give you good, easy recipes. They also have helpful information on budgeting, shopping, meal planning, and nutrition and can help you understand and plan menus for special diets.

Some frozen dinners provide well-balanced meals, but these are often expensive. Many, however, are low in vitamins and high in salt and lack the fiber older people need to prevent constipation.

Mealtimes

Seat the person comfortably, in as close to a normal eating position as possible. Be sure that possible distractions (such as a television or needing to use the toilet) are taken care of. Some people do better with someone else at the table; others are distracted by this.

The dining area should be well lit so that the person can easily see their food. Use a plate that contrasts with the placemat or tablecloth and with the food. (For example, it is easier to see a white plate if it is on a bright blue placemat.) Avoid glass if the person has difficulty seeing it. Avoid dishes with patterns if the person is confused by them. If they are confused by having condiments (salt, pepper, sugar, for example) on the table, remove them. If they are confused by having several eating utensils to choose from, put out only one. Some people do better in a dining room or kitchen where there are many subtle cues like food smells that remind them to eat. Allow people to feed themselves as much as possible.

Some people are unable to decide what to eat when several different foods are on their plate. If that is true of your relative, limit the number of foods you put in front of them at one time. For example, serve only the salad, then only the meat. Having to make choices often leads to playing with food. Don't put salt, ketchup, or other condiments where the person who has dementia can reach them and mix them inappropriately into their food. Season their food for them. Be sure their food is cut into pieces that are small and tender enough to be eaten safely; people who have dementia may forget to chew or fail to cut up meats properly because their hands and brain no longer work together.

Messiness

As people develop problems with co-ordination, they may become messier and begin to use their fingers instead of eating utensils. It is almost always easier to adjust to this than to fight it. It usually means they are no longer able to use eating utensils. Use a plastic tablecloth or placemats. Serve meals in a room in which the floor can be easily cleaned. Don't scold when they use their fingers. Eating with fingers postpones the time when the person will need more help from you. Serve things that are easy to pick up in bite-sized pieces.

People who are able to use a fork or spoon will be more successful eating from a dish with sides. You can purchase a scoop plate or a plate guard (which attaches to a plate) from a medical supply store. Use fairly heavy dishes (they slip less).

Dycem (available online and from medical supply stores) placed under a plate will keep it from slipping. Plates with suction cups are also available. Utensils with large (thick) handles are easier for people with arthritis or coordination problems to use. You can purchase these or build up your own spoon and fork handles with foam rubber. (Do this to your own pens and notice how much less tiring writing is.)

Some people who have dementia will agree to wear a smock over their clothing. Others will be confused or offended by it. If you try this, use a smock or large apron rather than a bib.

> As people develop problems with coordination, they may become messier and begin to eat with their fingers instead of utensils. It is almost always easier to adjust to this rather than to fight it.

Some people lose the ability to judge how much liquid will fill a glass and overfill glasses. They will need your help. To prevent spilling, don't fill glasses or cups full.

Fluids

Be sure that the person gets enough fluid each day. Even people with mild cognitive impairment may forget to drink, and inadequate fluid intake can lead to other physical problems (see pages 101–2). Determine with a health care professional the appropriate amount of fluid the person should drink each day.

Always check the temperature of hot drinks. People may lose the ability to judge temperature and burn themselves as a result.

> Be sure that the person gets enough fluid each day

If the person does not like water, offer juices and frequently remind them to take a few sips. If possible, they should not have more than one cup of coffee, tea, or caffeinated cola in a day. Caffeine is a diuretic, which increases the volume and frequency of urination and, as a result, takes fluids from the body.

A Pureed Diet

If the person is on a pureed diet, use a blender or a baby food grinder. You can puree normally prepared foods in it. This saves time and money. Home-cooked foods will be more appealing to the person than baby foods.

Spoon-Feeding

If you need to spoon-feed the person with dementia, put only a small amount of food on the spoon at a time. Wait until the person swallows before giving them the next bite. Late in the disease you might have to remind them to swallow.

Problem Eating Behaviors

Forgetful people who are still eating some meals alone may forget to eat, even if you leave food in plain sight. They may hide food, throw it away, or eat food after it has spoiled. These are signs that the person can no longer manage alone and that you must make new arrangements. You may manage for a time by phoning at noon to remind them to eat lunch, but this is a short-term solution. People who live alone and have mild cognitive impairment or dementia are frequently malnourished. Even if they appear overweight, they may not be eating the proper foods. A poor diet can worsen their ability to think.

Many of the problems that arise at mealtime involve catastrophic reactions. Make mealtime as routine and regular as possible, with as little confu-

sion as you can arrange. This will help prevent catastrophic reactions. Fussy or messy eaters do better when things are calm.

Check that dentures are tight fitting. If they are loose, it may be safer to leave them out until they can be adjusted.

People who have dementia often lack the judgment to avoid burning themselves. Check the temperature of foods. Food heated in a microwave oven may be too hot in spots. Stir thoroughly.

Make mealtime as routine and regular as possible, with as little confusion as possible

---

People who have dementia may develop rigid likes and dislikes and refuse to eat certain foods. Such people may be more willing to eat familiar foods, prepared in familiar ways. If the person never liked a particular food, they will not like it now. New foods may confuse them. If the person insists on eating only one or two things, and if all efforts at persuasion or disguising foods fail, you will need to ask the doctor about vitamins and diet supplements.

Hoarding Food

Some people save food and hide it in their room. This is a problem if it attracts insects or mice. Some people will give this up if they are frequently reassured that they can have a snack at any time. Leave a cookie jar where the person who has dementia can find it and remind them where it is. Some families give the person a container with a tightly fitting lid to keep snacks in. You may need to remind them to keep the snacks in the container. Others persuade the person to "trade" their old, spoiled food for fresh food.

If the person has a complicating illness that requires a special diet, such as diabetes, it may be necessary to put foods they should not eat where they cannot get them and allow access only to those foods they should have. Remember, many people with dementia lack the judgment to decide responsibly between their craving and their well-being. Because a proper diet is important to their health, you may have to be responsible for preventing them from getting foods they should not have, even if they vigorously object. A locksmith can put a lock on the refrigerator door if necessary. Childproof locks will secure cabinets.

Nibbling

Some people seem to forget that they have eaten and will ask for food again right after a meal. They may want to eat all the time. Try setting out a tray of small, nutritious "nibbles" such as small crackers or cheese cubes. Perhaps they will take one at a time and be satisfied. If weight gain is a problem, put out carrots or celery.

Eating Things They Should Not Eat

People who have dementia may be unable to recognize that some things are not good to eat or not good in large quantities. You may need to put out of sight foods like salt, vinegar, oil, or Worcestershire sauce, large amounts of which can make a person sick. Some people will eat nonfood items like soap, the soil in planters, washing machine pods, or sponges. This probably re-

sults from damage to perception and memory. If such behavior occurs, you will need to keep these objects out of sight. Many people do not develop this problem, so we do not recommend removing these objects unless a problem does occur.

Not Eating or Spitting Out Food

Some of the medications given to people who have dementia make the mouth and throat dry, making many foods unpalatable or hard to swallow. Your pharmacist can tell you which drugs have this effect. This may cause the person to not eat or to spit out food. Mix food with juice or water, and offer the person a sip of water with each bite.

Sometimes the mouth and throat can be so dry as to be painful and can make the person cranky. Offer fluids frequently.

Not Swallowing

Sometimes people with dementia carry food around in their mouths but don't swallow it because they have forgotten how to chew or swallow. This is an apraxia (see pages 39–40) and is best handled by giving the person soft foods that do not require much chewing, such as chopped meat, gelatin, and thick liquids.

If they do not swallow pills, crush them and mix them with food. Check with your pharmacist first since some medications should not be crushed.

Malnutrition

People who have dementia can easily become malnourished, even when their caregivers are doing the best they can. Malnutrition and dehydration contribute to people's overall poor health, increase their suffering, and shorten their lives. Malnutrition affects the way the entire body functions, including how quickly a person recovers from an illness and how quickly a wound heals. It is possible to be overweight and still not be getting needed protein, minerals, or vitamins. People who have difficulty swallowing or who have had a stroke are especially at risk of malnutrition.

> Malnutrition affects the way the entire body functions, including how quickly a person recovers from an illness and how quickly a wound heals

In the past, many residents of nursing homes became malnourished or did not receive adequate amounts of fluid. If your relative is in a nursing home, insist that the staff evaluate their nutritional status regularly and treat any problems.

Weight Loss

People who have dementia lose weight for all the same reasons that other people do. Therefore, if someone is losing weight and is not on a diet, the first step is to consult their doctor. Weight loss often indicates a treatable problem or a disease unrelated to the dementia. Do not assume that it signals a decline. It is important that the physician search carefully for any contributory illness. Is the person constipated? Does the person have cancer, heart failure, or another medical condition that causes weight loss? Is the person depressed? Depression can account for

weight loss even in a person who has dementia. Poorly fitting dentures and sore teeth or gums can contribute to weight loss. Weight loss very late in the illness may be a part of the disease process itself. Certainly, all other possible causes should be considered.

When a person is still eating and yet losing weight, they may be pacing, agitated, or so active that they are burning up more calories than they are taking in. Offer nutritious, substantial snacks between meals and before bedtime. Some health care professionals think that several small meals and frequent snacks help prevent this kind of weight loss.

Sometimes all that is needed to get a person to eat better is a calm, supportive environment. You may have to experiment before you find the arrangement that best encourages the person to eat. Be sure the food tastes good. Offer the person their favorite foods. Offer only one thing at a time, and do not rush them. People who have dementia often eat slowly. Frequently offer snacks. Gently remind them to eat.

Eating problems are common in assisted living facilities and nursing homes. Most people eat better in a small group or at a table with one other person in a quiet room. Sometimes it is best if the nursing facility sets aside space to serve a few people who have dementia away from a large, noisy dining room. Sometimes nursing home staff members are too rushed to coax a person to eat; a familiar family member may have better success. Homemade goodies may be more appealing than institutional food. One person who had dementia ate better when her back was gently stroked while she was being fed.

Another person who had dementia responded to a low dose of medication that calms behavior, given one hour before meals.

You may give a person who is not eating well a high-calorie, liquid diet supplement like Ensure or Sustacal. You can purchase these by the case from most pharmacies and discount warehouses. They contain vitamins, minerals, calories, and proteins the person needs. They come in different flavors; the person may like some flavors or products better than others. Offer this as the beverage with a meal or as a "milkshake" between meals. Consult the doctor about using these products.

Choking

Sometimes people who have dementia have difficulty coordinating the act of swallowing and choke on their food. If the person has difficulty changing facial expression or has had a stroke, they may also have trouble chewing or swallowing. When this occurs, it is important to guard against choking. Do not give the person foods that they may forget to chew thoroughly, such as small hard candy, nuts, carrots, chewing gum, or popcorn. Soft, thick foods are less likely to cause choking. Easy-to-handle foods include chopped meat, soft-boiled eggs, canned fruit, and frozen yogurt. Foods can be pureed in a blender. Seasoning will make them more appealing. You can mix a liquid and a solid (for example, broth and mashed potatoes) to make swallowing easier.

If the person has trouble swallowing, be sure they are sitting up straight with their head slightly forward—never tilted back—when they eat. The person should be sitting in the same position in which people would usually sit at a table. They should remain sitting for fifteen minutes after they eat.

Do not feed a person who is agitated or sleepy.

Learn the Heimlich maneuver; it can save the life of a choking person

Foods like cereal with milk may cause choking. The two textures—solid and liquid—make it hard for some people to know whether to chew or swallow.

Some fluids are easier to swallow than others. If a person tends to choke on fluids like water, try a thicker liquid like apricot or tomato juice. A nurse can help you cope with this problem.

First Aid for Choking

A nurse or the Red Cross can teach you a simple technique that can save the life of a choking person. It takes only a few minutes to learn this simple skill. Everyone should know how to do it.

If the person appears to be choking but can talk, cough, or breathe, *do not interfere*. Encourage them to keep coughing. If the person cannot talk, cough, or breathe (and may point to their throat or turn bluish), *you must help them*. If they are in a chair or standing, stand behind them, then reach around them and lock or overlap your two hands in the middle of their abdomen (belly) below the ribs. Pull hard and quickly, back and up (toward you). If the person is lying down, turn them so that they are face up, put your two hands in the middle of their belly, and push. This Heimlich maneuver will force air up through the throat and cause the food to fly out like a cork out of a bottle. (You can practice where to put your hands, but you should not push hard on a breathing person.)

When to Consider Tube Feeding

People who have dementia stop eating for many reasons. They may have difficulty swallowing due to an apraxia, ulcers in the esophagus, an esophageal obstruction (narrowing), or overmedication. They may dislike the food being offered, not recognize it as food, lose the sense of feeling hungry or thirsty, or be sitting in an uncomfortable position. They may have cancer or depression, both of which can cause people to stop eating and can occur even in a person with advanced dementia. People who have dementia may stop eating when they are experiencing a concurrent illness; they *may* resume eating when they recover. However, some people who have dementia reach a point in their illness when they have lost the ability to chew even soft food or to swallow.

Whenever a person who has dementia loses a significant amount of weight, good care requires that a physician carefully review the person's medical status, even if the dementia is very advanced. Then, if the weight loss cannot be stopped, you and the doctor are left with an ethical dilemma. Should you allow the insertion of a feeding tube directly into the stomach (a gastrostomy tube or PEG tube)? Or should you allow the person who has dementia to die? This decision is different for each person and family.

It is helpful if the family has talked about this issue before it arises or as soon as the person begins to lose weight or have difficulty swallowing. It is important to discuss all aspects of the decision to place a feeding tube with a physician who knows the person well. There is no evidence that gastrostomy tubes prolong the lives of people who have dementia. There is no evidence that they lower the risk of aspirating stomach contents into the lungs or prevent pneumonia when aspiration does occur.

> While the circumstances are different for each person, there is no evidence that gastrostomy tubes prolong the life of people who have dementia, lower their risk of aspiration, or prevent pneumonia

Many physicians believe that a gastrostomy tube (a tube that goes through the abdominal wall and opens directly into the stomach) is more comfortable for the person who has dementia than the previously used nasogastric tube (a tube that goes through the nose, down the esophagus, and into the stomach). Patients are less likely to pull out gastrostomy tubes, and these tubes need to be changed less often. PEG tubes are put in place from within, that is, the person undergoes an endoscopy, in which a gastroenterologist places a flexible tube with a camera at the end through the person's mouth, down the esophagus, and into the stomach and then pushes the feeding tube through the stomach wall and abdominal wall to the outside. Because there is an opening through the abdomen, there is a slight risk of an adverse outcome, such as infection. If the person with dementia cannot sign the consent form for this procedure, someone else will be required to sign the form. Feeding a person through a gastrostomy or PEG tube usually takes place over many hours. Machines are available that can regulate the rate of flow, although gravity is often all that is needed. A visiting nurse can show you how to manage the tube at home.

People who have dementia sometimes try to pull out PEG tubes and occasionally succeed. We do not know whether this means they find the tube uncomfortable or whether they think that it does not belong there. Or it may happen because they are restless. People who pull out their tubes may have their hands restrained, further adding to their discomfort, but often covering the tube when it is not in use will lessen this risk.

We know very little about the psychological experience of the person who has dementia who stops eating and is not tube fed, but our clinical experience suggests that discomfort is very uncommon. Most experts agree that dehydration itself somehow diminishes or abolishes the experiences of thirst and hunger, but we cannot be sure that this is true. While knowledge gained from people dying from other causes may not apply to people who have dementia, cognitively normal individuals who have recovered from severe dehydration do not report feelings of discomforting thirst. In the end, you and your family must make the decision you feel most comfortable with. If the person has previously written or stated a preference, this should help guide your decision, but ultimately it is the family member or guardian with medical decision-making power who makes the decision unless a MOLST form has been prepared (discussed in detail on page 255).

Exercise

Remaining physically fit is an important part of good health. We do not know all the ways that exercise contributes to good health, but we do know that it is important for both you and the person who has dementia to get enough exercise. We do not know the relationship between tension and exercise, either, but many people who lead intense, demanding lives are convinced that physical exercise enables them to

handle pressure more effectively. Perhaps exercise will refresh you after the daily burdens of caring for a chronically ill person.

Several studies have found that people with dementia who exercise regularly are calmer and do less agitated pacing. Some studies have observed that motor skills seem to be retained longer if they are used regularly. Exercise is a good way to keep a person involved in activities because it is often easier for people who have dementia to use their bodies than to think and remember. Perhaps the most important fact is that sufficient exercise seems to help people sleep at night and keep their bowel movements regular.

You may have to exercise with the person who has dementia. The kind of exercise you do depends on what you and they enjoy. There is no point to adding an unpleasant exercise program to your life. Consider what the person did before they developed dementia, and find ways to modify that activity so that it can continue. Sometimes an exercise activity can also be a time for you and the person who has dementia to share closeness and affection without having to talk.

How much exercise can an older person safely do? If you or the person who has dementia has high blood pressure or a heart condition, check with the doctor before you do anything. If both of you can do normal walking around the house, climb steps, and shop for groceries, you can carry out a moderate exercise program. Always start a new activity gradually and build up slowly. If an exercise causes either of you stiffness, pain, or swelling, do less of it or change to a gentler activity. Check the person's feet for blisters or bruises if you begin walking.

Walking is excellent exercise. Try to take the person outside for a short walk in all but the worst weather. The movement and the fresh air may help them feel and sleep better. If the weather is too rainy or cold, drive to an indoor shopping mall. Make a game of "window shopping." Be sure both of you

have comfortable, low-heeled shoes and soft, absorbent cotton socks. You may gradually build up the distance you walk, but avoid steep hills. It may be easier for a forgetful person to walk the same route each day. Point out scenery, people, smells, and so on as you walk. Don't worry about repeating the same conversation day after day.

An exercise program may be a good time for you and the person who has dementia to share closeness without having to talk

---

Dancing is good exercise. If the person enjoyed dancing before becoming ill, encourage some sort of movements to music.

If the person played golf or tennis, they may be able to enjoy hitting the ball around long after they become unable to play a real game.

People who have dementia often enjoy doing calisthenics as part of a group, for example, in a day care setting. If you are doing exercises in a group or at home, try having them imitate what you are doing. If they have trouble with specific movements, try gently helping them move.

If people are able to keep their balance, standing exercises are better than those done sitting in a chair. However, if balance is a problem, do the same exercises while sitting in a chair.

If the person becomes bedfast because of an acute illness, ask the doctor or the physical therapist to help you get them moving again as soon as possible. This may postpone the time when they become permanently bedfast.

Even people who are confined to bed can exercise. However, exercises for seriously chronically ill people must be planned by a physical therapist so that they do not aggravate other conditions and are not dangerous to a person who has poor coordination, poor balance, or rigid muscles.

Exercise should be done at the same time each day, in a quiet, orderly way so it does not create confusion that would add to the person's agitation. Follow the same sequence of exercises. Make the exercises fun and encourage the person to remember them. If the person has a catastrophic reaction, stop and try again later.

When people have been sick or inactive, they may become weak and tire more easily. Joints may become stiff. Regular, gentle exercise can help keep their joints and muscles in healthy condition. When stiffness or weakness is caused by diseases such as arthritis or by an injury, a physical or occupational therapist can plan an exercise program that may help prevent further stiffness or weakness.

> **Exercise should be done at the same time each day, in a quiet, orderly way**

If the person has any other health problems, or if you are planning a vigorous exercise program, discuss this with your physician before you begin. You should notify your doctor of any new physical problems and of marked changes in existing ones.

Recreation

Recreation, having fun, and enjoying life are important for everyone. An illness that causes dementia does not mean an end to enjoying life. It may mean that you will need to make a special effort to find things that give pleasure to the person with dementia.

As the person's illness progresses, it may become more difficult to find things they can still enjoy. In reality, you may already be doing as much as you can and adding an "activity" program may further exhaust you and add to the stress in the household. Instead, look for things you can still do that both of you will enjoy.

Consider an adult day care program or an in-home visitor program. The sheltered social setting of adult day care may provide just the right balance of stimulation and security. If the person with dementia is able to adjust to the new setting, they may enjoy the camaraderie with other people who also have memory problems. Some in-home visitor programs offer occupational or recreational therapy services. These professionals can help you plan exercises or activities the person will enjoy. Both in-home visiting and day care offer social activities and opportunities for success and fun. If at all possible, involve the person in such a program.

People who have dementia often lose the ability to entertain themselves. For some, idleness leads to pacing or other repetitive behaviors. The person may resist your suggestions of things to do. Often, this is because they do not understand what you are suggesting. Try beginning an activity and then inviting them to join you. Select simple, adult activities rather than childish games. Select an activity that will be fun rather than one that is supposed to be "therapeutic." Look for things that the person will enjoy and that they will succeed at (like sanding wood, playing with a child, cranking an ice cream maker).

The amount of activity a person is able to tolerate varies widely. Plan activity when the person is rested. Help whenever the person becomes anxious or irritable, and break the activity down into simple steps.

Even individuals with severe impairments can enjoy familiar songs

Previously enjoyed activities may remain important and enjoyable even for people who have serious impairment. However, the things the person used to enjoy, such as hobbies, guests, concerts, or going out to dinner, can become too complicated to be fun for someone who is easily confused. These must be replaced by simpler joys, although it can be hard for family members to understand that simple things can now give just as much pleasure.

Music is a delightful resource for many people. Even individuals with a severe impairment usually retain the capacity to enjoy old, familiar songs. Some people will sing only when someone sits close by and encourages them. Others may be able to use a CD player or radio with large knobs. People are sometimes still able to play the piano or sing if they learned this skill earlier.

Music is a source of pleasure for many people

Some memory-impaired people enjoy television. Others become upset when they cannot understand the story. Television triggers catastrophic reactions in some people. Some people enjoy videos or cable channels that specialize in old movies.

Many people who have dementia enjoy seeing old friends, although they sometimes become upset. If this happens, try having only one or two people visit at a time instead of a group. It is often the confusion that comes from several people visiting at once that is upsetting. Ask visitors to stay for shorter periods, and explain to them in advance the reason for the person's forgetfulness and other behaviors.

Some families enjoy going out to dinner, and many people who have dementia retain most of their social graces. Others embarrass the family by their messy eating. It is helpful to order for the person and select simple foods that can be eaten neatly. Remove unnecessary glasses and eating utensils. Some families have found that it helps to discreetly explain to the wait staff that the person has dementia and cannot order for themselves.

Consider the hobbies and interests the person had before they became ill, and look for ways they can still enjoy these. Often, for example, people who liked to read will continue to enjoy leafing through newspapers, magazines, and books after they can no longer make sense of the text. Sometimes a person puts away a hobby or interest and refuses to pick it up again. This often happens with something a person had done well before but now has difficulty with. It can seem degrading to encourage a person to do a simplified version of a once mastered skill unless they particularly enjoy it. It may be better to find new kinds of recreation.

Everyone enjoys experiencing things through the senses. You probably enjoy watching a brilliant sunset, smelling a flower, or tasting your favorite food. People who have dementia are often more isolated and may not be able to seek out experiences to stimulate their senses. Try pointing out a pretty picture, a singing bird, or a familiar smell or taste. Like you, the person will enjoy certain sensations more and others less.

Many families have found that people who have dementia enjoy a ride in the car.

People who have always enjoyed animals may respond with delight to pets. Some cats and dogs seem to have an instinctive way with people who have cognitive impairments.

Some individuals enjoy a stuffed animal or doll. A stuffed toy can be either childish and demeaning or comforting; much depends on the attitude of the people around the person

who has dementia. Our opinion is that people should be allowed to have stuffed toys if they seem to enjoy them.

Touch can be an effective way of communicating long after the person can no longer understand what is being said

---

As the dementia progresses and the person develops trouble with coordination and language, it is easy to forget their need to experience pleasant things and to enjoy themselves. Never overlook the importance of hand-holding, touching, hugging, and loving. Often when there is no other way we can find to communicate with a person, a simple touch or hug will elicit a positive response. Touch is an important part of human communication. A backrub or a foot or hand massage can be calming. You may enjoy just sitting and holding hands. It's a good way to share some time when talking has become difficult or impossible.

Meaningful Activity

Much of what we do during the day has a purpose that gives meaning and importance to life. We work to make money, to serve others, to feel important. We may knit a sweater for a grandchild or bake a cake for a friend. We wash our hair and clothes so we will look nice and be clean. Such purposeful activities are important to us—they make us feel useful and needed.

When the person who has dementia is unable to continue their usual activities, you need to help them find things to do that are important to them and still within their abilities. Such tasks should be meaningful and satisfying to them—whether they seem so to you or not. For example, folding and refolding towels might have meaning for some people but not for others. Seeing themselves as "volunteers" rather than as "patients" is important to some people. This provides both a sense of worth and the benefit of participation. The person may be able to spade a garden for you or the neighbors, or to peel vegetables or set the table when they are no longer able to prepare a complete meal. People can wind a ball of yarn, dust, or stack magazines while you work. Encourage the person to do as much as they can on their own, although you can simplify tasks for them by breaking them down into steps or doing part of the task yourself.

Most experts urge people who have dementia to exercise or do things that keep their minds active. There is some evidence that staying mentally and physically active can help postpone the onset of dementia for *people who do not have thinking impairment*. In addition, once an illness that causes dementia has begun, keeping physically and mentally active may slow progression. Even more importantly, it can improve the quality of life for the person who has dementia.

Pushing people to do things that upset them is not helpful

It is important to consider the effect that any particular activity has on the person. Activities should be enjoyable, even if they are simple, such as petting the dog, talking with others, taking a walk, or sitting outside. If the person repeatedly shows signs of being upset, including irritability, stubbornness, crying, or refusing to do the activity, then it has become a stressor rather than a pleasure. Pushing a person to do things that upset them is not helpful.

Personal Hygiene

The personal care needs of people who have an illness that causes dementia depend on the type and extent of the brain damage. They may be able to care for themselves in the early stages of the disease but gradually begin to neglect themselves and eventually need total help.

Problems often arise over getting people to change their clothes or take a bath. "I already changed," the person may tell you, or they may turn the tables and make it sound as if you are wrong to suggest such a thing.

A daughter says, "I can't get her to change clothes. She has had the same clothes on for a week. She sleeps in them. When I tell her to change, she says she already did or she yells at me, 'Who do you think you are, telling me when to change my clothes?'"

A husband relates, "She screams for help the whole time I am bathing her. She'll even open the window and yell, 'Help, I'm being robbed.'"

•

A person who has an illness that causes dementia may become depressed or apathetic and lose any desire to clean themselves up. They may be losing the ability to remember how much time has passed: to them it doesn't *seem* like a week since they changed clothes. To have someone telling them they need to change their clothes may embarrass them. (How would you feel if someone came up to you and told you that you should change your clothes?)

Dressing and bathing are intensely personal activities. We each have our own individual ways of doing things. Some of us take showers, some take tub baths; some of us bathe in the morning, others bathe at night. Some of us change clothes twice a day, some, every other day. But each of us is quite set in our own way of doing things. Sometimes when a family member begins to help the confused person, the helper inadvertently overlooks these established habits. The change in routine can be upsetting. A generation or two ago, many people did not wash and change as frequently as we do today. Once a week may have been the way the person did things in their childhood.

We begin to bathe and dress ourselves as small children. It is a basic indicator of our independence. Moreover, bathing and dressing are private activities. Many people have never, as an adult, completely bathed and dressed in front of anyone else. Having other people's hands and eyes on one's naked, aging, not-so-beautiful body can be

an acutely uncomfortable experience for some. When we offer to help with something a person has always done for themselves—something everybody does for themselves and does in private—it is a strong statement that this person is not able to do things for themselves any longer, that they have, in fact, become like a child who must be told when to dress and must have help.

> **When bathing and dressing become difficult, look for ways to simplify the decisions a person must make**

Changing clothes and bathing involve making multiple decisions. A person must select among many socks, shirts or tops, and pants or skirts. When people begin to realize they can't do this, and when looking at a drawer full of blue, green, and black socks becomes overwhelmingly confusing, it can be easier just not to change.

Factors such as these often trigger catastrophic reactions involving bathing and dressing. Still, you are faced with the problem of keeping this person clean. Begin by trying to understand the person's feelings and need for privacy and independence. Know that the behavior is a product of their brain impairment and not deliberately offensive. Look for ways to simplify the number of decisions involved in bathing and dressing without taking away independence.

Bathing

When a person refuses to take a bath, part of the problem may be that the activities associated with bathing have become too confusing and complicated; for others it is anxiety or the fact that the caregiver must intrude into the person's private space. Look for ways to reduce these factors. Be calm and quiet, and simplify the task. Wrap the person in a robe or towel and help them wash under it. Try to follow as many of the person's old routines as possible while you encourage them to bathe, and at the same time simplify the job for them. Lay out the person's clothes and towels and start the bathwater. If a man has always shaved first, then showered, then eaten breakfast, he is most likely to cooperate with your request if you time his bath before breakfast.

Be calm and gentle when you help with a bath. Avoid getting into discussions about whether a bath is needed. Instead, tell the person *one step at a time* what to do in preparation for the bath:

- Avoid saying, "Dad, I want you to take a bath right after breakfast." ("Right after breakfast" means he has to remember something.)

- Avoid responding to "I don't need a bath" by saying, "Oh yes you do. You haven't had a bath in a week." (You wouldn't like to have him say that to you, especially if you couldn't remember when you last had a bath.)

- Try instead, "Dad, your bathwater is ready." "I don't need a bath," he may respond. "Here is your towel. Now, unbutton your shirt." (His mind may focus on the buttons instead of the argument. You can gently help him if you see him having difficulty.) "Now stand up. Undo your pants, Dad." "I

don't need a bath," he may say again. "Now step into the tub."

•

One daughter drew her father's bath, got everything ready, and then, when he wandered down the hall, said, "Oh, look at this lovely bath water. As long as it is here, why not take a bath? It would be terrible to waste it." Her father, who had always pinched pennies, yielded.

•

One wife told her husband, "As soon as your bath is over, you and I will eat those good cookies Janie brought."

•

Some families have found that the person who has dementia will let an aide in uniform or another family member bathe them.

Think over the person's lifelong bath habits: did they bathe or shower? In the morning or at night?

If all else fails, give partial baths or sponge baths. Watch the person's skin for rashes or red areas.

Bathing should be a regular routine, done the same way at the same time of day. The person will come to expect this and may put up less resistance. If bathing continues to be difficult, it is not necessary for the person to bathe every day.

Many accidents occur in the bath. Assemble everything in advance and *never turn away or leave the person.* Always check the temperature of the bath or shower water, even if the person has been successfully doing this for themselves. The ability to gauge safe temperatures can be lost quite suddenly.

Never leave the person alone in the tub. Use only two or three inches of water. This way the person feels more secure, and it is safer. Put a rubber mat or nonskid decals on the bottom of the tub to prevent slipping. Avoid using bubble bath or bath oils that can make the tub slippery. These can also contribute to vaginal infections in women.

<hr>

Never turn away from or leave the person in the bath

<hr>

It can be difficult to get a person in and out of a tub, especially if they are clumsy or heavy. An unsteady person can slip and fall while stepping over the side. An unsteady person may also fall while standing in the shower. Install grab bars that the person can use to help themselves in and out of the tub or shower and that they can hold on to while they bathe. Grab bars are essential for safe care. Use a bath seat in either a tub or shower. A bath transfer bench straddles the side of the tub. You help the person swing their legs over the rim, and then they slide along the bench so that they are sitting on the bench inside the walls of the tub. (See the next section for locating bath supplies.) Many families have told us that a bath seat and a handheld hose greatly reduce the bath time crisis. You have control of the water (and the mess). The seat is safer, and the controlled flow of water is less upsetting to the person. Bath seats reduce people's anxiety because they feel more secure, and it reduces your need to bend and stretch. The hose makes rinsing the person and washing their hair much easier.

People can often continue to wash themselves if you gently remind them one step at a time of each area to wash. Sometimes it is embarrassing for a family member to make sure that the genital area is thoroughly washed, but rashes can develop there, so see that this is done. Be sure that you or the person who has dementia has washed in folds of flesh and under breasts.

Use a bath mat that will not slip for the person to step out onto, and be sure there are no puddles on the floor. It may be helpful to replace bath mats with bathroom carpeting that does not slip, soaks up puddles, and is washable. For people who still dry themselves, check to see that they haven't forgotten some areas. If you dry the person, be sure they are completely dry. Use body powder, baby powder, or cornstarch under women's breasts and in creases and folds of skin. Cornstarch is an inexpensive, odorless, and non-allergenic substitute for talcum powder. Baking soda is an effective substitute if the person resists using a deodorant.

While the person is undressed, check for red areas of skin, rashes, or sores. If any red areas or sores appear, ask your physician to help you manage them. Pressure sores, also called decubitus ulcers, develop quickly on people who sit or lie down much of the time. Use body lotion on dry skin.

Locating Care Supplies

Many websites, big-box stores, drugstores, and medical supply companies carry the products we recommend, including bath supplies, toilet safety frames, commodes, Dycem, grab bars, incontinence supplies, canes, wheelchairs, and devices to build up the handles on eating utensils and toothbrushes. Supplies come in a variety of designs to fit different bathrooms and different needs. Ask if Medicare, Medicaid, or your major insurance provider will cover any supplies. A pharmacist can help you select the products that will be best for your needs.

A toilet safety frame provides a set of bars that fit around the toilet and help people lower themselves onto and lift themselves off the toilet. These bars also help to prevent people from toppling sideways.

Raised (built-up) toilet seats make it easier for people to get on and off the seat and easier to transfer a person from a wheelchair to the toilet. The seat should fasten securely to the toilet so it does not slip when the person sits on it. Padded (soft) toilet seats are more comfortable for the person who must sit for some time. This is especially important for the person who develops pressure sores easily.

You can rent portable commodes that can be placed near a person's bed or on the ground floor so that the person does not have to climb stairs. A variety of urinals and bedpans are also available.

Towel rods and the toothbrush or soap holder in many homes are often glued to the wall or fastened only into the drywall. They may come loose if a person grabs them for balance or to lift themselves up. Make sure that these items are installed by someone knowledgeable about carpentry to ensure they are anchored into the stud in the wall. Make sure they are designed for sturdiness.

Dressing

Lay out a clean outfit for the person who has trouble making choices. Laying out clothes in the order in which they are put on may also help. Put away out-of-season or rarely worn clothing so they do not add to the decisions the person must make. If all the person's socks go with all of their pants, they don't have to decide which pair to wear with what.

If the person refuses to change clothes, avoid getting in an argument. Make the suggestion again later.

Hang ties, scarves, or accessories on the hanger with the shirt or dress they go with. Eliminate belts, scarves, and other accessories that are likely to be put on wrong.

As the disease progresses, it becomes difficult for the person with dementia to put clothes on right side out and in the correct sequence. Buttons, zippers, shoelaces, and belt buckles become impossible to manage. If the person can no longer manage buttons, replace them with Velcro, which you can purchase in a fabric store. People can often manage this after their fingers and brain can no longer cope with buttons. One wife, sensitive to her husband's need to continue to dress himself independently, bought him clothes that were reversible. She bought attractive T-shirts that didn't look bad if they were worn backward, pants with elastic waistbands, and tube socks. (Tube socks don't have heels, so it takes less skill to put them on.) Slip-on shoes are easier than shoes with laces or ties. Women can wear reversible, slip-on shirts and reversible, wraparound, or elastic-waistband skirts and pants. Loose-fitting clothing is easier to manage.

You can find clothing designed for ease of dressing people who have dementia and those in wheelchairs on the internet.

Select clothing that is washable and that doesn't need ironing; there is no reason to add to your workload. Avoid clothing with "busy" patterns that are difficult to match.

Underwear is difficult for a person who has dementia to manage. Buy soft, loose-fitting underwear. It won't matter if they are put on backward or wrong side out. If you must put a bra on a woman, ask her to lean forward to settle her breasts in the cups. Pantyhose are difficult to put on, and knee socks are bad for people with poor circulation. Short cotton socks may be best to wear at home.

Tell the person, one step at a time, what to do or what you are doing. Go with what works. If the person is dressed oddly, let it be.

Grooming

Have the person's hair cut in a style that is easy to wash and care for. Avoid a style that requires blow drying or curling. People who have always gone to the hairdresser or barbershop may still enjoy doing so. If this is too upsetting an experience, it may be possible to arrange for a hairdresser or barber to come to your home.

It may be safer (and easier on your back) to wash the person's hair in the kitchen sink rather than the tub, unless you have a hose attachment in the bathtub. Invest in a hose attachment

for the sink. Be sure you rinse their hair well. It should squeak when rubbed through your fingers.

You will need to trim fingernails and toenails or check to see that they can still do this themselves. Long toenails can curl back against the toes and become quite painful.

Encourage the person to get dressed and to take pride in their appearance. Moping around in a bathrobe will not help their morale. If a woman has always worn makeup, it may be good for her to continue to wear simple makeup. It is not difficult for a caregiver to put blush and lipstick on a woman. Use pastel colors and a light touch on an older woman. Skip the eye makeup.

When the bathing and dressing are finished, encourage the person to look in the mirror and see how nice they look (even if you are exhausted and exasperated). Have the rest of the family compliment them also. Praise and encouragement are important in helping people continue to feel good about themselves, even when a task they have always been able to do, such as dressing, has become too much for them.

Oral Hygiene

With all the other chores of caring for a chronically ill person, it is easy to forget what we can't see, but good oral hygiene is important for the person's comfort and health. People who appear to be able to care for themselves in other ways may, in fact, be forgetting to care for their teeth or dentures.

Make oral care a part of a regular, expected routine and do it calmly so that you will encounter less resistance. Select a time of day when the person is most cooperative. If the person becomes upset, stop and try again later.

Because you want the person to be as independent as possible, you can assume the responsibility of remembering but letting the person do as much of the actual care as possible. One reason people stop caring for their teeth or dentures is that these are complicated tasks with many steps and they become confused about what to do next. Early in the illness, you will need to remind the person to brush their teeth. Later you will need to instruct them step by step. As they become more confused, simplify your instructions by breaking the activity into distinct steps: instead of "Brush your teeth," say, "Hold the toothbrush," then "I will put on the toothpaste," then "Put it in your mouth," and so on. It may help to have the person imitate you. Remind the person to rinse and spit. When you must brush the person's teeth for them, experiment with different-shaped brushes and try standing behind them.

Dentures are particularly troublesome. If they don't fit just right or if a person is not applying the denture adhesive properly, they interfere with chewing. The natural response is to stop eating those things that are difficult to chew. This can lead to inadequate nutrition or constipation. Dentures should be in place when a person is eating. If they don't fit properly or are uncomfortable, insist that the dentist fix them. If a person forgets to take out their dentures and clean them, or if they refuse to let you do it,

they can develop painful sores on their gums, which can further interfere with eating a proper diet.

> **To help the person remain as independent as possible, you should assume the responsibility of remembering while letting the person do as much of their own self-care as possible**

If you take over the care of the person's dentures, you must remove them daily, clean them, and check the gums for irritation. A dentist can show you how to do this.

Check the person's mouth for sores and be alert to changes in chewing or eating that might indicate dental problems. Find a dentist who has experience with people who have memory problems. There are many dentists who are gentle and patient and able to continue the person's dental care.

Healthy teeth or properly fitting dentures are critically important. People who have dementia tend not to chew well and to choke easily. Dental problems make this worse. Even mild nutritional problems caused by sore teeth can increase the person's confusion or cause constipation. Sores in the mouth can lead to other problems and can increase the person's impairment (see page 107).

Incontinence (Wetting or Soiling)

People who have illnesses that cause dementia may begin to wet themselves or have bowel movements in their clothing. This is called, respectively, urinary incontinence and bowel (or fecal) incontinence. The two are separate problems, and one often occurs without the other. There are many causes of incontinence that are treatable, so it is important to begin by having a doctor assess the problem.

Urinating and moving one's bowels are natural human functions. However, ever since childhood we have been taught that these are private activities. Many of us have also been taught that they are nasty, dirty, or socially unacceptable. In addition, we associate caring for our own bodily functions in private with independence and personal dignity. When another person has to help us, it is distressing for both the helper and the person being helped. Often, too, individuals find the urine or bowel movements of others disgusting and may gag or vomit when cleaning up. It is important for both family members and professional caregivers to be aware of their own strong feelings in these areas.

Urinary Incontinence

Urinary incontinence has many causes, some of which respond well to treatment. Ask yourself the following questions.

If the person is a woman, is she "leaking" rather than completely emptying her bladder, especially when she laughs, coughs, lifts something, or makes some other sudden exertion? Light pad incontinence products are inconspicuous under clothing and give a person confidence to continue to go out in public. Men may "dribble." There are also light pads designed for men. Do accidents happen only at certain times of day, such as at night? (It is helpful to keep a diary for several days of the times the accidents occur, the times the person successfully uses the toilet, and the times the person eats or drinks.) How often does the person urinate? Is the urination painful? Did the incontinence begin suddenly? Has there been a change in medication in the past month? Has the person's confusion suddenly gotten worse? Does the incontinence occur occasionally or intermittently? Is the person living in a new place? Is the person urinating in improper places, such as in closets or in flower pots? (This is different from the person who wets themselves and their clothing wherever they happen to be.) Do accidents happen when the person cannot get to the bathroom on time? Are they happening on the way to the bathroom?

When urinary incontinence occurs before the late stages of Alzheimer disease (each disease is different), it is usually not directly caused by the disease. You may be able to solve the problem.

Whenever incontinence begins, you should check with a doctor. You can help the doctor diagnose the problem by having the answers to the questions listed above. If the person has a fever, report this to the doctor at once. Do not let a physician dismiss incontinence without carefully exploring all potentially treatable causes.

Urinary incontinence may be brought on by chronic or acute bladder infections, uncontrolled diabetes, an enlarged prostate, dehydration, medications, and many other medical problems (see Chapter 6). "Leaking" can be caused by an inflexible bladder, a weakened sphincter muscle, or other conditions that are potentially treatable.

It might seem that giving less fluid would reduce incontinence, but this can be dangerous because it can lead to dehydration. A first step in addressing incontinence is to be sure that the person is getting enough fluid to stimulate the bladder to work. Both too little and too much fluid can be bad. If you are uncertain how much fluid the person should have, ask your doctor or nurse. A doctor or nurse can also determine whether the person is dehydrated.

As the illness progresses, the person may not experience or may be unable to respond correctly to the feeling of needing to urinate or may be unable to get up and get to the toilet in time. You can solve this problem by regularly reminding the person to go to the bathroom.

If the problem is that the person moves slowly or uses a walker or is clumsy and cannot get to the bathroom in time, say, "Do you want to go to the bathroom before you sit down?" If the person must walk a distance to go to the toilet, try renting a portable com-

mode, which brings the toilet closer to the person. You can also simplify clothing so the person can manipulate it easier and faster. Try Velcro instead of zippers or buttons. Can the person easily get up out of their chair? If they are sunk in a deep chair, they may not be able to get up in time. Remind them before it is too late.

> **Medication changes in the prior month might be causing new onset urinary incontinence**

Sometimes people cannot find the bathroom. This often happens in a new setting. A clear sign or a brightly painted door occasionally helps. People who urinate in wastebaskets, closets, and flower pots may be unable to locate the bathroom or unable to remember the appropriate place. Some families find that putting a lid on the wastebasket, locking closet doors, and taking the person to the bathroom on a regular schedule help.

Purchase washable chair cushion covers. Slide them on over a large garbage bag to waterproof cushions. If you have a favorite chair or rug that you are afraid will be damaged, take the easy way out and put it where the person will not use it.

Sometimes people need help but are either unable to or embarrassed to ask for it. Restlessness or irritability may be an indication that the person needs to be taken to the toilet. Learn what the person's cues mean and be sure that sitters or other caregivers know also.

If the person is incontinent at night, limit the amount of fluid they drink after supper unless there is some medical reason why they need extra fluid. (The rest of the day, be sure they are getting plenty of fluids.) Get them up once at night. It may be helpful to get a bedside commode the person can use easily, especially if they have trouble moving around. Night-lights in the bathroom and bedroom help too. Buy a waterproof mattress cover before accidents begin, and use waterproof pads for the bed (see below for incontinence wear).

Falls often occur on the way to the bathroom at night. Make sure there are adequate lights and no throw rugs, that the person can get out of bed, and that they have slippers that are not slick-soled or floppy.

Plan a regular schedule for toileting the person who no longer manages alone. This will minimize the frequency of accidents, reduce skin irritations, and make life easier for both of you. An interval of every two hours is often most successful at preventing incontinence. As long as the person is ambulatory, you may be able to manage incontinence this way even late in the illness.

A diary will provide you with the information you need to prevent many accidents. If you know when the person usually urinates (for example, immediately on awakening, or about 10:00 a.m., an hour after they have had their juice), you can take them to the toilet just before an accident would occur. This is, in fact, training yourself to their natural schedule. Many families find that they can tell when the person needs to go to the bathroom. They may become restless or pick at their clothes. If the person does not give you clues, routinely take them to the toilet every

two hours. While it may be embarrassing to ask the person to go to the bathroom, this routine will save the person the humiliation of wetting themselves.

Certain nonverbal signals that tell us it is time or not time to urinate may influence some people with an impairment. Taking down one's underpants or opening one's fly or sitting down on a toilet seat can be clues to "go." Dry clothes and being in bed or in public are signals to "not go." (Some people are unable to urinate when there are "no go" clues, such as in the presence of another person or when using a bedpan.) Pulling down underwear when undressing a woman may cause her to urinate. You may be able to use such nonverbal clues to help a person go at the right time.

One man urinated every morning as soon as he put his feet on the floor. If this is what is happening, you may be able to be prepared and catch the urine in a urinal. People may also be inhibited and unable to go when you are in the bathroom with them or if you ask them to use a commode in a room that is not a bathroom. It is often this involuntary "no go" response that leads families to say, "He wouldn't go when I took him and then he wet his pants. I think he is just being difficult." Make the person comfortable and then step out of the room.

Sometimes, if a person has trouble urinating, it may help to give them a glass of water with a straw and ask them to blow bubbles. This seems to help the urine start. Ask a nurse to show you how to press gently on the bladder to start the flow of urine.

Sometimes a person asks to go to the bathroom every few minutes. If this is a problem, have the doctor see the person to determine whether there is a medical reason why the person feels they need to urinate frequently. A urinary tract infection or certain medications can give a person this feeling or can prevent them from completely emptying their bladder. (If the bladder is not completely empty, the person will soon feel the need to urinate again.)

Many causes of incontinence can be controlled

Some doctors and nurses may dismiss incontinence as inevitable. It is true that some people who have dementia will eventually lose independent control of their elimination functions, but many do not, and many causes of incontinence can be controlled. Even when the person has lost independent function, there is much you can do to make your workload easier and to reduce their embarrassment. If you are having problems, ask for a referral to a nurse or physician who has experience managing incontinence in people who have dementia. Avoid using a catheter to permanently manage urinary incontinence if possible.

Bowel Incontinence

Bowel (or fecal) incontinence, like urinary incontinence, should be discussed with a doctor. Abrupt onset or temporary incontinence may be the result of an infection, diarrhea, irritable bowel syndrome, medication, eating foods that stimulate the bowel to evacuate, constipation, or a fecal impaction (see Chapter 6).

Be sure that the bathroom is comfortable and that the person can sit without discomfort or instability long enough to move their bowels. Their feet should rest on the floor, and they should have something to hold on to. A toilet safety seat will give a person something to hold and will encourage someone who is restless to stay put. Try giving them something to do or letting them listen to music.

Learn when the person usually moves their bowels and take them to the bathroom at that time.

Avoid reprimanding the person who has accidents. Consult your physician if the person may be constipated or have an impaction (see also page 103).

Keep disposable adult washcloths on hand in case of a bowel accident. Skin-cleansing products that liquefy stool and reduce odors make gentle cleaning much easier.

Cleaning Up

A person who remains in soiled or wet clothing can quickly develop irritated skin and sores. Watch for these. Keeping the skin clean and dry is the best protection against skin problems. The skin must be washed after each accident. Powder will keep the skin dry. There are creams that protect the skin from moisture and that help skin irritations. Use only creams designed for the perineal area (the area between the anus and genitals).

The personal care of an incontinent person can seem degrading to them and unpleasant or disgusting to you. Therefore, some families have made a deliberate effort to use the cleanup time as a time to express affection. This can help to make a necessary task less unpleasant.

There is apparel available for incontinent people. Should you use it? Professionals disagree over the use of incontinence wear. Some think that "diapers" are demoralizing and encourage infantile behavior. Some find that scheduled toileting is easier than managing incontinence wear. The answer lies in your own feelings about this and in the incontinent person's response. Incontinence clothing may make things easier for you and more comfortable for the person who has dementia. You may choose to use it only at nighttime. Nursing homes or residential homes should not routinely use diapers as a cost savings without considering the impact of the practice on the individual. We believe a toileting schedule is ideal when it works, but we recognize that some people who have dementia resist it and others are incontinent even when a schedule is tried. The doctor or nurse will help you decide what is right for you.

Some families use cleanup as a time to express affection; this can help to make a necessary task less unpleasant

---

Disposable adult diapers and plastic outer pants are sold online and in grocery stores, big-box stores, and drugstores. Some are more comfortable and stay on better if regular underpants are worn over them. Because of the negative feeling about the word *diaper*, these products are advertised as "adult briefs" or "incontinence wear." There are many choices. Some are made so that one size fits all; others are sized by the hip or waist measurement. Some are designed for men, others for women. Some are for people who are bedfast. Some are disposable, and others have a disposable liner. Adult disposable washcloths are available for cleaning up and are much more convenient than having to launder extra cloths.

Garments and pads are labeled for the amount of urine they will hold. A full bladder may empty eight to ten ounces (about one cup) of urine. You may have to experiment to find the style and absorbency that works best for you. Garments that don't fit or that are too saturated may leak. Don't expect the garment to hold more than one urination.

Several products consist of outer, washable underpants that hold a disposable pad. The ideal is a soft, cool material in which the absorbent pad tends to draw urine away from the crotch so that the person's skin feels dry. It is helpful if the garment is designed so that the pad can be changed without lowering the garment and so that the garment can be lowered for toileting.

The legs of the underpants should fit snugly, to prevent leakage, but should not bind. Adult briefs may leak around the legs of a thin person. Families have found that using a toddler-size diaper plus the absorbent section of an adult brief helps. Using a safety pin to attach the brief to the undershirt of a bedfast person will help contain a bowel movement. Some briefs have greater absorbency in the front (for men), while others are more absorbent toward the back. Experiment to find the one that works best.

You should wash your hands thoroughly with soap each time you provide care for a person since you can transmit infection to the person you are caring for, to yourself, and to others. Use disposable hand wipes for emergencies. Keep bottles of hand sanitizer in the bathroom, kitchen, and areas in which the person is cared for.

In large cities, there are adult diaper services that save you the burden of washing these garments if you do not want to use disposable items.

Disposable pads are available to protect bedding, and you can also buy rubberized flannel sheets. These are much less unpleasant than the rubber sheets used in the past.

Plastic underpants or rubber sheets need to be shielded by a layer of cloth next to the skin. Without the protection of the cloth, plastic causes moisture to stay in contact with the skin and leads to irritation and rawness.

Problems with Walking and Balance, and Falling

As dementia progresses, the person may become stiff, walk awkwardly, and have difficulty getting out of a chair or out of bed. They may develop a stooped or leaning posture or a shuffling walk. They will need close supervision when their risk of falling is increased.

•

A family member writes, "His steps are very slow now. As he walks, he often raises his feet high, for he has little sense of space. He clutches door frames or chairs. Sometimes he just grasps at the air. His gaze is unfocused, like that of a blind man. He stops in front of mirrors, and he talks and laughs with the images there."

•

A wife says, "He sometimes falls down. He trips over his own feet or just crumples up. But when I try to lift him—and he is a big man—he yells and struggles against me."

•

Any of these symptoms *may* be caused by medications. Discuss with the doctor any change in walking, posture, stiffness, repetitive motions, or falling. The doctor should make sure that there is not a treatable cause for the change, such as medications or delirium. These same symptoms will occur when the dementia has damaged the areas of the brain that control muscle movements. But do not assume that this is the cause until the doctor has eliminated other causes, including stroke, arthritis, and muscle disease. If the person has had a small stroke or has symptoms of parkinsonism or weakness due to inactivity, physical therapy might help.

Watch for the time when the person starts to trip, can no longer safely negotiate stairs, or has other difficulties walking. If a person is unsteady on their feet, have them take your arm, if they will, rather than you grasping theirs. Hold your arm close to your body. This maximizes your ability to keep your balance. Or you may steady someone by walking behind them and holding their belt.

Put away scatter rugs, which may slide when the person steps on them. Install handrails, especially in the bathroom. If the person slips on the hardwood stairs, apply anti-slip adhesive treads to them or pad them with secured rug pieces. Staple or tack down rug edges. Be sure that chairs or other furniture that the person tends to lean on are sturdy. You can find foam shaped to pad sharp corners on the internet or you can make your own.

Some people are unsteady and fall when they first get out of bed. Have the person sit on the edge of the bed for a few minutes before standing and walking. Many slippers and shoes have slick soles that can cause falls. Some people will stumble more in crepe-soled shoes. Others benefit from the grip crepe gives. Some people can learn to use canes or walkers. Others cannot learn this new skill. If the person cannot learn to use a device properly, it is safer for them not to use it.

> It is safer to call 911 for help after a fall than to risk injury to the person who has fallen or their caregiver

When you help a person, it is important that you not hurt yourself or throw yourself off balance. A physical therapist or visiting nurse can show you ways to assist a person without strain.

Avoid leaning forward or bending over when you lift. If you must bend to lift something or someone, bend at the knees, not at the waist. Take your time; accidents happen when you rush yourself or the person who has dementia. If you lift a person, lift from under their arms, in the armpits. Avoid pulling a person up out of bed by their arms. Avoid trying to put an awkward or heavy person into the back seat of a two-door car.

When a person falls, do the following:

- Remain calm.

- Check to see if they are visibly injured or in pain.

- Avoid triggering a catastrophic reaction.

- Watch the person for swelling, bruises, signs of pain, agitation, drowsiness, and increased distress.

- Call 911 or the doctor if any of these symptoms appear or if you think there is any chance that they hit their head or otherwise hurt themselves.

Instead of trying to get her husband up when he fell, one wife trained herself to sit down on the floor with him. (Obviously this took an effort to calm her own distress.) She would pat him and chat with him gently until he calmed down. When he was relaxed, she was able to encourage him to get himself up one step at a time rather than having to lift him.

For *both of you*, it is safer for you to call 911 for help rather than to risk injury trying to get a person up after a fall. Emergency personnel tell us that this is part of their job and that they are glad to respond.

Becoming Chairbound or Bedfast

As dementia progresses, some people gradually lose the ability to walk. This begins with occasional stumbling and falling, progresses to taking smaller and smaller steps, and develops, usually after years, into being unable to stand. Eventually the person may not be able to straighten their legs to the floor when held upright by others. This is sometimes called an apraxia of gait (see pages 39–40).

In contrast to this gradual progression, an abrupt loss of the ability to stand or walk or the sudden onset of falling suggests that the person has another illness or has had an adverse reaction to a medication. These possibilities should be investigated promptly by a physician.

The gradual loss of the ability to walk or stand in a person who has dementia is usually the result of progressive brain damage; the person has "forgotten" how to walk. Keeping people as active as possible helps to maintain their muscle strength and general health, but there is no evidence that exercise or activity can postpone or prevent the loss of the ability to walk due to dementia.

Even when a person cannot walk, they may be able to sit up. Sitting in a chair much of the day enables them to continue being a part of the family or to participate in care center activities. If the person has a tendency to fall forward or out of the chair, you can prop them up with pillows (ask for a physical therapy consultation to show you how) or, very rarely, use a waist restraint. Alternatives to lap restraints include "lap buddies" and lounge chairs or Geri Chairs (you can rent or purchase these from medical supply stores). When a lounge chair is kept in the reclined position, it protects the person from falling forward. You may prop the person with pillows so that they are comfortable. You may want to move the person from one chair to a different chair or to bed as a way of changing their position. Use pieces of "egg-crate" foam (available from a medical supply store or a store that sells bedding) to cushion them. A lap buddy is a piece of foam that sits on a person's lap and under the arms of a chair. It is easier to remove than a lap restraint and is therefore safer.

Some people eventually become unable to sit. They usually have contractures—stiffened tendons that do not allow their joints to open or extend fully. Contractures may be postponed or reduced by keeping people physically active and by physical therapy, but they can occur late in any progressive disease that causes dementia or following a stroke, even when the person's joints are moved and exercised by others.

When people who have dementia are no longer able to move voluntarily and are confined to bed, they require almost constant physical attention. They are at high risk of developing pressure sores, also called bedsores (see page 101), and of getting food, saliva, and other substances into their lungs because they cannot swallow or because they are lying down.

People who have dementia and are bedfast should be carefully turned from one side to the other every two hours, if possible. Your doctor may recommend more frequent turning. Care must be taken to avoid putting undue pressure or weight on any one part of the body because many people have brittle bones and fragile skin. Satin or silk sheets and pajamas can make it easier to move someone who cannot move independently. When people are lying on their side, they should be propped up with a pillow. It is sometimes necessary to place a pillow or pad between the knees to prevent sores from forming. The skin must be kept clean and dry.

Moving a totally bedfast person requires skill and training. Visiting nurses and physical therapists can be helpful in teaching you how to move and turn the person.

Wheelchairs

If the time comes when the person needs a wheelchair, your doctor or a visiting nurse can give you guidance in selecting and using one. You can get information about how to best maneuver wheelchairs from medical equipment stores and the internet. Wheelchairs can be uncomfortable for people who sit in them for long periods. The seats of many chairs are hard and can cause pressure sores. Chairs that do not support the body correctly can cause muscle and nerve damage as well. Sometimes people slump in the chair or are left sitting with an arm hanging so that their fingers go numb. The right kind of chair can help avoid these problems.

There are different kinds of wheelchairs. A qualified person should help you select a chair that is comfortable and supports the user. You will also need a chair that meets your needs in weight (can you lift it?), portability (will you need to take it in the car?), and width (will it go through your doorways?). Ask a physical therapist or nurse to show you how to help someone in and out of the chair and how to support the person correctly.

You may have to advocate strongly to get Medicare to pay for a wheelchair or electric scooter

Medicare Part B (and Medicare Advantage Plans) will pay for one wheelchair (for each person) that is properly fitted according to a physical therapist's prescription. A prescription-fitted wheelchair can reduce pain, pressure sores, and other problems. The Medicare website (www.medicare.gov) lists the eligibility requirements. Families tell us that they have had to advocate strongly to have wheelchairs and electric scooters paid for. Ask your doctor or health care provider whether Medicare will cover other durable medical equipment that the person needs and that has been ordered by the physician.

Changes You Can Make at Home

There are many changes you can make at home that might make life easier for you and for the person who has dementia. As you read or as you talk to other families about dementia, you will hear many suggestions. While they may help, gadgets are not the total solution. When you consider changes, ask yourself whether you can live with them comfortably. Also, remember that people who have dementia may not be able to learn even simple new things and sometimes cannot adjust to minor changes. You might purchase a new phone that is easy for you to operate, only to find that the person who has dementia cannot learn to use it. Or you might rearrange the furniture and then realize that the change upsets rather than calms the person.

Remember that no single suggestion will work in all situations. Look for ideas that make sense to you and are affordable. Usually, you will not need expensive "Alzheimer" devices. Some of these products and medical supplies, like walkers and wheelchairs, may be available secondhand. We discuss devices that help you manage wandering in Chapter 7.

Gadgets that make life easier for older people. These include recliners, special cushions for thin people or those with sensitive skin, heating pads that shut off automatically, clip-on lights for areas that are dim, magnifying glasses for people with vision problems, and amplifiers and lights that alert people with hearing problems to sounds such as the phone or the doorbell.

Many devices are available to enlarge the size of eating utensil handles, pens and pencils, and other items that must be grasped. There are also long reaching devices for getting things off the floor or down from a high shelf. There are several devices for opening jars. These are usually advertised in media aimed at an older audience and may be available online or at the drugstore.

Devices that record phone calls. Cell phones identify the phone numbers of incoming calls and the caller's name if they are in the phone's contact list. The call log ("Recents" or "Recent calls") tells you who has called recently in case the person with dementia forgets to tell you about calls. Answering machines attached to landlines can be set to record all calls. This allows you to monitor calls the person might forget to tell you about.

Gadgets that turn on the lights. Solar-powered lights will turn on outside at dusk. Motion-sensor lights will turn on when a person moves around at night. (Such a light in the bathroom may help the person you're caring for find their way without your having to get up.)

Gadgets that provide sound. Headphones will allow you to listen to music while the person who has dementia watches television (or vice versa). Wireless headphones can also be used to listen to the television, which may be helpful for people who cannot otherwise hear it.

Gadgets for security. Consider a home security system. It can make you feel safer, can include smoke and fire detectors, and can be set to beep whenever a door or window is opened. This will alert you if the person who has dementia tries to go outside. Consider getting a personal security device that you wear and that will call for help if you cannot reach a phone.

Gadgets that monitor sounds. Originally designed for parents of babies, these systems enable you to hear what is going on while you are in another room or out in the yard. You place a small transmitter in the person's room or pocket and carry a small receiver with you that picks up the sounds of whatever the person is doing.

Devices to watch and record videos. The choice of available videos is almost unlimited, whether using a television, tablet, or computer. Some people who have dementia enjoy watching films (especially from their own era). Home movies can be converted to digital format so that family members can reminisce together.

You can record yourself giving a message to the person, for example, "Carlos, this is Daniela, your wife. I have gone to work. Mrs. Lambe will be with you until I come home at 6:00. She will fix your lunch and then you will go for a walk. I want you to stay with her. I love you. See you at 6:00." The person who has dementia can watch this video message as often as they want, and the temporary caregiver can play it if the person gets anxious.

Should Environments Be Cluttered or Bare?

How cluttered should the person's environment be? People who have dementia often have difficulty focusing on one thing in a cluttered area or room. Order, routine, and simplicity are generally very helpful to the person who has trouble concentrating or thinking. However, some environments are so barren as to result in sensory deprivation and disorientation. Some people urge families to put away many things; others say that people who have dementia need stimulation. Some people argue that pictures on the wall or wallpaper cause

hallucinations or disorientation. How do you know what is right? The answer depends on the individual person and the kind of clutter or interest the room offers.

Observe the person who has dementia. Do they tend to grab at everything in the bathroom? Do they put their hands into serving dishes or play with the condiments in the center of the table? Do they seem unable to decide what food to eat first or what eating utensil to pick up? If you observe these things, try simplifying. Remove unnecessary things from the bathroom; leave serving dishes in the kitchen or put only one item of food on their plate at a time. Occasionally a person will talk to the pictures on the wall or try to pick the flowers off the wallpaper. However, most people will not do this. One woman in a nursing home was proud of the wallpaper "her husband put up." Some people cannot recognize their reflection in a mirror and become upset when they see a "stranger" in the room. If a picture or mirror is distressing the person, remove it. There is no reason to remove a mirror or picture if the person just talks to it and is not distressed by it.

In general, people, animals, noise, and action in a room are more distracting than the decor. If the person is restless or irritable or has difficulty paying attention when you communicate with them, consider reducing these distractions, but be sure that plenty of meaningful, focused, one-to-one interactions are provided in their place.

Things a person has to choose between (such as several bottles of shampoo in the shower or several kinds of food on a plate) cause more problems than things that are "just there," like several cushions on the sofa. If the person stacks the pillows or carries them around, there is no need to put them away. Remove things only if they are causing a problem.

Assisted living facilities and nursing homes may not offer enough stimulation, interest, or environmental cues. Whatever the setting, observe the person's response to it. People who pace, fiddle, or repeat the same thing over and over may stop if they are helped to do an activity they can focus on.

There are many ways we can help a person function by changing their physical environment. For example, as people age, they often need more light to see; therefore, be sure that there is enough light. People who have dementia are doubly disabled because they may not think to turn on a lamp or go over to the window for light. Reduce glare from windows and lamps. Glare confuses the already thinking-impaired person. Colors with considerable con-

trast might be easier to see than pastels or colors similar in intensity. To the person with some visual impairment, it may be impossible to see light-colored food on a white plate. If the bathroom rug is deep blue, the person may have more success targeting the white toilet than if the rug is also white.

There are many ways you can change the environment to help a person remain active and engaged

The environment can also be used to keep the person away from certain areas. Just as color can be used to help people notice things, it can be used to hide things. Paint a door (frame, baseboard, and all) to match the adjoining walls if you want the person to ignore it.

Hearing aids magnify background noise, and people who have dementia often cannot learn to compensate for this. Eliminate background noise wherever possible.

CHAPTER 6

Medical Problems

People who have illnesses that cause dementia can also have other diseases, ranging from relatively minor problems, like the flu, to serious illnesses. They may not be able to tell you they are in pain (even if they are able to speak well), or they may neglect their bodies. Cuts, bruises, and even broken bones can go unnoticed. People who sit or lie for long periods of time may develop pressure sores. Their physical health may gradually decline. *Correcting even minor physical problems can greatly help people who have dementia.*

You may have experienced a feeling of mental "dullness" when you were sick. This phenomenon can be worse in people who have dementia, who seem to be especially vulnerable to additional troubles. The person's confusion and behavioral symptoms may worsen. A delirium (see page 305) can be brought on by other conditions (flu, minor cold, pneumonia, heart trouble, reactions to medications, and many other things), and it may look like a sudden worsening of the dementia. However, the delirium (and the symptoms) usually goes away when the condition is treated. You should routinely check for signs of illness or injury and call them to the attention of their nurse or doctor.

People who have difficulty expressing themselves may not be able to answer "yes" or "no" when you ask them specific questions such as, "Does your head hurt?" Even people who still express themselves well may fail to recognize or may be unable to report feeling sick or being in pain or may not be able to tell you where the problem is. The person may not be able to tell the difference between something serious and something minor. They will not remember having told you and will not remember your reassurances, so repeated comforting is usually helpful.

> **Correcting even minor physical ailments can greatly help someone who has dementia**

All indications of pain or illness must be taken seriously. It is important to find a medical professional who is gentle, who understands the person's condition, and who will properly evaluate general medical problems. Do not let a doctor or nurse dismiss a person because they have dementia or are "old." Insist that their symptoms be evaluated and their pains diagnosed and relieved. Because of the person's vulnerability to delirium, it is wise to check with the doctor about even minor changes because they might indicate the presence of a new medical problem.

Keep in mind that concurrent illness and pain are often overlooked in residential homes and nursing facilities. You may need to advocate aggressively for the person who has dementia.

> **When a person changes suddenly, ask yourself: Has the person had even a minor fall? Have they moved their bowels in the last seventy-two hours? Have they had a medication change within the past month? Are they suddenly not moving an arm or leg? Are they wincing in pain?**

Signs of illness include the following:

- abrupt worsening of behavior (such as refusal to do things they were previously able and willing to do)

- fever (a temperature over 100 degrees F). When taking a temperature, use a forehead thermometer (some take only a few seconds to register). These are available in drugstores or online. People who have dementia may bite an oral thermometer, so don't use a glass one. (Glass thermometers are no longer sold in the United States because of the danger posed by the mercury inside.) Older people may not have a significant fever even when they are seriously ill. *Lack of a fever does not mean that the person is well.*

- new flushing or paleness

- a rapid pulse (over one hundred beats per minute) that is not obviously associated with exercise. A normal pulse for most people is sixty to one hundred beats per minute. Have a nurse show you how to find the pulse in the wrist. Count for twenty seconds and multiply by three. It is helpful to know the person's normal resting pulse rate.

- vomiting or diarrhea

- changes in the skin (it may lose its elasticity or look dry or pale)

- dry, pale gums or sores in the mouth

- thirst or refusal of fluids or foods

- a change in personality, increased irritability, or increased lassitude or drowsiness

- headache

- moaning or shouting

- sudden onset of convulsions, hallucinations, or falls

- becoming incontinent

- swelling of any part of the body (check especially the hands and feet)

- coughing, sneezing, signs of respiratory congestion, or difficulty breathing

Ask yourself the following questions: Has the person had even a minor fall? Have they moved their bowels in the last seventy-two hours? Have they had a recent change (within the past month) in medication? Are they suddenly not moving an arm or leg? Are they wincing in pain? Do they have other health problems, such as heart disease, arthritis, or a cold?

If a person begins to lose weight, this may indicate the presence of a serious disease. It is important that a health care professional determine the cause of any weight loss. A person who has lost 10 percent of their weight needs to be seen by a physician or nurse as soon as possible. This is true even if they are overweight (but not dieting).

Pain

Families ask whether people suffer pain as part of an illness that causes dementia. As far as we know, Alzheimer disease does not cause pain, and vascular dementia causes pain only very rarely. People who have dementia do have pain from other causes, such as stomach cramps, constipation, hidden sprains or broken bones, sitting too long in one position, flu, arthritis, pressure sores, bruises, cuts, sores or rashes resulting from poor hygiene, sore teeth or gums, and clothes or shoes that rub or are too tight.

Indications of pain include a sudden worsening of behavior, moaning or shouting, not moving body parts or crying out when a particular part of the body is touched, refusal to do certain things, and increased restlessness. All signs of pain must be taken seriously. If the person cannot tell you where or whether they are in pain, a health care professional may have to search for a specific site and cause of the pain.

Falls and Injuries

People who have dementia frequently become clumsy, fall out of bed, bump into things, trip, or cut themselves. It is easy to overlook serious injuries for several reasons:

- Even seemingly minor injuries can result in broken bones or other serious injuries in older people because of increased vulnerability due to other common diseases, such as osteoporosis.

- The person may continue to use a fractured limb.

- People who have dementia may not tell you they are in pain.

- The person may forget that they have fallen. A bruise may not be evident for several days. Even minor head injuries can cause bleeding within the skull; this must be treated promptly to avoid further brain damage.

We suggest you routinely check the person for cuts, bruises, and blisters that may be caused by accidents, falls, pacing, or uncomfortable clothing. The feet, hips, and mouth are frequently overlooked sites of pain. Changes in behavior may be your only clue to an injury.

Pressure Sores

Pressure sores (decubitus ulcers), also called bedsores, develop when a person sits or lies down for long periods of time. They can also be caused by tight clothing, swelling, or poor nutrition. Older people's skin may be quite vulnerable to pressure sores. Pressure sores begin as red areas and can develop into open sores. They are more common over bony areas of the body: heels, hips, shoulders, shoulder blades, spine, elbows, knees, buttocks, and ankles. Fragile skin can easily be torn and bruised, even during routine washing. You must watch for red spots or bruises, especially over the tailbone, hips, heels, and elbows. If any reddening appears, make sure the person does not lie on that spot. Continue to turn the person so other sores do not form. Contact your health care professional or visiting nurse. Prompt attention can prevent an area of minor redness from progressing to something more serious.

Encourage the person to change position. Ask them to turn to look at you, go for a walk, set the table. Ask them to come into the kitchen to check that dinner is cooking correctly or to come to the window to see something.

People who are no longer able to move or who are bedfast or chairbound are at high risk of developing pressure sores. Develop a schedule in which you move the person who has dementia from one side to the other or change their position every two hours.

If the person does not change position enough, try to protect vulnerable areas. Medical supply stores and websites sell "flotation" cushions that the person can sit or lie on. There are air cushions, water cushions, gel pads, foam pads, and combinations of these. Select cushions or pads that have soft, washable covers and shields to protect against spills and odors. Websites and stores also sell heel and elbow pads (made of a synthetic fleece-like material) that protect these bony areas. Use these *in addition* to frequent turning.

Dehydration

Even people who can walk and appear to be able to care for themselves may become dehydrated. Because we assume that they are caring for themselves, we may not be alert to the signs of dehydration. Watch for this problem especially in people who have vomiting, diarrhea, or diabetes or are taking diuretics (water pills) or heart medications. Symptoms of dehydration include thirst or refusal to drink; fever; flushing; rapid pulse; a dry, pale lining of the mouth; dry, inelastic skin; dizziness or light-headedness; and confusion or hallucinations.

The amount of fluid a person needs varies with the individual and with the season. People need more fluids during the summer months. If you are uncertain whether the person is getting enough fluid, ask your doctor how much they should be drinking.

Pneumonia

Pneumonia is an infection of the lungs caused by bacteria or viruses. It is a frequent complication of dementia, but it may be difficult to diagnose because symptoms such as fever and cough may be absent. Delirium may be the earliest symptom, so pneumonia should be suspected when a person who has dementia worsens suddenly. People who choke frequently or who are bedfast are particularly vulnerable to pneumonia.

Influenza and COVID-19

Older people are particularly vulnerable to viral and bacterial infections. The seasonal "flu," or influenza, kills upward of 60,000 people annually in the United States, many of them over age 70. Bacterial pneumonia, which is very treatable in younger people, is also a common cause of death in people over age 70.

In 2020, COVID-19 was added to the list of diseases to which older people are especially vulnerable. Since most people with dementia fall into this age group, COVID-19 has wreaked havoc in long-term care facilities and among elders with dementia living at home.

Limiting visitors, serving meals in a person's room rather than in a facility dining room, social distancing, and wearing masks—all appropriate steps to take in an epidemic of infectious disease—can be frightening, not understandable, and anxiety provoking for people with dementia. These preventive actions can seem especially threatening and incomprehensible to people with impaired memory and judgment.

You can help lessen a person's distress with phone and video conferencing and by frequently reminding the person that there is an epidemic, that their safety is the goal of these actions, and that family and friends still love them even though they cannot visit. Supportive listening can help reduce anxiety, especially when it is followed by a reminder of why these things are happening. People with prominent memory loss might need to be reminded why these things are happening every time you interact with them.

Constipation

When people are forgetful, they may not be able to remember when they last moved their bowels, and they may not understand the cause of the discomfort that comes from constipation. Some people move their bowels less frequently than others. In general, people should have a bowel movement every one to three days.

Constipation can cause discomfort or pain, which can make the person's confusion worse. Constipation can lead to a bowel impaction, in which the bowel becomes partially or completely blocked by stool and the body is unable to rid itself of wastes. You should consult a doctor or nurse if you suspect this. (A person can have a partial impaction even if they have diarrhea because diarrhea can run around the impaction.)

Constipation can cause discomfort or pain, which can make the person's confusion worse

---

Many factors contribute to the development of constipation. One important factor is that most Americans eat a diet high in refined, easy-to-prepare foods and low in fiber-containing foods that encourage bowel activity. Often when a person has dementia or their dentures fit poorly or their teeth hurt, they make further changes to their diet that aggravate the problem of constipation. Reduced fluid intake can lead to hard stool that causes or worsens constipation. The muscles of the bowel that move wastes along are believed to be less active as we age, and when we are less physically active, our bowel is even less so. Some drugs and some diet supplements (given to people who are not eating) tend to increase constipation. Ask the pharmacist whether the drugs the person is taking can cause constipation.

If a person has dementia, you cannot assume they are able to keep track of when they last moved their bowels, even if they seem to have only a mild impairment or if they tell you they are taking care of themselves. A person who is living alone may have stopped eating foods that require preparation. They may be eating too many highly refined foods, such as cake, cookies, and so forth. It may be impossible to find out how regularly their bowels move. If you suspect that they may be becoming constipated, you will need to keep track for them. Do this as quietly and unobtrusively as possible so that you do not inadvertently make them feel that you are "taking over."

Most people are private about their bodily functions, and a person who has dementia can react angrily to your seeming invasion of their privacy. Also, keeping track of someone else's bowel movements is distasteful to many of us, and we tend to avoid doing it. These two feelings can conspire to cause a potentially serious problem to be overlooked.

When a person who has dementia appears to be in pain or has a headache, do not overlook constipation as a possible cause. If the person complains of bloating or "gas," constipation may be the problem. In the midst of providing care for a person who has dementia, it is easy to forget to keep track of bowel movements. If you think the person may be constipated, you may want to talk this over with a health care professional. They can quickly determine whether the person's bowels are working properly, and if they are not, they can help manage the problem.

Regular or frequent use of over-the-counter laxatives is not recommended. Instead, increase the amounts of fiber and water in the diet, and help the person exercise more (perhaps a daily walk). Most people should drink at least six glasses of water or juice every day unless they are on a fluid-restricted diet, but the necessary amount varies from person to person. Increase the amounts of vegetables (try putting them out as nibbles), fruits (including prunes and apples, as more nibbles or on cereal), whole-grain cereals (bran, whole-grain bread, whole-grain breakfast cereal), salads, beans, and nuts in their diet. Bran flakes and other whole-grain cereals make a good snack. Wheat or oat bran can be stirred into juice.

> **When a person who has dementia appears to be in pain or complains of a stomachache or headache, consider the possibility of constipation**

Ask your doctor whether you should add more fiber by giving psyllium preparations (sold under various brand names, such as Metamucil and Citrucel) or fiber-containing pills or bars. Do not use any such product without medical supervision.

Medications

Medications are a two-edged sword. They may play a vital part in helping the person who has dementia stay well, control pain, sleep better, control distress, or prevent health problems from developing. At the same time, people who have dementia (and older people in general) are susceptible to overmedication and to reactions from combinations of drugs. This includes over-the-counter medications, supplements, and supposed memory enhancers. A sudden increase in agitation, a slow, stooped walk, falling, drowsiness, incontinence, apathy, increased confusion, leaning, stiffness, or unusual mouth or hand movements may be a side effect of medication. Dizziness, light-headedness, headache, nausea, vomiting, diarrhea, loss of appetite, constipation, restless legs or cramps, change in heartbeat, change in vision, and skin rash or redness are also common side effects and should be called to the doctor's attention.

Doctors cannot always eliminate all the side effects of a medication and at the same time maintain the needed benefits, but sometimes a lower dose or a similar medication can be given that will treat the problem without—or with fewer—side effects. You and the health care professional must work together to achieve the best possible balance. Occasionally people are prescribed behavior-controlling medications to help them through some phases of their illness. However, because these can cause serious side effects, including more confusion and even death, they must be used cautiously.

Drugs that treat behavioral symptoms should be used as a last resort when other approaches have failed or when they are targeted to very specific symptoms, such as hallucinations, suspicions, severe depression, and severe irritability. Drugs do not work well for controlling aimless wandering or restlessness, occasional distress, or broken sleep. Whenever the health care professional is considering starting or raising the dosage of a behavior-modifying drug, ask whether there are any nondrug approaches that can be tried first (see Chapters 3, 7, and 8). Could you respond more

calmly to their behavior or divert their attention before problems develop? Could you tolerate more restlessness on their part if you had more time to yourself? If such a drug is absolutely necessary, ask whether it can be given so that it has its strongest effect at the person's worst time of day.

Your pharmacist is highly trained in the effects and interactions of drugs. Pharmacies can print out a list of all the person's medications, and the pharmacist can go over the list and review potential drug interactions and side effects with you. Since much of the responsibility for medications falls to the caregiver, you should pay particular attention to all medications the person who has dementia is taking. Here are some ways you can help.

Be sure that all the medical professionals involved in the person's care know about all the medications the person is taking. Some combinations of drugs can make the person's confusion worse.

When a health care professional is considering starting or raising the dosage of a behavior-modifying drug, ask what nondrug approaches can be tried first

---

Ask the pharmacist to print out a list of all the medications the person is prescribed and take this with you to all doctor appointments. Also bring all over-the-counter medications even if you do not think of them as "drugs." Ask the pharmacist if any of the medications should be listed on the ID bracelet the person who has dementia wears.

Whenever a new drug is prescribed, ask the health care professional to review all the medications to see whether any can be discontinued. This will help reduce the risk of drug interactions. Ask the clinician to start the new drug at as low a dose as possible and to increase the dose later if necessary. People who have brain injuries like dementia often develop side effects at low or regular adult doses. Ask whether this drug stays in the body the shortest amount of time and whether another, similar drug would have fewer side effects.

> *Never* assume that a forgetful person can manage their own medications

Ask what side effects to watch for. Side effects can appear even three weeks or a month after a person begins taking a new drug or an increased dose of a medication that they been taking for a long time. By then, you and the clinician may not attribute new symptoms to the medication. Ask if there are any possible side effects that you should report to your doctor immediately.

Some insurance plans cover only some drugs of each type. If possible, select a plan that includes the medications the person needs.

Some drugs must be taken before meals, some after. Some have a cumulative effect (that is, they gradually build up their effectiveness) in the body, and some don't. Older people and people who have dementia are especially sensitive to incorrect dosages, so it is imperative that you make sure the person receives their medications in the amounts and at the times prescribed. If a medication makes the person drowsy, ask if it can be given at bedtime, when it will help their sleep, and not in the morning, when they should be active.

Find out what you should do if you miss a dose or accidentally give a double dose.

Some people who have dementia do not understand why you want them to take a medication and may have a catastrophic reaction. Avoid arguing about it. Next time, tell the person one step at a time what is happening: "This is your pill. Dr. Allen gave it to you for your [reason for medication]. Put it in your mouth. Drink some water. Good." If the person becomes upset, stop immediately and try again later to give the medicine. Some people will take pills more easily if you routinely put each dose in a cup instead of handing the person the whole bottle.

People who have dementia may fail or refuse to swallow pills. They may carry the pill around in their mouth and spit it out later. You may find the pills much later on the floor. Getting the person to drink something with the medication helps. If this continues to be a problem, ask the doctor if the medication is available in another form. Capsules or a liquid may be easier to swallow than pills. Sometimes pills can be crushed and mixed into food (applesauce works well). Ask the pharmacist whether it is okay to crush the pills. If you are not sure whether the person actually took the pill, find out from the doctor or pharmacist what you should do. If pills are going on the floor, be sure that children and pets don't find them.

Never assume that a forgetful person is able to manage their own medications. If you must leave the person alone, put out one dose for them and take the bottle away with you. Even people who have mild memory impairment or individuals with no memory problems can forget whether they have taken their pills.

When you are tired or upset, you may forget the person's pills. Drugstores and health food stores sell plastic containers with compartments labeled for each day of the week. You can tell at a glance whether today's pills have been taken. (This device is helpful for *you:* do not expect the person who has dementia to be able to use it.) Newer electronic devices keep track of when pills were taken and can provide automatic reminders. You can ask the pharmacist for easy-to-open pill bottles if the childproof ones are difficult for you to open. However, childproof caps may keep a person who has dementia from taking pills they should not.

Store medications where the forgetful person cannot reach them.

This section has been written to meet the needs of families caring for someone at home. But even when a person is in an assisted living facility or nursing home, check in regularly with the medication nurse about what the person is receiving. Let them know that you expect to be notified of all medication changes. Be aware that there is a high rate of medication errors in these facilities. Follow the same suggestions discussed above: whenever there is a change in the person, ask about medications as a possible cause.

Dental Problems

Regular dental checkups are an important element of good dementia care. Painful cavities, abscesses, and sores in the mouth may be hard for you to find, and people with dementia may not be able to tell you about them. They may refuse to let you look in their mouth. Even mildly forgetful people may neglect their teeth or dentures and develop oral infections. The person's teeth must be pain free, and dentures must fit well. Poor teeth or ill-fitting dentures can lead to poor nutrition, which can significantly add to the person's problems. Oral problems can increase confusion or worsen behavior. If the person is in a residential or nursing home, be sure that arrangements are made for continued dental care.

People who have dementia tend to lose dentures and partial plates. Ask the dentist to consider alternatives that cannot be removed and lost. Because people who have dementia have a shortened life expectancy, treatments that last for many years may be less important than ease of management (for example, a fixed crown versus a removable bridge).

Many people resist going to the dentist. Look for a dentist who understands people who have dementia and who is patient and gentle. Geriatric dentistry provides special training relevant to the care of people who have dementia. If the dentist recommends a general anesthetic during dental care, carefully weigh the need for the care against the risks of the anesthetic.

Before the person enters a nursing home or residential care facility, ask the dentist or denturist to put the person's name on their dentures (don't do this yourself). Sometimes dentures get mixed up, and this will ensure that the facility can identify them.

Vision Problems

Sometimes it appears that people with dementia cannot see well or are going blind. They may bump into things, pick their feet up very high over low curbs, be unable to pick up food on their fork, or become confused or lost in dim light. One of several things may be happening. Such behavior is often a result of the brain damage, but the person may have a problem with their eyes, such as farsightedness or cataracts. Have the problem checked by an optometrist or ophthalmologist. A correctable vision problem should be corrected, if possible, so that the impaired brain can receive the best possible information from the eyes. If their eyes and brain are not seeing well and not thinking well, the person will be even less able to make sense of their environment and will function more poorly. Do not let a health care professional dismiss vision problems because a person is "senile." Even if the clinician cannot help, they should explain to you what the problem is.

People who have dementia may be less able to distinguish between similar color intensities. Thus, light blue, light green, and light yellow may look similar.

A white handrail on a pale wall may be hard to see. It may be hard for some people to tell where a light green wall joins a blue-green carpet. This problem may cause the person to stumble into walls.

Some people have difficulty with depth perception. Prints and patterns may be confusing. A black-and-white bathroom floor can look as if it is full of holes. It may be difficult to know whether one is close enough to a chair to sit down, or to judge how high a step or a curb is, or to see where to step on the stairs. Glare from windows tends to mask the details of objects near the window. Older eyes may adjust more slowly to sudden changes from bright light to darkness or vice versa.

When the brain is not working well, the person will be less able to compensate for these vision problems, but you can help them. We all need to see as well as possible so that we can function at our best. Paint a handrail dark if the wall is light. Paint baseboards dark if the walls and floor covering are light. The dark line will help the person see the change from floor to wall.

Increase the light in rooms in the

daytime and the evening and leave night-lights on at night. Install lights in dark closets.

People who have dementia can also lose the ability to *know* what they see. In this instance the eyes work alright but the brain is no longer able to correctly use the information the eyes tell it. For example, the person may bump into furniture not because they have a visual acuity problem but because their brain cannot recognize that there is something in front of them. When this is the case, what seems like a vision problem may be part of the dementia. This condition is called agnosia and is discussed in Chapter 8. When problems are caused by agnosia, the ophthalmologist will not be able to help. In fact, ophthalmologists and optometrists often have trouble testing the vision of a person with thinking or language impairments. Obviously, when agnosia is the problem, it will do no good to tell the person to watch where they are going. They will need increasing care to protect them from injuries they cannot avoid, and you may need to check frequently for cuts and bruises.

For people who lay their glasses down and forget where they are, it often helps to have them wear their glasses on a chain. Keep the old glasses, or buy the person a spare pair in case they lose them. Carry the prescription and your own with you if you go out of town. With the prescription in hand, you can replace lost or broken glasses with less trouble and expense.

If the person wears contact lenses, you may need to replace them with glasses before they reach the point where they are unable to manage contact lenses. If they continue to wear the lenses, you must watch for irritations of the eye and be sure they care for their lenses properly.

Hearing Problems

Failing to hear properly deprives the brain of information needed to make sense of the environment. Hearing loss can cause or worsen forgetfulness, suspiciousness, and withdrawal (see "Misinterpretation" in Chapter 8), and it may increase the risk of developing Alzheimer disease, so correct any hearing loss if possible. An audiologist can determine the cause of the hearing loss and help you select an appropriate hearing aid. As with vision problems, it can be difficult for people to separate problems in thinking from problems in hearing. People who have dementia develop problems understanding what is said to them (see page 36). An audiologist should be able to distinguish between this and the type of hearing loss that can be corrected. If not, consult an expert in memory disorders such as a neuropsychologist.

Because people who have dementia cannot learn easily, they may not be able to adjust to hearing aids. Hearing aids amplify background noises and feel like a foreign object in one's ear. This can be upsetting to the wearer who can't remember the purpose of the hearing aid. You should try to purchase a hearing aid with the agreement that you can return it if it does not work out.

If the person uses a hearing aid, you must be responsible for it and must check regularly to see that the batteries are working or that the hearing aid is fully charged.

In addition to correcting hearing loss with a hearing aid, here are some other things you can do:

- Reduce background noises, such as noise from appliances, the television, or several people talking at once. It is difficult for people who have dementia to distinguish between these sounds and what they want to hear.

- Sit or stand by the person's "better" ear when speaking to them.

- Give the person clues to where sounds are coming from. It can be hard to locate and identify sounds, and this may confuse the person. Remind them, "That is the sound of the garbage truck."

- Use several kinds of clues at one time: point, speak, and gently guide the person, for example.

Dizziness

Dizziness is a common problem in later life and is a side effect of many medications. People who have dementia may be unable to compensate for their loss of balance or unable to tell you that they feel dizzy. They may refuse to move around or may fall as a result of feeling dizzy. If you suspect dizziness, ask the person directly if they feel light-headed or as if the room is spinning. Observe whether the person

> If you suspect dizziness, notify the person's doctor or nurse right away since the poor balance that it causes increases the risk of a serious fall

seems unsteady. Nausea may be a symptom of dizziness. Because dizziness increases the risk of a serious fall, notify the doctor or nurse right away.

Visiting the Doctor

Visits to doctors or other health care professionals can turn into an ordeal for you and the person who has dementia. Here are some ways to make them easier.

The person may not be able to understand where they are going or why. This, combined with the bustle of getting ready to go, may trigger a catastrophic reaction. Look for ways to simplify things.

Some people do better if they know in advance that they are going to the doctor. Others do better if you avoid an argument by not bringing up the doctor visit until you are almost there. Instead of saying, "We have to get up early today. Hurry with your breakfast because today is your visit to Dr. Chen, and she has to change your medicine," just get the person up with no comment, serve their breakfast, and help them into their coat. When you are almost there, say, "We are seeing Dr. Chen today."

Rather than get in an argument, ignore or downplay objections. If the person says, "I am not going to the doctor," don't say, "You have to go to the doctor," but try changing the subject instead, saying something like "We will get an ice cream while we are downtown."

> Ask for a doctor's appointment at the person's best time of day. If the person who has dementia is likely to become upset in the car, take someone else with you who can drive or comfort them.

Plan trips in advance. Know where you are going, where you will park, how long it will take, and whether there are stairs or elevators. Allow enough time without rushing, but not so much time that you will be early and have a longer wait. Ask for an appointment at the person's best time of day. Take someone with you to drive while you comfort the person who has dementia.

Talk to the receptionist or nurse. They may be able to tell you whether there will be a long wait. If the office is crowded and noisy, they may be able to arrange for you to wait in a quieter place. Take along some snacks, a bottle of water, or some activity the person enjoys doing. If the receptionist knows that you will have a long wait, you may be able to take a short walk if you check in frequently. Never leave a person who has dementia alone in the waiting room. The strange place may upset them, or they may wander away.

In very rare circumstances, the doctor may prescribe a sedative for the person to take before the visit, but sedatives can cause many additional problems. Usually, being calm and matter-of-fact and giving the person simple information and reassurance are all that is needed. On rare occasions the visit might have to be abandoned.

If the Person with Dementia Must Enter the Hospital

People who have dementia are likely to have other medical illnesses. They may need to be hospitalized. This can be a trying time for you and the person who has dementia. The illness that caused the hospitalization may also cause a temporary decline in the person's cognitive function. The unfamiliar environment, the confusion of a busy hospital, and new treatments may cause a further decline in function and cognition. It is not unusual for people who have dementia to become agitated, scream, or strike out in such circumstances. Additional behavior-controlling medications should be avoided if at all possible because they can further impair thinking and worsen behavior. Usually the person will gradually return to their earlier level of functioning after the hospitalization unless a new brain injury has occurred. If they do not, have the medical team review medications and other new treatments.

> **There are some things you can do to make a hospital stay easier, but recognize that you cannot completely prevent problems. It is important that you not become exhausted yourself.**

There are some things you can do to make a hospitalization easier, but recognize that you cannot completely prevent problems. *It is important that you not become exhausted yourself.*

Talk to the doctor in advance of the person's admission. Make sure all physicians involved in their care know that the person has dementia, and ask about how the dementia may complicate the hospitalization. Ask if part or all of the treatment can be done on an outpatient basis. This may be difficult, but it shortens the time the person must be in a strange setting. If you do this, arrange for home nursing for the first few days.

At admission, talk to the nursing staff. Let them know that the person has dementia. Urge them to tell the person where they are as frequently as possible and to be calm and reassuring with them. Write out things the nurses need to know, and ask that your notes be put in the chart. Mention things that will help the person feel more comfortable and will enable the staff to be supportive, such as nicknames, family whom they might ask about, things they will need to have done for them (like filling out the menu and opening milk cartons), and how toileting is managed.

Hospitals are often short-staffed, and nurses frequently work under pressure. They may not be able to spend as much time with the person as they would like. They may not be trained to work with people who have dementia.

> **We recommend that you hire a sitter to stay with the person in the hospital whenever you or other family members cannot be there**

It is usually comforting for the person to have someone they know with them as much as possible and to accompany them to tests and treatments. A family member can help with meals, see that the person gets enough fluid, and reassure them about what is going on. Most hospitals will let family members stay overnight with patients who have dementia or delirium. *But,* sometimes a family member's own anxiety and nervousness upsets the person who has dementia or delirium or gets in the way of the staff. Calmness is contagious, and so is nervousness. The person will be influenced by your feelings. You may want to ask someone else they know to spend time with them, to give you a break. If you cannot go with the person for tests, explain to the staff how important it is to comfort and reassure them.

When a person who has dementia is hospitalized, we recommend that you stay with the person full-time or hire sitters around the clock. Today, most hospitals will help you find a sitter or provide one as part of the hospital stay. If possible, schedule visits so that children, family, or understanding close friends can be with the person. Familiar clothing, a familiar blanket, and large photos of family members will help reassure the person. Some families write the person a letter that nurses can use to reassure them when they are anxious. It might read like this:

Dear Mom: You are in the hospital because you broke your hip. You will be coming back home to our house soon. Ted or I will come to see you every night right after you have your supper. The nurses know you have trouble remembering things and they will help you. I love you. Your daughter, Maria.

Restraints should be used only as a last resort when there is a significant risk that the person will be harmed, for example, by pulling out tubes or dressings. Having a twenty-four-hour attendant is the best way to avoid the use of restraints.

Do not be alarmed if the person's confusion worsens in the hospital. In most cases the person's level of impairment will later return to what it was before the hospitalization.

Seizures, Fits, or Convulsions

The majority of people who have illnesses that cause dementia do not develop seizures. Because they are so uncommon, you are not likely to have to face this problem. However, seizures can be frightening for you if you are not prepared to deal with them. Various diseases can cause seizures. Therefore, if the person does have a seizure, it may not be related to the dementia.

There are several types of seizure. With a generalized major motor or tonic-clonic seizure (the kind we usually associate with a fit or seizure), people become rigid, fall, and lose consciousness. Their breathing can become irregular or even stop briefly. Their muscles will become rigid and begin to jerk repetitively. They may clench their teeth tightly. After some seconds the jerking will stop and the person will slowly regain consciousness. They may be confused, sleepy, or have a headache. They may have difficulty talking.

Other types of seizure are less dramatic. For example, just a hand or an arm may move in a repetitive manner, or the person may be unresponsive to voice or touch for several seconds or minutes. These are referred to as partial seizures.

A single seizure is not life-threatening. Most important, remain calm. Do not try to restrain the person. Try to protect them from falling or banging their head on something hard. If they are on the floor, move things out of the way. If they are seated, you may be able to ease them to the floor or quickly push a sofa cushion under them to soften their fall if they should fall out of the chair.

Do not try to move the person or to stop the seizure. Stay with them and let the seizure run its course. Do not try to hold their tongue, and do not try to put a spoon in their mouth. Never force their mouth open after their teeth are clenched; you may damage their teeth and gums. Loosen clothing if you can. For example, unfasten a belt, a necktie, or buttons at the neckline.

When the jerking has stopped, be sure the person is breathing correctly. If they have more saliva than usual, turn their head gently to the side and wipe out their mouth. Let them sleep or rest if they wish. They may be more confused or irritable or even combative after the seizure. They may know something is wrong but will not remember the seizure. Be calm, gentle, and reassuring. Avoid restraining them, restricting them, or insisting on what they should do.

Take a few minutes after the seizure to relax and collect yourself. If the person has a partial seizure, nothing else needs to be done immediately. If the person wanders about, follow them and try to prevent them from hurting themselves. When this type of seizure ends, they may be temporarily confused, irritable, or have trouble talking.

You may be able to identify warning signals, such as specific repetitive movements, that indicate that a seizure is about to start. If so, make sure the person is moved to a safe place (out of traffic, away from stairs or stoves, and so on) when the warning signs occur.

Any person who has had a first-time seizure should be taken to an emergency room to determine the cause of the seizure. You should stay with the person until the seizure is over and you have had a chance to collect yourself. Then call an ambulance. Seizures are preventable. If seizures occur repeatedly or frequently, the doctor may decide to prescribe medication to decrease the likelihood of further seizures.

If the person who has dementia is being treated for seizures, they should be taken to an emergency room if they have multiple seizures over a short period of time, if the seizure continues for more than a few minutes, or if you suspect that the person has hit their head or injured themselves in some other way.

Seizures are frightening and unpleasant to watch, but they are usually not life-threatening, and they are not indications of insanity or danger to others. They can become less frightening as you learn how to respond to them. Find a nurse or an experienced family member with whom you can discuss your distress and who can knowledgeably reassure you.

Jerking Movements (Myoclonus)

People who have Alzheimer disease occasionally develop quick, single, jerking movements of their arms, legs, head, or body. These are called myoclonic jerks. They are not seizures. Seizures are repeated movements of the same muscles, while myoclonic jerks are single thrusts of a body part.

Myoclonic jerks are not a cause for alarm. They do not progress to seizures. The only danger they present is accidentally hitting something and causing an injury. At present there are no established treatments for the myoclonus associated with Alzheimer disease. Drugs can be tried, but these usually have significant side effects and offer little improvement.

Death of the Person Who Has Dementia

Whenever you have the responsibility for an ill or elderly person, you face the possibility of that person's death. You may have questions you are reluctant to bring up with their doctor. Often, thinking about such things in advance will help relieve your mind and make things easier if you have to face a crisis.

The Cause of Death
In the final stages of a progressive illness that causes dementia, so much of the nervous system is failing that the rest of the body is profoundly affected. For this reason, the dementia is the cause of death. The *immediate* cause of death may be a complicating condition, such as pneumonia, dehydration, infection, or malnutrition, but the *actual* cause of death is often the dementia. The most common cause of death, occurring in 40 to 60 percent of people with dementia, is pneumonia.

Some people will die from stroke, heart attack, cancer, or other causes even though they also have Alzheimer disease. These deaths can come at any time, so some people are alert, able to walk, and fairly functional up until their death.

Dying at Home
Families sometimes worry that the ill or elderly person will die at home, perhaps in their sleep, and that they will find them. Because of this, a caregiver may be afraid to sleep soundly or may get up to check on the person several times a night.

•

One daughter said, "I don't know what I would do. What if one of the children found her?"

•

Perhaps you have heard of someone who found a husband or a wife dead, and you wonder how you would handle this. Most families find it reassuring to plan in advance what they would do first, second, and third, such as the following:

- When the person dies, you can dial 911 or the local emergency number. Emergency personnel or paramedics usually will arrive promptly. In many jurisdictions, paramedics are required to begin resuscitation efforts unless specific forms have been filled out. If you do not want resuscitation to happen, you may not want to call them right away.

- You can select a funeral director or mortician in advance. When death occurs, you only have to call.

- If the person is in hospice care, you may only need to call the hospice nurse, who can then call the funeral director.

- Discuss in advance with your clergy and physician whether they can respond to an emergency call late at night.

- Some people want a little time to say goodbye; others do not. If you do, the thing to do first might be to sit with the person a little while, and then call someone.

> **Most families find it reassuring to plan in advance what they will do first, second, and third when the person dies**

Some families value the peacefulness and privacy that death at home allows, but families often worry about what dying looks like and about what to

do. If you want the person to be able to die at home, a hospice nurse can show you what care is needed and give you guidance on how to conserve your own energy.

Hospice and Palliative Care

Hospice programs enable people to die either at home or in special hospice facilities that offer comfort without aggressive medical interventions. The staff take steps to keep the person comfortable and can provide some services such as in-bed bathing, but they do not try aggressive medical interventions unless these are aimed at improving comfort. Hospice programs are a valuable resource to families.

Hospice care is covered by Medicare in all states, by Medicaid in most states, and by most insurance plans and health maintenance organizations (HMOs). For a patient to be admitted to hospice care, Medicare requires that an attending physician and the hospice medical directors certify that the person is terminally ill, that is, that they are expected to die within six months. Medicare recognizes the special problems associated with Alzheimer disease, and individuals may receive hospice care for more than six months. Contact your local hospice program for admission.

Palliative care provides many of the same supports and philosophy of hospice care but without the specific benefits that hospice legislation mandates. Both hospice and palliative care seek to maximize quality of life, minimize discomfort and pain, support the family, and help organize supportive services such as visiting aides and funeral arrangements.

Many states now have specific forms that stop the person from being transported to a hospital at the end of life. For individuals and families who have decided that a death at home is desirable, these forms prevent misunderstandings when 911 is called.

Dying in the Hospital or Nursing Home

Some families are comforted to know that professionals are in charge at this time, and so they choose a nursing home or a hospital (if the person is eligible for hospital care). Bedside care of a totally dependent person is hard work and is emotionally draining. Do not feel bad if this is not for you. You may be better able to give loving reassurance if someone else is providing the physical care.

Plan end-of-life care in advance, no matter where the person with dementia is living

---

Whatever choice you make is the right one for you, but whatever the setting, it is important to do some advance planning. Families have told us that unless you plan in advance, you may have little control over what takes place, and things may be done very differently from the way you and your family member would have wished. Most of these problems revolve around how much and what kinds of life-sustaining interventions should be used. You must have a durable power of attorney for health care (see pages 254–56). Have this handy and bring it to the hospital.

When Should Treatment End?

When a person has a chronic, terminal illness, their family faces the question of whether it would be better to allow their life to end or to prolong it for a few days or weeks. This is a difficult question, one that doctors, judges, and clergy struggle with, as do seriously ill people and their families. Each of us must make the decision based on our own background, beliefs, and experiences and what we understand to have been the wishes of the ill person.

Most jurisdictions provide MOLST forms that list a person's wishes for care at the end of life. These documents allow a seriously ill person to designate what treatments they do and do not want when death is near.

In many states, laws have been passed to identify who should make health care decisions for a person who has been declared incompetent by one or two health professionals (states vary in who is allowed to make such a declaration). All states now allow for an individual to designate the person they wish to be their substitute decision maker if they become incompetent. This is referred to as a *durable power of attorney for health care*. Ideally, the person who is designated to be the substitute knows the ill person's wishes and will make the health decisions that the person most likely would have wanted. These documents often contain written descriptions of the person's specific wishes if certain health issues arise. Most states also have laws that identify a hierarchy of individuals who are designated to make a substituted decision for a person who has not identified a substitute decision maker in advance. Usually they identify the spouse as the first decision maker, the parents as the second (if a spouse is not available), and children as the third. Courts can appoint a *guardian of the person* if there has been no designation in advance.

Many primary care physicians now discuss wishes about end-of-life care when people become Medicare eligible and during routine office visits. Because people change their minds, it is important to discuss any changes in wishes with your doctor.

There are no "good" or "bad" choices. Ideally, a person will receive the care they would have chosen had they remained competent. We describe some of the options to help family members and surrogates select the kind of care that will be right for their loved one. Some families want to be sure that everything possible has been done. Others have felt hassled or upset by medical interventions they did not want.

Occasionally a physician, social worker, or nursing home has strong opinions about life support and resuscitation and will push those opinions regardless of your wishes. This is occurring much less often now than in the past but is still a possibility. Ask your physician and the residential facility or nursing home what steps they will take if a person is close to death. Will they routinely transfer the person who has dementia to a hospital? Will they honor the person's wishes regarding continuing or stopping treatments that might not benefit them? What procedures, if any, do they consider "routine" and carry out without the explicit consent of the substitute decision maker? Will

they discourage you from being present in the person's room around the time of death? Will they allow a *do not hospitalize* order to be written if that is the wish of the person who has dementia or their substitute? Will the hospital automatically try resuscitation? Are they open and responsive to your questions, or do they avoid your questions or strongly state their own positions?

> **Ask the physician and facility if they will honor the person's wishes for end-of-life care if the person is close to death**

You might ask a member of your religious community or a friend to help you make the necessary phone calls to ask these questions. If there is a local hospice organization, its staff may be able to tell you what the usual practices in your community are.

Provide the hospital, nursing home, or residential home with a medical directive detailing the end-of-life care you want the person to receive, along with a copy of your durable power of attorney or guardianship papers. Request that these instructions be placed in the person's chart. Make one copy for the doctor and one copy for the nursing home or residential home to send with the person to the hospital, and sign each copy. Ask the doctor and the nursing home or residential home directly whether it will honor these instructions. Go with the person to the hospital if possible. A copy of the person's living will, MOLST form, and advance directives should be placed in the chart (see page 277).

Occasionally, a family feels so strongly opposed to the care available in a hospital or long-term care facility that they transfer their family member to another facility or take the person home to die.

What Kind of Care Can Be Given at the End of Life?

When a person has a chronic, terminal illness, the person's family must often make decisions about when to allow treatment and when to accept the declining course of the disease. There are few right or wrong answers, but because of the severity of the illness, the person who has dementia is almost never able to participate in the decision-making. The questions that families most often face include whether to hospitalize the person, whether to do blood work, whether to insert a feeding tube or give only the food or fluids they will take, and whether to treat concurrent illnesses with antibiotics or surgery. (You may have faced similar issues earlier in the illness, such as whether to restrain an ambulatory person who might fall.)

As you make these decisions, be cautious about accepting strong, matter-of-fact opinions from "experts." Like the rest of us, professionals can easily confuse personal values with facts in this emotion-laden topic.

When you consider questions about life-support interventions for terminally ill people, such as feeding tubes, ventilators (breathing machines), treating illnesses such as pneumonia with antibiotics, or surgery for acute problems, recognize that there is often no absolutely right answer. It is sometimes difficult to know whether an abrupt decline is part of the dementia or whether, if treated, the person might continue to live comfortably for some time. It can be difficult to determine when a person who has dementia is "terminally ill" and to predict when a person who has late-stage dementia will die. These uncertainties add to the family's burden. Neither you nor the doctors may be able to say whether an intervention will help or will be distressing to a person who has dementia and who is close to death.

> The common illnesses that cause dementia are gradually progressive. Difficult decisions can arise at any point in the disease.

We often cannot know for sure how the person experiences treatments—whether the person who has a severe dementia is frightened by feeding tubes, bathing and turning, or restraints or whether the lack of food or fluids is painful. When a person who has dementia tries to pull out tubes, we do not know whether they do so because the tube is frightening or because it is uncomfortable. It is risky to generalize about people who have dementia from what we know about people who are dying from other illnesses. What we do know is that pain perception appears to be intact in most people who have dementia, so individuals with late-stage dementia do experience discomfort and pain. Even if they cannot express it directly with words, people who have dementia do show by their behavior that they are uncomfortable or experiencing pain. They look distressed, wince when moved or touched, or cry. We also know that they can be soothed and calmed by gentle touch or softly spoken words.

The illnesses that cause dementia are gradually progressive, and you may have to make difficult decisions several times in the course of the illness. Each decision must be made separately. For example, when pneumonia causes an ambulatory and apparently content person to stop eating, you may decide to use tube or intravenous feeding for a while. Later in the illness, you might decide not to use tube feeding if they stop eating.

Everyone should identify a substitute decision maker (or a group of decision makers) for themselves since we are all at risk of becoming suddenly or gradually unable to make medical decisions for ourselves

---

Pain medication can be given even when a decision has been made not to use antibiotics, tube feeding, or other physical treatments, but pain medications often carry risks—they can impair a person's drive to breathe, for example. This is rarely a problem when these medications are used carefully, and the relief of pain and suffering that results is one of the positive interventions we can make at the end of life. Explicitly discuss this issue with the person's physician and nurses. Decisions will be easier if you weigh the ethical issues *after* you have obtained the best medical information available. Research by us has shown that the quality of life of people with late-stage dementia is better when they are receiving appropriate pain medication.

•

Mrs. Allen's children argued among themselves over whether it was against their religion not to give her food through a tube. She tried to pull out the tube and seemed frightened. When the doctor told them that there is no scientific evidence that the tube would extend her life, they found it much easier to decide not to use tube feeding but to give her small spoonfuls of ice chips from time to time to moisten her mouth.

•

Ask your physician how likely it is that the person will return to some previous level (that of a week or month ago, for instance) if given a certain treatment. Is it likely that the person's death will be delayed by hours, days, or months by the proposed intervention? What are the available alternatives? Are there any other interventions that might be less distressing?

Who makes the decision? Sometimes the person who has dementia has left a written statement about their wishes for life-prolonging care. Even more often, people have told their families how they wish to be cared for or have made statements such as "I never want to be kept alive the way Mabel was." It is most helpful if, at an early stage before the disease becomes advanced, the person has discussed their wishes with the person who will make substitute decisions for them in case they become incapacitated. In fact, we urge all readers to identify a substitute decision maker (or a group of decision makers) in case they become suddenly or gradually unable to make medical decisions for themselves.

You should arrive as early as possible at an agreement with the rest of the family on the kind of care to give. Health care providers usually honor a patient's previous statement of their wishes or the request of the person with legal responsibility for the patient's care. Health care providers are often reluctant to give palliative care when the family members are in disagreement.

> **Talking things over before an emergency arises can significantly lessen anxiety and dread as death approaches**

It can be difficult for family members to discuss these challenging issues. Some people may refuse to talk about them; others may become angry. Some feel that it is wrong to "plan" for a death. However, talking things over often relieves feelings of anxiety and dread as death approaches and allows for clear and direct communication with the medical team. Waiting until there is an emergency situation that demands a decision can adversely affect the life of the ill person. If there are disagreements among family members, show this section to your family members and ask your physician, social worker, or clergyperson to help coordinate a family discussion. Suggest that family members not bring up old disagreements but focus on this issue.

The death of the person who has dementia, even after a very long illness, may be painful for you, and the practical tasks surrounding death are likely to be distasteful. Nevertheless, arranging a gentle and dignified death is one way you can give love and care to the person who has dementia and grieve in the way that is right for you without intrusions from strangers.

CHAPTER 7

Managing the Behavioral and Neuropsychiatric Symptoms of Dementia

The things people who have dementia do and experience can be the most distressing part of their illness. These symptoms are referred to by various terms: *behavioral symptoms*, *noncognitive symptoms*, *neuropsychiatric symptoms*, and *psychological symptoms*. Chapters 3 and 8 discuss some of the common behavioral and emotional symptoms, including overreacting, irritability, anger, and agitation. They also discuss why people act as they do: *Dementia damages the brain. As a result, the person becomes unable to make sense of what they see and hear.* Not being able to make sense of things leads to confusion. This confusion may make the person with dementia frightened and anxious. This is why they sometimes insist on "going home," why they lash out in anger at you or resist care, why they believe that someone is stealing their money or trying to poison them. Most of these behaviors are not under their control, and they usually are trying as hard as they can. Other symptoms result more directly from the brain damage. We know that people with brain injuries also experience false beliefs, hallucinations, and explosive

behaviors, even when their memory and perception are normal.

Here are some general guidelines for managing difficult symptoms. Ask yourself if this behavior could result in harm to someone—you, the person who has dementia, or someone else. Or is the behavioral symptom making life intolerable for others (yourself, other residents, or staff), even though it is not dangerous?

If the behavior is potentially harmful, then you probably need to find a way to stop it. Occasionally this means using medication, but most of the time this is not necessary. Because many of the drugs used to treat behavioral and neuropsychiatric symptoms have serious, even fatal, side effects, they should be avoided whenever possible. If the behavior or neuropsychiatric symptom is not dangerous, you should strongly consider letting it continue. The behavior may be easier to tolerate if you get away from the person once in a while.

Some families tell us that the person who has dementia does some things that create serious problems. Do not assume that you will face all or even most of the symptoms listed in this chapter. But if you do face such problems, one of the first places to seek help is a support group, such as those offered by dementia support agencies like the Alzheimer's Association, by long-term care facilities, and by local social support agencies. It was from families dealing with dementia that we learned many of the suggestions we make in this book. Some support groups have telephone helplines and websites and publish newsletters. These are excellent sources of information and help. The national Alzheimer's Association and the National Institute on Aging have excellent websites with links to downloads and printouts of helpful information and advice.

You will solve problems better when you are not worn out

One husband does not call these behavioral symptoms "problems." He calls each difficulty a "challenge." This helps him approach it with a positive outlook. You will find that you solve problems better when you are not exhausted, so make sure you take time for yourself.

The Six *R*'s of Behavior Management

Behavioral symptoms have different causes in different people, and different solutions will work in different households. Some families have found the following six *R*'s helpful in thinking through a behavioral symptom.

The Six *R*'s of Behavior Management

1. **Restrict**. The first thing we often try is to get the person to stop whatever they are doing. This is especially important when the person might harm themselves or someone else. But trying to make the person stop may upset them more.

2. **Reassess**. Ask yourself these questions: Might a physical illness or drug reaction be causing the behavioral symptom? Might the person be having difficulty seeing or hearing? Is someone or something upsetting them? Could the bothersome person or object be removed? Might a different approach avoid upsetting the person who has dementia?

3. **Reconsider**. Ask yourself how things must seem from the point of view of the person who has dementia. Many of the symptoms of dementia—such as memory impairment, the inability to comprehend or express language, the inability to do things that one has done since childhood, and an unawareness of the extent of impairment—can lead directly or indirectly to behavioral difficulties. When you try to bathe or dress someone who does not understand that they need help, they may become upset. The person might

feel that their privacy is being invaded or that someone is trying to harm them rather than help them. The resulting anxiety is understandable when they can't make sense of things that are going on.

4. **Rechannel**. Look for a way that the behavior can continue in a safe and nondestructive manner. The behavior may be important to the person in some way that we cannot understand. One man who had been a mechanic continued to take things apart around the house, but he could not put them back together. His wife had some old automobile parts steam cleaned and gave them to him. He was able to enjoy taking them apart for several months, and he left the household appliances alone.

5. **Reassure**. When the person has been upset, fearful, or angry, take time to reassure them that things are all right, that they are safe, and that you still care for them. While the person may not remember the reassurance, they may retain the feeling of having been reassured and cared for. Putting your arm around the person or hugging them is a way of reassuring them. Say something like "We had a fuss, but it's over." Take time to reassure yourself as well. You are doing the best you can with a demanding and difficult job. Give yourself a pat on the back for surviving one more challenge. If possible, find some time away from the person to regain your energy.

6. **Review**. Afterward, think over what happened and how you managed it. You may face this symptom again. What can you learn from this experience that will help you next time? What led up to this behavior? How did you respond to it? What did you do right? What might you try next time?

Concealing Memory Loss

People with a progressive dementia can become skillful at hiding their declining abilities and forgetfulness. This is understandable since many people are afraid of "having Alzheimer's." In addition, many people with Alzheimer disease have, as part of the illness, a reduced ability to recognize their impairments.

This tendency to hide limitations can be distressing for families. The family members living with a person who has dementia may know that the person is impaired yet receive no support or understanding from others who cannot see the problem. Friends may say, "He looks and sounds perfectly all right. I don't see anything wrong, and I don't see why he cannot remember to call me." Even family members may not be able to differentiate between real memory loss and plain contrariness.

If the person has been living alone, family, neighbors, and friends may be unaware for a long time that something is wrong. When a person does not recognize their memory problems, they may manage for years until a crisis occurs. Families are often shocked and distressed by the extent of the problem when they finally learn of it.

In a person who has dementia, personality and social skills may remain the same as they have always been while memory and the ability to learn new information are being lost

---

You may wonder what people who have dementia are still able to do for themselves and what needs to be done for them. If they are still employed, have responsibility for their own money, or are driving, they may not realize or may be unwilling to admit that they can no longer manage these tasks as well as they once could. Some people in these situations recognize that their memory is slipping, but many don't. People cope with declining abilities in different ways. Some don't want to admit that anything is wrong, while others find relief and comfort in talking about what is happening to them. Listen to their thoughts, feelings, and fears. Your attentiveness can be comforting and can give you a chance to correct misconceptions.

Others may successfully conceal their impairment by keeping lists. Or they may use conversational devices such as saying, "Of course I know that," to cover their forgetfulness. Some

people become angry and blame others when they forget things. Some people stop participating in activities that they have always enjoyed. One woman said, "I have dementia. My memory is terrible." But when her family found out that she had sent a bad check to the IRS, she insisted that she would never make a mistake like that. Her family could not understand how she could know about her forgetfulness and yet "lie" about the check. Families often ask why a person forgets one thing and remembers another. It can be difficult to understand the quirks of memory, but it is likely that this woman was honestly trying as hard as she could. Memory is complex, and contradictions like this are common. The person cannot help themselves.

A frequent characteristic of dementia is that personality and social skills appear nearly intact while memory and the ability to learn new information are declining. As a result, many people can conceal their illness for a long time. One can talk with such a person about routine matters and fail to recognize that their memory or thinking is impaired. Psychological testing or an occupational therapy evaluation can be helpful in such situations because the evaluation will give you a realistic measure of how much you can expect from the person and what they can still do. Because dementia can be so deceiving, even to people close to the affected person, the assessment of a professional can help you and your family make realistic plans for future care. These professionals may also talk over their findings with the person who has dementia and show them ways they can remain as independent as possible.

Wandering

Wandering is a common and frequently serious behavioral symptom. Wandering behavior can make it difficult to manage a person at home. It can make it impossible for day care centers, residential care homes, or nursing homes to care for a person. The person is endangered when wandering onto busy streets or into strange neighborhoods. In addition, becoming disoriented and lost is likely to make the person even more frightened.

Because some people do not understand dementia, strangers who try to help the individual may think they are drunk or seeking attention. When wandering occurs at night, it can deprive the family of needed rest. However, it can often be stopped or at least reduced.

A person who has begun to wander away from home or who gets lost running errands should no longer live alone

---

A person who has begun to wander away from home or who gets lost running errands should no longer live alone. This is a signal to you to provide a safer living arrangement for the person.

Because it appears that there are different kinds of wandering and different reasons why people who have dementia wander, identifying the cause or causes of the behavior may help you plan a strategy to manage it.

Why People Wander

Wandering may result from being disoriented or feeling lost. Sometimes a person sets out on an errand, such as going to the store, makes a wrong turn, becomes disoriented, and gets completely lost trying to find the way back. Or they may go shopping with you, lose sight of you, and get lost trying to find you.

Wandering often increases when a person moves to a new home, begins a day care program, or for some other reason is in a new environment.

Some people wander around intermittently for no apparent reason. Some wandering behavior appears aimless and can go on for hours. It appears different from the wandering associated with being lost or with being in a new place and is often not associated with distress.

Some people develop an agitated, determined, "driven" pacing. If this occurs regularly, it gets on everyone's nerves. It can become dangerous if the person becomes determined to "get away." This seemingly incomprehensible pacing may be associated with the damage to the brain.

Some people wander at night. This can be dangerous for the person who has dementia and exhausting for you.

Most of us can sympathize with the person's experience of becoming disoriented. We may have lost our car at a parking lot or gotten "turned around" in a strange place. For a few minutes we feel unnerved until we get hold of ourselves and work out a logical way to find out where we are. The person with memory impairment is more likely to panic, is less able to "get hold of themselves," and may feel that they must keep their disorientation a secret.

> **Like other behavioral symptoms, wandering is not a behavior that the person can control**

When wandering increases following a move to a new home or some other change in the environment, it may be because the person with memory impairment is unable to learn their way around the new setting. They may not be able to understand that they have moved and may be determined to go "home." The stress of such a change may undermine their remaining abilities and make it even harder for them to learn their way around.

Aimless wandering may be the person's way of saying, "I *feel* lost. I am searching for the things I feel I have lost." Sometimes wandering behavior is the person's way of trying to communicate feelings.

·

Mr. Griffith was a vigorous man of 60 who kept leaving the day care center. The police would pick him up several miles away, hiking down the highway. Mr. Griffith always explained that he was going to Florida. Florida represented home, friends, security, and family to Mr. Griffith.

·

Wandering may be the person's way of expressing restlessness, boredom, or the need for exercise. It may help to fill the need of an active person to be "doing something." Wandering may signal a need to use the toilet.

A constant or agitated pacing or a determination to get away may be difficult to manage. Sometimes this is a catastrophic reaction. Something may be upsetting or frightening the person. They may not be able to make sense out of their surroundings, may be misinterpreting what they see or hear, or may be having frightening hallucinations. Sometimes this agitated wandering appears to be a direct result of the brain damage. It is hard to know exactly what is happening to the brain, but we do know that brain function can be seriously and extensively disrupted. Remind yourself that this is not a behavior that the person can control.

Night wandering can also have various causes, from simple disorientation to a seemingly incomprehensible part of the brain injury (see page 134).

The Management of Wandering

The management of wandering behavior depends on its cause or causes. If it appears to be aimless and is not associated with distress or harm, then allowing it to happen might be best.

If the person is getting lost and if you are sure they can still read and follow instructions, a pocket card may help them. Write *simple* instructions on a card that the person can carry in their pocket and refer to if they are lost. You might put at the top of the card the written reminder "Stay calm. Don't walk away." You might write on the card "Call home" and put the phone number, or write "Ask someone to show you to the men's clothing department and stay there. I will come for you." You may need different cards for different trips. This can make it possible for a person who has mild dementia to help themselves.

It is essential that you get the person an ID bracelet with their name and your phone number on it, along with the statement "memory impaired." A bracelet that is securely fastened (so the person cannot take it off) and too small to slip off is probably safer than a necklace. This information will help anyone who finds the person if they get lost. You can have an inexpensive bracelet engraved in a store that engraves mugs, key rings, and the like. Have a "memory impaired" bracelet made *now* if there is any possibility that the person will wander or get lost. This is so important that some clinics require that their clients who have dementia have such identification. A lost, confused person will be afraid and upset, and this can cause them to resist help. A person with dementia may be ignored by the people around them or thought to be crazy. Under stress, the person may function more poorly than they usually do.

> **It is essential that you get the person a bracelet with their name and your phone number on it**

You can purchase bracelets with medical information on them from pharmacies or online. You may want the person to wear one, especially if they have a heart condition or some other serious health problem. You can order a MedicAlert bracelet reading "Alzheimer disease" or "dementia/memory impaired." These bracelets also have a phone number that can be called for further information about the person. MedicAlert maintains a trust fund to help low-income families pay for bracelets. Several similar products are also available.

Some forgetful people will carry a card in their pocket or wallet that gives their name, address, and phone number. Others, supplied with such a card, will lose it or throw it away. ID cards are worth trying but are not a substitute for a bracelet.

There are several invaluable devices for locating a person who has wandered away. Cell phone apps, chips that can be inserted into the sole of a shoe, and watches and bracelets with location finders are available. One wife was able to let her husband walk in their enclosed neighborhood long after he was unable to find his way home because he always carried his phone, which had a family tracker app on it. She could always locate him if he went for a walk, and she knew he couldn't leave the neighborhood.

To reduce increased wandering when the person moves to a new environment, you may want to plan in advance of the move to make it as easy as possible for the person who has dementia. If they are still able to understand and participate in what is going on around them, it may help to introduce them gradually to their new situation. If they are moving to a new home (see page 56), involve them in planning the move and visit the new setting several times before the move. When a person's impairment makes it impossible for them to understand what is happening, it may be easier not to introduce them gradually but simply to make the move as quietly and with as little fuss as possible. Each person is unique. Try to balance the person's need to participate in decision making with their ability to understand and remember. If you have a choice, make a move early in the illness as it will probably be easier for the person to adjust and learn their way around.

If you are considering a day care center, we urge you to do so early in the illness (see Chapter 10). Day care centers have found that people with dementia often adjust best when (1) they do not stay long the first few visits, (2) the caregiver stays with them the first few times, and (3) someone from the program visits them at home before the transition. Leaving a person who has dementia alone to adjust or asking the family not to visit at first may add to the person's panic.

When a person who has dementia finds themselves in a new place, they may feel lost, worry that you cannot find them, or decide that they are not supposed to be there. Reassure them often about where they are and why. "You have come to live with me, Father. Here is your room with your things in it," or "You are at the day care center. You will go home at 3:00."

When we give this advice, families sometimes tell us, "It doesn't work!" It doesn't work in the sense that the person may continue to insist that they don't live there and may keep trying to wander away. This happens because they are memory impaired and not able to remember what you told them. They need to be gently and frequently reassured about their whereabouts. It

takes time and patience to help them accept the move and gradually come to feel secure. People with dementia also need this frequent reassurance that you know where they are. A gentle reassurance and your understanding of their confusion help reduce their fear and the number of catastrophic reactions they have. Our experience with people who are hospitalized and have dementia is that frequent gentle reassurance and reminders about where they are help them become comfortable (and easier to manage). However, it may take several weeks of reassurance and reminders when someone moves to a new living environment.

Because changes in their environment may make the person's behavior or wandering worse, it is important to carefully consider the impact that a change might have. You may decide that a vacation or an extended visit is not worth upsetting the person. The change of scenery might be relaxing and stimulating for you, but it can take away the support that the person who has dementia feels when they are in a familiar place.

For wandering that seems to be aimless, some professionals suggest exercises and scheduled activities to help reduce this restlessness. Try taking the person for a walk each day. You may have to continue an activity plan for several weeks before determining whether it is making a difference. (If a person is physically active, be sure they are eating enough to provide them with the energy they need. Not eating enough may add to their confusion.)

When wandering seems to be the person's way of saying "I *feel* lost" or

"I am searching for the things I feel I have lost," you can help by surrounding the person with familiar things (for example, pictures of their family). Make them feel welcome by talking with them or by taking time to have a cup of tea with them.

Distract the person who has wandered rather than confront them

Agitated pacing or a determined effort to wander away is sometimes caused by frequent or almost constant catastrophic reactions. Ask yourself what may be happening to cause the catastrophic reactions (see page 28). Does this behavior happen at about the same time each day? Does it happen each time the person is asked to do a certain thing (like take a bath)? Review the way people around the person are responding to the wandering. Does their response increase the person's restlessness and wandering? If you must restrain a person or go after them because of the risk of harm, try to distract them rather than directly confronting them. Tell them you will walk with them. Then lead them around in a big circle. Usually they will accompany you back into the house. Talking calmly can reassure them and prevent a catastrophic reaction that will change aimless wandering into a determination to get away. Wandering can often be reduced by creating an environment that calms the person.

•

When Mrs. Dollinger came into the hospital, she had been making constant, deter-

mined efforts to leave the nursing home. In the hospital, which was also a strange place, the nurses had much less difficulty with her.

In both places Mrs. Dollinger felt lost. She knew this was not where she lived and she wanted to go home. Also, she was lonely—she wanted to go back to her job, where her fogged mind remembered friends and a sense of belonging. So she wandered toward the door. The overworked nursing staff at the nursing home would yell loudly to her, "Come back here." After a few days, one of the other residents in the home began to "help." "Mrs. Dollinger escaped again!" she would shout. The noise confused Mrs. Dollinger, who doubled her efforts to get out. This brought a nurse on the run. Mrs. Dollinger would panic and run away as fast as she could, straight into a busy street. When an attendant caught her arm and held her, Mrs. Dollinger bit him. This happened several times, exhausting the staff and precipitating almost constant catastrophic reactions. The family was told that Mrs. Dollinger was unmanageable.

In the hospital, Mrs. Dollinger headed for the door almost at once. A nurse approached her quietly and suggested they have a cup of tea together (distraction rather than confrontation). Mrs. Dollinger never stopped wandering to the door, but her vigorous effort to escape and assaultive behavior did stop.

•

If you think the person is wandering because they are restless, try giving them some active task like dusting, folding clothes, or stacking books. Adult day care that provides both companionship and things to do can be a great help for those who wander.

Medications are often ineffective in managing wandering and should be avoided because they may increase the person's confusion and the risk that they will fall. Indeed, antipsychotic drugs can actually make wandering worse. *They should be used only after all nondrug interventions have failed and only if there is a meaningful risk of harm or severe distress in the person who has dementia.*

Changing the environment to protect the person is an important part of coping with wandering. One family found that the person who had dementia would not go outside if he did not have his shoes on. Taking away his shoes and giving him slippers kept him inside.

There are many products on the market that will help you manage the person's wandering safely. In fact, there are so many devices that you should be wary of "Alzheimer wandering devices" that cost a lot but may be of limited use. Enrolling the person in the Wandering Support for a Safe Return program is one step you can take to minimize the risk of a bad outcome if they do wander away. This service is a collaboration between the Alzheimer's Association and the MedicAlert Foundation.

Wandering can often be reduced by creating an environment that calms the person

---

Before you invest in a wandering management system, there are several things you should consider. (We are addressing personal residences only here, not adult day care, residential care, or nursing homes.) Consider the behavior of the person who has dementia: do they go outside only occasionally, or is their wandering determined or dangerous? Consider yourself: how much of your own stress is caused by trying to keep tabs on them? Much of the value of a system to prevent wandering or to alert you to wandering is to relieve you of the constant burden of monitoring the person. Consider the costs of a system and the alternatives: if you depend on homemade and less expensive devices, will they really work? Will a system designed to prevent wandering really work? Will you and other family members use the system you set up? If the system you use does not really work to keep the person safe, based on the person's individual behavior, it can be dangerous. If you are lulled into relying on a system and it fails, this is worse than you constantly monitoring the person.

To help you decide what you need, consider these categories of helpful devices:

- things that lock or secure the home so that the person cannot go out

- things that make the home safe for the person who wanders around inside

- systems that alert you that the person is moving around or trying to leave

- things that allow you to communicate with the person

- things that help if the person does wander away

Use a combination of approaches to make the person's home secure. Many of the available devices are inexpensive.

A handy person can install most of them using supplies sold in hardware stores. It is not necessary to invest in a fancy, expensive system.

Things that lock or secure the home so that the person cannot go out. Go around your home or the part of your home that you want to make safe. Perhaps you need only to make the person's bedroom completely secure or only the bedroom, family room, and kitchen. Perhaps it is wisest to secure the whole residence. Window and door locks may be simple flip-up or pin locks, but use more than one on each door and window. The person who has dementia may not find them both. If possible, put locks where the person will not notice them. There is an inexpensive plastic gadget available at hardware stores called a childproof doorknob. It slips over the existing doorknob. *You* can still open the door, but the person who has dementia may not be able to figure out how to operate it. It is handy for closet doors that you don't want the person to enter. Remember to lock patio doors and basement doors. Select window locks that allow you to open the window a little so that fresh air can come in. Secure doors and windows leading to balconies and the garage.

But locks alone do not ensure safety. Even the most sophisticated locks will not stop a person who is determined to leave or who figures out the locks. Also, you must remember to use the security devices you install, and tell other family members that they must use them as well.

Things that make the home safe for the person who wanders around inside. You can't watch the person every

minute. They may get up and wander around while you sleep. You should consider having an electrician put a switch on the stove so that it cannot be turned on. Secure closets and drawers where unsafe items are kept, and keep the person out of certain rooms. We discuss these things on pages 61–63.

Systems that alert you that the person is moving around or trying to leave. These provide a backup to locks and allow you to be out of the room or go to sleep without being constantly alert to the possibility that the person will slip out. The simplest, but somewhat unreliable, is a bell that jingles when the door is moved. A door or window alarm can sound a chime or turn on a light in the room where you are sleeping so that you will be wakened if the person who has dementia is moving around or tries to go out. A motion detector in the area where they are likely to be moving around or in their room when they might get out of bed can be wired to ring a bell or turn on a light in the room where you are sleeping. Motion detectors are available that react to a person's moving around but not to pets. These are inexpensive, available at hardware stores, and easily installed.

A pressure-sensitive pad or mat (sold for Alzheimer wandering) by the person's bed or chair that is connected to a chime will alert you when the person steps on it in order to get up. A tab system (also sold for Alzheimer wandering) is a cord that connects a chair with the clothing of the person who has dementia. It sounds an alarm when the connection is broken. If the noise frightens the person, some other solution should be sought.

A motion-detector light will turn on lights so that the person can find their way around at night.

A baby monitor or dementia-specific monitor will allow you to listen to the person while you are nearby (in the yard or in another room).

Things that allow you to communicate with the person. An inexpensive and easily installed intercom system will allow you to speak to and reassure the person when you are in another room.

Things that help if the person does wander away. Despite your best efforts, the person who has dementia may wander away. *Be prepared.* Register them with the Wandering Support for a Safe Return program. Have a current picture of the person available to give to the police or others who might search for them. GPS-based apps can be downloaded onto cell phones. Specially designed bracelets, watches, and running shoes that have embedded GPS technology can help quickly locate people who have dementia who will carry a phone or wear these apparel items.

If the person does go outside, be alert to hazards in the neighborhood, such as busy streets, swimming pools, and dogs. The person may no longer possess the *judgment* to protect themselves from these things. You may want to take a walk through the neighborhood in which the person lives and look around for things that are dangerous to someone who no longer has the ability to assess their surroundings appropriately. At the same time, you may want to alert people in the neighborhood to the problem, reassuring them that the person is not crazy or dangerous but just disoriented.

The person can be their own worst hazard. When they look healthy and act reasonable, people tend to forget that they may have lost the judgment that would keep them from stepping over the side of a swimming pool or in front of a car.

Other people are also a hazard to the person who has dementia and who wanders. In addition to those who don't understand the signs of dementia, there are those who are cruel and vicious, who harass, torment, or rob older and frail people. Unfortunately, there seem to be enough such people, even in the "nicest" neighborhoods, that you need to recognize these hazards and protect the person from them.

There are physical devices to restrain a person in a chair or bed that should be used only as a last resort. A "lap buddy" (see page 93) will keep most people seated. Other devices include Posey brand restraints and the Geri Chair. The decision to use a restraint should be made jointly between you and the health care professional who knows the person best. A restraint should be used *only if there is a high level of risk of harm and all other possibilities have been tried.* In our experience the risk of harm from wandering is often exaggerated, and restraints often make the person more restless and distressed. (We are addressing here the use of restraints at home. The use of restraints in a residential care home or nursing home involves other issues and is discussed in Chapter 15.)

A Geri Chair is like a recliner with a tray on it that prevents the person from getting up. It will elevate a person's feet. A person can eat, sleep, and watch television in a Geri Chair. These chairs can be rented or purchased.

> **Physical devices that make it difficult for a person to get out of a chair or bed should be used only as a last resort**

You may reach a point when the wandering behavior is more than you can manage or when the person who has dementia cannot be kept safely in a home setting. If this time comes, you will have done all you can and will need to plan realistically for institutional care for them. Many residential care places will not accept anyone who has dementia and who is agitated, combative, or a wanderer. See Chapter 15 for a discussion of placement issues.

Sleep Disturbances and Night Wandering

Many people who have dementia are restless at night. They may wake to go to the bathroom and become confused and disoriented in the dark. They may wander around the house, get dressed, try to cook, or even go outside. They may "see things" or "hear things" that are not there. Few things are more distressing than having your much-needed sleep disrupted night after night. Fortunately, there are ways to reduce this behavior.

Older people seem to need less sleep than younger people. People who have dementia may not be getting enough exercise to make them tired at night, or they may doze during the day. Often it seems that the internal "clock" within the brain is damaged by the disease that is causing the dementia. Some nighttime behavioral symptoms may be in response to dreams that the person cannot separate from reality.

If the person naps during the day, they will be less tired at night. Try to keep them occupied, active, and awake in the daytime. Often people who have dementia are not very active and don't get much exercise. It may be helpful to develop a regular activity program, for example, a long walk in the late afternoon. This may make the person tired enough to sleep better at night. Some families find that taking the person outside in the fresh air and sunlight, especially in the morning, helps. A car ride makes some people sleepy. Day care centers are one of the best ways to keep a person active during the day.

See that the person has used the bathroom before going to sleep. Older people may not see as well in the dark, and this may add to their confusion. As our eyes age, it becomes more difficult to distinguish dim shapes in poor light. The person who has dementia may misinterpret what they see and therefore believe they see people or are in some other place. This can cause catastrophic reactions. Leave night-lights on in the bedroom and the bathroom. Night-lights in other rooms may also help the person orient themselves at night. Try renting a commode that can sit right beside their bed.

Many of us have had the experience of waking from a sound sleep and momentarily not knowing where we are. This experience may be magnified for the person who has dementia. Your quiet reassurance may be all that is needed.

Be sure the sleeping arrangements are comfortable—that the room is neither too warm nor too cool and that the bedding is comfortable. Duvets and quilts are less likely to tangle than blankets and sheets.

> **Nighttime behavioral symptoms may be a response to dreams that the person cannot separate from reality**

If the confused person gets up in the night, speak softly and quietly to them. When you are awakened suddenly in the night, you may tend to respond irritably and speak crossly. If you do, it may trigger a catastrophic reaction that will get everybody up in the middle of the night. Often all that is needed is to remind the person gently that it is still nighttime and that they should go back to bed. A person will often go back to sleep after using the bathroom or having something to drink. Encourage them to go back to bed, and sit with them quietly while they drink. Softly playing music will quiet some people. Try using room-darkening shades and quietly remind the person that it is dark and the shades are drawn, and therefore it is time to stay in bed.

Sometimes a person who will not sleep in their bed will sleep in a lounge chair or on a sofa. If the person gets up in the night and gets dressed, they may sit back down again and fall asleep in their clothes if you don't interfere. It may be better to accept this than to be up part of the night arguing about it.

If the person does wander at night, you must examine your house for safety hazards. Arrange the bedroom so they can move around safely. Lock the window.

Can the person turn on the stove or start a fire while you are sleeping? Can they unlock the outside doors and exit? Can they fall down the stairs? A substantial gate across the stairs (not one that can be climbed over) may be essential in houses where a person who has dementia sleeps.

Finally, if these measures fail and your sleep is markedly disrupted, a cautious trial of a sedative-hypnotic medication may help. However, you cannot simply give the person a sleeping pill and solve the problem. Because sedatives affect the chemistry of the brain, they can set off a series of interacting problems that cause more difficulties.

> **If the person gets up in the night, gets dressed, and then sits down and falls back asleep, there is no harm in accepting this behavior rather than trying to change it**

Older people, including those who are well, are more susceptible to the side effects of drugs than are younger people. Side effects of sedatives are numerous, and some are serious. Sedatives may make a person dizzy. People who have dementia are more sensitive to drugs than well people are. Older people are more likely to be taking other drugs that can interact with a sedative or to have other illnesses that can be aggravated by a sedative.

Sedative medications may make the person sleep in the daytime instead of at night, or they may cause a hangover effect that worsens cognitive functioning during the day. This can make the person even more confused, more vulnerable to falls, or incontinent. Paradoxically, sedative medications may even interfere with sleep. Each person is different; what works for one may not work for another.

The effect of the sedative may change—for many reasons—after it has been used for a while. Your doctor may have to try first one drug and then another, carefully adjusting the dosage and the time at which it is given. Drugs may not make the person sleep all night. Therefore, it is important that you do all you can with non-medication approaches to help the person sleep. Although we strongly discourage the use of sedative medication, these drugs are occasionally necessary for a person with dementia living at home, especially if the medication is the only way that you, the caregiver, can get some rest. In the nursing home, on the other hand, staffing should be adequate enough to allow the use of other interventions. Sleep medications, even the newer ones, do not help many people who have dementia, and they worsen memory and behavior in some people.

•

Mrs. Huang was up most of the night. She thought she still ran a grocery store and

had to get the fresh produce at 3:00 a.m. Her daughter, who worked all day in the grocery store, was exhausted. The doctor pointed out that sleep disturbances in general and this lifelong habit were difficult to change.

No one thing helped much, but by combining many small interventions the family was able to manage. They kept Mrs. Huang up later and increased her involvement in daily life. They had her take care of the baby, even though there had to be another adult present at all times. They used a short-acting sedative, and they hung blackout curtains, which Mrs. Huang remembered from the war. Many small changes and teamwork got the family through this difficult time until Mrs. Huang forgot about getting the produce and began sleeping longer.

•

People who have dementia may have an unrelated sleep disorder such as sleep apnea. Loud snoring and periods of gasping for air while sleeping are signs of sleep apnea. Unfortunately, people with dementia are rarely able to cooperate with the breathing masks used to treat the disorder. Restless legs syndrome, which is a precursor to Parkinson disease in some people, can also cause difficulty falling asleep. It can be helped by medication.

Worsening in the Evening ("Sundowning")

S ome people who have dementia seem to have more behavioral symptoms in the evening. The reasons for this vary from person to person but include afternoon fatigue, afternoon caregiver fatigue, loss of the usual patterns of hormonal secretion that follow a twenty-four-hour cycle, lessened stimulation later in the day, and, least likely, lowered light levels later in the day (the source of the label *sundowning*). A whole day of trying to cope with confusing perceptions of the environment may be tiring, so a person's tolerance for stress is lower at the end of the day. You are also more tired and may subtly communicate your fatigue to the person who has dementia, causing catastrophic reactions.

Plan the person's day so that less is expected of them at the times when they are not at their best

If a person's symptoms are worse in the evening, there are several things you can try: increase afternoon stimulation and activity, have them take an afternoon nap, determine whether you are doing something different in the afternoon or early evening that places pressure on the person, and expose the person to more daytime light. Frequently reminding the person where they are and what is happening may help.

Plan the person's day so that fewer things are expected of them in the evening. A bath (which is often difficult), for example, might be scheduled for morning or midafternoon if this works better.

There may be more things happening simultaneously in the house in the evening. This may overstimulate an already confused and tired person. For example, are you turning on the television during meals? Are more people in the house in the evening? Are you busy preparing dinner and less available to the person? Are children coming in? Being tired may make it harder for the person who has dementia to understand what is going on and may cause them to have catastrophic reactions.

If possible, try to reduce the number of things going on around the person at their worst time of day, whenever that is, or try to confine the family activity to an area away from them. It is also important to try to plan your day so that you are reasonably rested and not too pressed for time at the point in the day you know is worst for the person. For example, if they regularly become most upset while you are cooking dinner, try to plan meals that are quick and easy, that are left over from lunch, or that you can prepare in advance. Eat the larger meal at midday.

·

Edna Johnson's father-in-law was at his worst just at the time her sons came in from school and her husband came home from work. The family had little money for respite care, and it seemed wasteful to use it when they were all at home, but they decided that peaceful family time was important. They hired a respite care worker, who took the elder Mr. Johnson to the park just before the family arrived home in the evening, stayed there with him during meal preparation, and brought him back in time for dinner.

·

Sometimes the trouble is that the person wants your constant attention and becomes more demanding when you are busy with other things. Perhaps you can occupy them with a simple task close to you while you work, or ask someone else in the family to spend some time with them.

You may want to talk to the doctor about changing the schedule for giving medications if other methods don't help change this pattern.

Periods of restlessness or sleeplessness may be an unavoidable result of the brain injury. While the term *sundowning* is widely used, some individuals are more restless or difficult to care for in the morning or early afternoon. No matter what time of day these difficult behaviors occur, reassure yourself that the person is not acting deliberately even if they are acting up at the times of day that are hardest for you.

Losing, Hoarding, or Hiding Things

Most people who have dementia put things down and forget where they put them. Others hide or collect things and forget where they hid them. Either way, the result is the same: just when you need them most, the person's dentures or your car keys have vanished and cannot be found.

First, remember that you probably cannot ask the person where they put them. They will not remember, and you may trigger a catastrophic reaction by asking them. There are several things you can do to reduce this behavioral symptom. A neat house makes it easier to locate misplaced items. It is almost impossible to find something hidden in a cluttered closet or drawer. Limit the number of hiding places by locking some closets or rooms.

Take away valuable items such as jewelry so they cannot be hidden and lost. Do not keep a significant amount of cash around the house. Make small, easily lost items larger, more visible, or locatable with a tracking chip. Tracking chips make it possible to locate objects they are attached to or sewn into. Put one on your key ring, glasses, wallet, and remote. When you click on the "find" button, a bell will ring, a light will appear on the lost item, or the phone app will locate the chip. Have a spare set of necessary items such as keys, eyeglasses, and hearing aid batteries.

Get in the habit of going through wastebaskets before you empty them. Check under mattresses, under sofa cushions, in shoes, and in everyone's dresser drawers for lost items. Ask yourself where the person used to put things for safe keeping. Where did they hide Christmas gifts or money? These are good places to look for lost dentures.

> To make it easier to find hidden things, limit the number of hiding places by locking some closets or rooms

Some people hoard or save food, dirty clothes, or other possessions (see page 69). Some people hoard things because they have always collected things. Others seem to need to "hold on" to something or to "keep things safe." If this happens occasionally, it is best to ignore it. If possible, when you clean up, leave a little of the person's "stash." They may feel less need to add to the collection than they would if they found their supply wiped out.

One daughter said, "I solved my problem when I decided that it was all right to keep the silver in a laundry hamper. Now I look for it there instead of carrying it back to the dining room several times a day."

Rummaging in Drawers and Closets

Some people with dementia rummage through dresser drawers or take everything out of closets, making a mess for you to clean up. It can be particularly upsetting when the person rummages through other people's things. If there are young people in the household, they especially will need a private and undisturbed place to keep their things. You may have to put a hard-to-open latch on some drawers and closets. You may need to put a lock on one drawer and put dangerous or valuable things in it, or you may decide to move such things to a safer place. Childproof latches may secure a door or a drawer. It may help to fill a top dresser drawer or a box on top of the dresser with interesting things for the person with dementia to sort through. This will give them a sense of purpose but allow you to secure the rest of the drawers. Select items that will interest the person: small tools and machine parts will appeal to one person, while sewing supplies will interest another.

Inappropriate Sexual Behavior

Sometimes people who have dementia take off their clothes or wander out into the living room or down the street undressed.

One teenage boy came home to find his father sitting on the back porch reading the newspaper. He was naked except for his hat.

Occasionally, people who have dementia will expose themselves in public. Sometimes they will fondle their genitals. Or they will fidget in such a way that their fidgeting reminds others of sexual behaviors.

One man repeatedly undid his belt buckle and unzipped his trousers. A woman kept fidgeting with the buttons of her blouse.

Sometimes brain damage will cause a person to demand sexual activities frequently or inappropriately. But much more common than actual inappropriate sexual behavior is the myth that old people commonly develop inappropriate sexual behaviors.

·

One wife who brought her husband to the hospital for care confessed that she had no problems managing him but that she had been told that, as he got worse, he would go into his "second childhood" and start exposing himself to little girls.

·

There is *no* basis to this myth. Inappropriate sexual behaviors in people with illnesses that cause dementia are uncommon. In a study of our patients with dementia, instances of such behavior were very uncommon.

Accidental self-exposure and aimless masturbation do sometimes happen. Disoriented people may wander out in public undressed or partially dressed simply because they have forgotten where they are, how to dress, or the importance of being dressed. They may undo their clothes or lift up a skirt because they need to urinate and have forgotten where the bathroom is. They may undress because they want to go to bed or because their clothing is uncomfortable. Urinary tract infections, itching, or discomfort may lead to handling the genital area. Check with your doctor.

Don't overreact to this behavior. Just lead the person calmly back to their room or to the bathroom. If you find the person undressed, calmly bring them a robe and matter-of-factly help them put it on. The man who sat on the porch undressed had taken off his clothes because it was hot. He was unable to recognize that he was outside, was in sight of other people, and was not in the privacy of his home. Most people who have dementia will never exhibit this kind of behavior because their lifelong habits of modesty remain intact.

Undressing or fidgeting with clothing can often be stopped by changing the kind of clothing the person wears. For example, use pants that pull on instead of pants with a fly in them. Use blouses that slip on or zip up the back instead of buttoning in front.

> **Most people who have dementia do not engage in inappropriate sexual behavior. If such behavior occurs, handle it matter-of-factly. It is a result of the brain injury.**

In our culture we have strong negative feelings about masturbation, and such actions are upsetting to most families. Remember that this behavior, when it occurs, is a result of the brain damage. It does not mean that the person will develop other upsetting sexual behaviors. The person is only doing what feels good; they have forgotten their social manners. If this occurs, try not to act upset, because it may trigger a catastrophic reaction. Gently lead the person to a private place. Try distracting them by giving them something else to do. If a person's fidgeting is suggestive or embarrassing, turn their attention to some other activity or give them something else to fidget with.

We know of no case in which a person who has dementia has exposed themselves to a child, and we do not wish to contribute to the myths about "dirty old men" by focusing on such behavior. However, should such an incident occur, react matter-of-factly and without creating any more fuss than is absolutely necessary. Your reaction may have much more impact on the child than the actual incident had. Remove the person quietly and explain to the child, "He forgets where he is."

Some people who have dementia have a diminished sex drive, and some have more interest in sex than they did previously. If a person develops increased sexuality, remember that, however distressing this is, it is a factor of the brain injury. It is not a factor of personality or a reflection on you or your prior relationship with them (see pages 7–9 and 226–28).

Occasionally a father may make inappropriate advances to his daughter. *This is not incestuous behavior.* While it can be terribly upsetting for everyone, it usually means only that he is unable to recognize familiar people. Probably he has mistaken his daughter for his wife. Daughters often look much like their mothers did when the mother was young. The person who has dementia may remember that time much more clearly than the present. Such gestures indicate that he does remember his wife and their marriage. Gently redirect him when this happens, and try not to be too distressed.

Don't hesitate to discuss upsetting sexual behavior with the doctor, a counselor, or even other families. They can help you understand and cope with it. The person you choose should be knowledgeable about dementia and comfortable discussing sexual matters. They may make specific suggestions to reduce the behavior. Also see "Sexuality" in Chapter 12 and "Sexual Issues in Nursing Homes or Other Care Facilities" in Chapter 15.

Repeating Questions

M any families find that people who have dementia ask the same question over and over and that this is extremely irritating. In part, this behavior may be a symptom of the fear and insecurity that is common in people who can no longer make sense out of their surroundings. The person may not remember things for even brief periods and have no recollection of having asked you before or of your answer.

Sometimes, instead of answering the question again, it is helpful to reas- sure the person that everything is fine and that you will take care of things. Sometimes the person is worried about something else, which they are unable to express. If you can correctly guess what this is and reassure them, they may relax. For example:

•

Mr. Rockwell's mother kept asking, "When is my mother coming for me?" When Mr. Rockwell told her that her mother had been dead for many years, she would either get upset or ask the question again in a few minutes. Mr. Rockwell realized that the question really expressed her feelings that she was lost, and he began saying, "I will take care of you." This obviously calmed his mother.

Mr. Rockwell might also try saying, "Tell me about your mother," or "Do you remember when your mother took us to the play?"

•

Repetitious Actions

An occasional and distressing behavior that may occur in people with a brain disease is the tendency to repeat the same action over and over.

•

Mrs. Weber's mother-in-law folded the laundry over and over. Mrs. Weber was glad the older woman was occupied, but this same activity upset her husband. He would shout, "Mother, you have already folded that towel five times."

•

Mrs. Andrews had trouble with baths. She would wash just one side of her face. "Wash the other side," her daughter would say, but she kept on washing the same spot.

•

Mr. Barnes paces around and around the kitchen in the same pattern, like a bear in a cage.

•

It seems as if the damaged mind has a tendency to "get stuck" on one activity and has difficulty "shifting gears" to a new activity. When this happens, gently suggest that the person do a specific new task, but try not to pressure them or sound upset because doing so can easily lead to a catastrophic reaction.

In the case of Mrs. Weber's mother-in-law, ignoring the problem worked well. As Mr. Weber came to accept his mother's illness, the behavior ceased to bother him.

Mrs. Andrews's daughter found out that gently patting her mother's cheek where she wanted her to wash next would get her out of the repetitious pattern. Touch is a very good way to get a message to the brain when words fail. Touch the arm you want a person to put in a sleeve, touch the place you want the person to wash next, place a spoon in the person's palm to cue them to hold it.

Mr. Barnes's wife found ways to distract him from pacing by giving him something to do. "Here, Joe, hold this," she would say, and hand him a spoon. "Now hold this," and she would take the spoon and give him a potholder. "Helping" enabled him to stop pacing. It kept him busy and perhaps also made him feel needed.

Distractibility

People who have dementia are often easily distracted. The person may look elsewhere or grab at other things while you are trying to get their clothes on. They may eat the food on someone else's plate, or they may walk off while you are talking to them. Part of our brain filters out things we do not want to pay attention to—this is how we "tune out" unimportant noises, for example. When dementia damages this ability, the person may be unable to ignore extraneous stimuli and be equally attracted to everything that is happening, no matter how unimportant some of it may be.

If you can identify the things that distract them—people, animals, and sudden noises are common distractions—you may be able to minimize the distractions so that the person can better focus on one activity, such as dressing. Put their plate a little farther from the other plates. Have fewer visitors at once, and visit in a calm, quiet area. If the person is distracted by the television or music playing, turn it off. Arrange for eating and other activities to take place where other people are not moving about and talking.

Clinging or Persistently Following You Around ("Shadowing")

Families tell us that people who have dementia sometimes follow the caregiver from room to room and become fretful if the caregiver disappears into the bathroom or the basement. Or the person who has dementia may constantly interrupt whenever the caregiver tries to rest or get something done. Few things can irritate one more than being followed around all the time.

This behavior can be understood when we consider how strange the world must seem to a person who constantly forgets. The trusted caregiver becomes the only security in a world of confusion. When a person cannot depend on themselves to remember the necessary things in life, one form of security is to stick close to someone who does know.

The memory-impaired person cannot remember that if you go into the bathroom, you will be right back out. To their mind, with their confused sense of time, it may seem as if you have vanished. A childproof doorknob on the bathroom door may help give you a few minutes of privacy. Sometimes, setting a timer and saying "I will be back when the timer goes off" will help. One husband got himself a set of headphones so he could listen to music while his wife continued to talk. (Then he got her a set because he discovered that she enjoyed the music.)

It is most important that you try not to let annoying behaviors such as these wear you down. You must find other people who will help care for the person so you can get away and do the things that relax you—go out for dinner or shopping, take a nap, or enjoy an uninterrupted bath.

Setting a timer and telling the person "I will be back when the timer goes off" may help when you leave the room

---

Using medication to stop behaviors like these is often unsuccessful, and the side effects can be disabling. Unless the behavior places the person who has dementia or someone else in danger, medication should be used only after other attempted solutions have failed.

Find simple tasks that the person can do, even if they are things that you could do better or things that are repetitious. Winding a ball of yarn, sorting coins, or stringing beads may make a person feel useful and keep them occupied while you work.

•

Mrs. Hunter's mother-in-law, who has dementia, followed Mrs. Hunter around the house, never letting her out of her sight and always criticizing. Mrs. Hunter hit upon the idea of having her mother-in-law fold the wash. Because Mrs. Hunter has a large family, she has a lot of wash. The older woman folds, unfolds, and refolds laundered items (not very neatly) and feels like a useful part of the household.

•

Is it unkind to give a person made-up tasks to keep them occupied? We don't think so, and neither does Mrs. Hunter. The person who has dementia needs to feel that they are contributing to the family, and they need to be active.

Complaints and Insults

Sometimes people who have dementia repeatedly complain, despite your kindest efforts. The person may say things like "You are cruel to me," "I want to go home," "You stole my things," or "I don't like you." When you are doing all that you can to help, you may feel hurt or angry when they say such things. When the person looks and sounds well, your first response may be to take the criticism personally. You can quickly get into a painful and pointless argument, which may cause them to have a catastrophic reaction and perhaps even scream, cry, and throw things at you, leaving you exhausted and upset.

If the person with dementia speaks unkindly, step back and think through what is happening. Even though they look well, they have an injury to their brain. Having to be cared for, feeling lost, and losing their possessions and independence may seem to them like cruel experiences. "You are cruel to me" may really mean "Life is cruel to me." Because they cannot accurately sort out the reality around them, they may misinterpret your efforts to help as stealing from them. They may not be able to accept, understand, or remember the facts of their increasing impairment, their financial situation, the past relationship they had with you, and all the other things you are aware of. For example, they know only that their things are gone and that you are there. Therefore, they feel that you must have stolen their things.

> **When you are criticized by a person who has dementia, your first response may be to take the criticism personally. Instead, step back and think through what is happening. Even though they may look well, the person has an injured brain.**

A wife contributed the following interpretations of the things her husband often said. Of course, we cannot know what a person who has dementia feels or means, but this wife has found loving ways to interpret and accept the painful things her husband says.

He says: "I want to go home."

He means: "I want to go back to the condition of life, the quality of life, when everything seemed to have a purpose and I was useful, when I could see the products of my hands, and when I was without the fear of small things."

He says: "I don't want to die."

He means: "I am sick, although I feel no pain. Nobody realizes just how sick I am. I feel this way all of the time, so I must be going to die. I am afraid of dying."

He says: "I have no money."

He means: "I used to carry a wallet with some money in it. It is not in my back pants pocket now. I am angry because I cannot find it. There is something at the store that I want to buy. I'll have to look some more."

He says: "Where is everyone?"

He means: "I see people around me, but I don't know who they are. These unfamiliar faces do not belong to my family. Where is my mother? Why has she left me?"

In coping with remarks such as these, avoid contradicting the person or arguing with them since those responses may lead to a catastrophic reaction. Try not to say, "I didn't steal your things," "You *are* home," or "I gave you some money." Try not to reason with the person. Telling them "Your mother died thirty years ago" will only confuse and upset them more.

> **Try not to reason with a person who is complaining. Instead, respond sympathetically by acknowledging the feelings behind the complaint.**

Some families find it helpful to ignore many of these complaints or to use distractions. Some families respond sympathetically to the feeling they think is being expressed: "Yes, dear, I know you feel lost," "Life does seem cruel sometimes," "I know you want to go home."

Of course, you may become angry, especially when you have heard the same unfair complaint over and over. To do so is human. Probably the person will quickly forget the incident.

Sometimes the person who has dementia loses the ability to be tactful. They may say, "I don't like John," and you may know they never did like that person. This can be upsetting. It helps for those involved to understand that the person who has dementia is unable to be tactful, that while they may be being honest, they are not being purposefully unkind.

Perhaps you can cope with such remarks, but what about other people? Sometimes people who have dementia make inappropriate or insulting remarks to others. These can range from naive directness, such as telling the sitter her haircut is terrible, to shouting at the neighbor who brings dinner, "Get out of my house! You're trying to poison us."

People who have dementia may tell casual friends or strangers stories such as "My daughter keeps me locked in my room." When you take the person to visit someplace, they may put on their coat and say, "Let's go home. This place stinks."

Each person who has dementia is different. Some will retain their social skills. In others, a tendency toward bluntness may develop into open rudeness. Some people who have dementia are fearful and suspicious, leading them to make accusations. Catastrophic reactions account for some of this behavior. The person who has dementia often misjudges the one they are speaking to or misjudges the situation.

•

A secretary was talking with a man who had dementia while the doctor spoke with the man's wife. He was obviously trying to make polite conversation, but he had lost the subtlety he once had. "How old are you?" he asked. "You look pretty old." When she answered another question with, "No, I'm not married," he said, "I guess no one would have you."

•

People chuckle at this sort of behavior in a small child because everyone understands that a child has not yet learned social norms. It will be helpful to you if most of the people around you understand that the person has an illness that causes dementia and affects their memory of good manners. Most people are now aware of Alzheimer disease. They should recognize that these behaviors are the result of specific diseases and that, while such behavior is unwelcome, it is not deliberate.

To those people who see you and the person who has dementia often, such as neighbors, friends, and perhaps familiar store clerks, you may want to give a brief explanation of the person's illness. When you make this explanation, you should reassure people that the illness does not make the person dangerous and that they are not crazy. Some caregivers have cards printed up that say something like, "Please pardon my family member who has Alzheimer disease. Although he looks well, this disease has destroyed his memory." You may want to add a few lines about the disease and how to find more information about Alzheimer disease.

If a person who has dementia creates

a scene in a public place, perhaps due to a catastrophic reaction, remove them gently. It may be best to say nothing. While this can be embarrassing, you do not necessarily owe strangers any explanation.

Distraction is a good way to get a person out of what might become an embarrassing situation. For example, if they are asking personal questions, change the subject. When they tell others that you are keeping them prisoner or not feeding them, try distracting them. Avoid directly denying the accusation as this can turn into an argument. If these are people you know, you may want to explain what happened later. If they are strangers, ask yourself whether it really matters what strangers think.

Sometimes there is a gossip or insensitive person in a community who may build on the inappropriate remarks of a person who has dementia. It is important that you not be upset by such gossip. Usually other people have an accurate estimate of the truth of such gossip.

Taking Things

People who have dementia may pick up things in stores and not pay for them or may accuse the cashier of stealing their money. One wife reported that her husband was stealing and butchering the neighbors' chickens. He did not realize that they were not his own and was proud to be helping with dinner.

If a person is taking things in stores, they may be doing so because they have forgotten to pay for them or because they do not realize that they are in a store. Several families have found that giving the person things to hold or asking them to push the shopping cart, so that their hands are occupied, will stop the problem. Before you leave the store, check to see if they have anything in their pockets. You may want to dress the person in something that has no pockets the next time you go shopping.

If the person continues to do this, you might ask your doctor for a brief letter explaining that the person has dementia and sometimes forgets that they have put things in their pockets. If they do take something and you discover it later, or if they are caught by store personnel, you can use the letter to help explain matters.

•

The wife of the man who took chickens had her clergyperson explain things to the neighbors and then arranged to replace any chickens that turned up on her dinner table.

•

Forgetting Phone Calls

Forgetful people who can still talk clearly often continue to answer a landline or their own cell phone. However, they may not remember to write down phone messages. This can upset friends, confuse people, and cause you considerable inconvenience and embarrassment.

You may want to discontinue your landline and use your cell phone as your primary phone. If some people still call you on the landline, have that number transferred to a cell phone account. However, some people who have dementia are able to use a telephone but not a cell phone, either because they have done so for many years or because the numbers are large and easy to press. If you still have a landline, consider an answering machine feature that records all calls.

If the person who has dementia has a cell phone and you are concerned about missing calls, you can check the call log to determine if they received calls that you should know about.

•

One husband writes, "I found out from the log on her phone that she called the dentist five times, probably about her upcoming appointment. Since I knew about it, I called them and told them how to manage that."

•

Demands

Mr. Cooper refused to stop living alone, even though it was clear to his family that he could not manage. Instead, he called his daughter at least once a day with real emergencies that sent her dashing across town to help out. His daughter felt angry and manipulated. She was neglecting her own family, and she was exhausted. She felt that her father had always been a self-centered, demanding person, and that his current behavior was deliberately selfish.

•

Mrs. Dietz lived with her daughter. The two women had never gotten along well, and now Mrs. Dietz had Alzheimer disease. She was wearing her daughter out with demands: "Get me a cigarette," "Fix me some coffee." The daughter could not tell her mother to do these things herself, because she started fires.

•

Sometimes people who have dementia can be demanding and appear to be self-centered. This is especially hard to accept when the person does not appear to be significantly impaired. If you feel that this is happening, try to step back and objectively evaluate the situation. Is this behavior deliberate, or is it a symptom of the disease? The two can look alike, especially if the person had a way of making people feel manipulated before they developed dementia. However, what is often happening with a person who has dementia is *not* something they can control. Manipulative behavior requires the ability to plan, a skill that many people who have dementia lose over time. Perhaps you are experiencing an old style of relating to others that is no longer deliberate. An evaluation by a health care professional can be helpful because it tells you objectively how much of such behavior is something the person can control.

> An evaluation by a health care professional can tell you objectively how much of an upsetting behavior is something the person can understand and choose to do or not do

Some demanding behaviors reflect the person's feelings of loneliness, fright, or loss. For example, when a person has lost the ability to comprehend the passage of time and to remember things, being left alone for a short time can make them feel that they have been abandoned. This may lead to their accusing you of deserting them. Realizing that this behavior reflects feelings of abandonment can help you not to feel so angry and can help you respond to the *real* symptom (for example, that they *feel* abandoned) instead of responding to what seems to you like selfishness or manipulation.

Sometimes you can devise ways for the person to continue to feel a sense of control over their life and mastery over their circumstances that are not so demanding of you.

•

Mr. Cooper's daughter was able to find an "apartment" for her father in a sheltered housing building, where meals, social services, and housekeeping were provided. This reduced the number of emergencies but enabled Mr. Cooper to continue to feel independent.

•

A medical evaluation confirmed for Mrs. Dietz's daughter that her mother could not remember her previous requests for a cigarette for even five minutes. After trying several things, the daughter realized that the stress of the relationship was too destructive and placed her mother in a residential care home. Others, who had not lived with Mrs. Dietz's abrasive personality, found her easier to care for.

•

Families often ask whether they should "spoil" the person by meeting their demands or whether they should try to "teach" them to behave differently. The best course is often neither of these strategies. Because they cannot control their behavior, you are not "spoiling" them, but it may be impossible for you to meet endless demands. Because the person has limited ability, if any, to learn, you cannot teach them. Scolding may lead to catastrophic reactions and make things worse.

If the person demands that you do things you think they can do, be sure that they really can do these things. They may be overwhelmed by what seems to you to be a simple task. Breaking a task down into multiple steps may make it possible for the person to do it.

Being specific and direct with the person often helps. Saying "I am coming to see you Wednesday" is more helpful than getting into an argument over why you don't visit more often. Say, "I will get you a cigarette when the timer goes off. Do not ask me for one until the timer goes off." Ignore further demands until then.

You may have to set limits on what you realistically can do. But before you set limits, you need to know the extent of the person's disability and what other resources you can mobilize to replace what you cannot do. You may need to enlist the help of an outside person—a nurse or a social worker who understands the disease—to help you work out a plan that provides good care for the person who has dementia without leaving you exhausted or trapped (see Chapter 10).

When demands make you feel angry and frustrated, try to find an outlet for your anger that does not involve the person who has dementia. Your anger can trigger catastrophic reactions, which may make the person even more stubborn and willful.

Stubbornness and Uncooperativeness

"Whatever I want him to do, he won't do it," said one daughter-in-law. Said another, "Whenever it's time to dress Dad, he says he has already changed his clothes. He won't go to the doctor, and whatever I serve for dinner he won't eat."

•

Families often suspect that a stubborn and uncooperative person who has dementia is deliberately trying to frustrate them. It is hard to know whether a person who has always been stubborn is now more so or whether the stubbornness is because of the dementia. Some people are more uncooperative than others by nature. However, this kind of behavior is usually at least partly caused by the illness.

If a person cannot remember when they last took a bath, they may be insulted when they are told to bathe. This is understandable.

The person may not understand what they are being asked to do (go to the doctor, help set the table), and so refuse to do it. Uncooperativeness may seem a safer course than risking making a fool of oneself. Sometimes a statement such as "I hate this food" really means "I am miserable."

Take the path of least resistance. Avoid arguments and accept whatever compromise is safe and works.

Be sure that requests are understood. "Can you smell our supper cooking? See the roast? It will be delicious. Have a seat. We'll be eating soon."

Focusing on a pleasant experience sometimes helps: "As soon as we leave Dr. Brown's office, we'll celebrate with a big ice cream cone."

If strategies like this do not work

(and sometimes nothing does), consider that the negative attitudes are often a part of the illness rather than a personal attack. The person may be too confused to *intend* to insult your cooking. Take the path of least difficulty. Avoid arguments and accept whatever compromise will work.

When the Person Who Has Dementia Insults the Sitter

When a family is able to arrange for someone to stay with the person who has dementia, they may become angry or suspicious, insult the sitter, not let them in, or accuse them of stealing. They may fire the sitter This can make it seem impossible for you to get out of the house. It may mean that the person can no longer live in their own home. Often you can find ways to solve the problem.

As with many other behavioral symptoms, this situation may arise out of the person's inability to make sense of their surroundings or to remember explanations. All they may recognize is that a stranger is in the house. Sometimes the presence of a "babysitter" means a further loss of their independence, which they may realize and react to negatively.

Make sure the sitter knows that it is you, not the person who has dementia, who has the authority to hire and fire. This means that you must trust the sitter absolutely. If possible, find a sitter the person already knows or introduce the person to the sitter gradually. The first time or two, have the sitter come while you remain at home. Eventually the person may become accustomed to

the idea that the sitter belongs there. This will also give you an opportunity to teach the sitter how you manage certain situations and to evaluate how well the sitter relates to the person who has dementia. Often the person will adjust to the presence of a sitter if both you and the sitter can weather the initial stormy period.

> Make sure the sitter knows that it is you, not the person who has dementia, who has the authority to hire and fire

Be sure the sitter understands the nature of the illness that causes dementia and knows how behaviors such as catastrophic reactions are handled. (Hiring a sitter is discussed in Chapter 10.) Try to find sitters who are adept at engaging the person's trust and who are clever about managing them without triggering a catastrophic reaction. Just as there are some people who are naturally good with children and others who are not, there are some people who are intuitively good with people who have dementia. However, they are often hard to find. If the person will not accept one sitter, try another. Ask yourself whether your reluctance to use a sitter is part of the problem.

Be sure the sitter can reach you, another family member, and the doctor in the event of a problem. Give them a list of numbers to call.

Introduce the sitter as a friend "who wants to visit with you" and not as a sitter. Or perhaps as a new "house-keeper." If the person is suspicious of the sitter, the doctor may be able to write a signed note to them reminding them to stay with the visitor. If there is no other alternative, medications that reduce suspiciousness might be tried very cautiously.

In all events, consider your own health. Even if a sitter does upset the person who has dementia, it is essential that you get out from time to time if you are to continue to be able to give care (see Chapter 10).

Using Medication to Manage Behavior

This chapter has suggested many ways to address behavioral symptoms. Ideally, medication would never be necessary to control these symptoms. In the past, drugs were overprescribed as treatments for behavioral and emotional symptoms of dementia, but antipsychotic and sedative medications have multiple serious side effects. Concern is greatest regarding the use of antipsychotic drugs because they significantly increase the risk of death in people who have dementia. As a result, these drugs should be used only when other reasonable interventions have been tried and not worked, *and* if there is a meaningful likelihood of harm or severe distress associated with the behavior or symptom. If antipsychotic or sedative drugs must be used, they are most effective when targeted to specific symptoms. They are not helpful when given for generalized or nonspecific reasons.

If the behavior is potentially dangerous to the person who has dementia or others or if the person has a condition for which there is a specific treatment, such as an antidepressant for depression, then medication might be tried before other approaches have failed. The medication should be tried for a specified period of time, usually weeks or a few months at most, and stopped if the problem is not improving.

CHAPTER 8

Symptoms Associated with Mood Change and Suspiciousness

Depression

People with memory problems may also be sad, low, or depressed. When a person has memory problems and is depressed, it is important that the correct diagnosis be made and the depression treated. Memory problems may improve when depression is treated, whether or not the depression is caused by the dementia.

Most people who have Alzheimer disease or other chronic illnesses are not depressed

When a person with an incurable disease is depressed, it can seem logical that they are depressed about the chronic illness. But not all people who have Alzheimer disease or other chronic illnesses are depressed. In fact, most are not, and many seem to be unaware of their problems. A certain amount of discouragement about being ill is natural and understandable, but a deep despondency or a continuing depression is neither natural nor necessary. Fortunately, this kind of depression responds well to treatment, so the person can feel better whether or not they also have an irreversible dementia.

•

Mrs. Sanchez was irritable and often whined about her health. She said she "just wanted to die," and she was losing weight. It seemed that there was never a time when she cheered up. Because she had a serious memory problem, the doctor said she had Alzheimer disease. A psychiatrist determined that she was also depressed. When her depression was treated with medication, her mood—and her memory—improved. She gained weight. From time to time the doctor had to change her medication to manage her depression. She gradually became more forgetful, and ultimately it was clear that she did have Alzheimer disease as well as depression. Treating her depression enabled her to live as full a life as possible and made caregiving much more pleasant for her family.

•

It is important that a mental health expert assess the person's depression and determine whether it is a response to a situation or the kind of despondency that will respond to medication, and then treat the depression appropriately. Indications of depression include frequent crying, weight loss, fatigue, a change in sleep patterns, feelings that one has done something bad and deserves to be punished, and a preoccupation with health problems that are not confirmed by a medical evaluation. People who are depressed often do not eat properly, causing nutritional problems that further impair them. They may also act nasty, stubborn, or hostile. The person may or may not say that they feel depressed.

It may be impossible for depressed people to "snap out of it" by themselves. Telling them to do so may only increase their feelings of frustration and discouragement. For some people, trying to cheer them up makes them feel that they are not understood.

You should encourage a depressed or discouraged person to continue to be around other people. If they have memory problems, be sure that the activities they try are things they can still do successfully and are of some use so that they can feel good about themselves for accomplishing something. Help the person avoid tasks that are too complicated. Even small failures can make them feel more discouraged about themselves. Have them help you set the table. If they don't have that much energy, have them set just one place. If that task is too complicated, have them set out just the plates.

If groups of people upset the person, encourage them not to withdraw completely but instead to talk with one familiar person at a time. Ask one friend to visit. Urge the friend to talk to the depressed person, to meet their eyes and involve them.

When a person is feeling discouraged, it may be helpful for them to talk over their concerns with a knowledgeable counselor, member of the clergy, physician, psychiatrist, or psychologist. This is possible only when the person can still communicate well and remember some things. *This person must be a professional who understands dementia and who will adjust the treatment accordingly.*

Complaints about Health

If the person often complains about health problems, it is important to take these complaints seriously and have a doctor determine whether there is a physical basis for them. (Remember that chronic complainers can get sick. It is easy to overlook real illnesses when a person frequently focuses on things that have no physical basis.) When you and the doctor are sure that there is no physical illness present, the doctor can treat the depression that is the underlying cause of the problem. Never let a physician dismiss a person as "just a hypochondriac."

Suicide

When a person is depressed, demoralized, or discouraged, there is always a possibility that they will harm themselves. While it may be difficult for a person who has dementia to plan a suicide, you do need to be alert to the possibility that they will injure themselves. If they have access to a knife, gun, power tools, solvents, medications, or car keys, they may use them to kill or maim themselves. Statements about suicide should always be taken seriously. Notify your physician.

Alcohol or Drug Abuse

Depressed people may use alcohol, pain pills, tranquilizers, or other drugs to try to blot out the feelings of sadness. These drugs can actually deepen the depression. For a person who has dementia, drugs can also further reduce their ability to function. You need to be especially alert to this possibility in someone who is living alone or who has used medications or alcohol in the past.

> If the brain impairment makes it impossible for the person to control their drinking, you have to provide this control for them

People who are heavy drinkers and who also develop dementia can be difficult for their families to manage. The person may be more sensitive to small amounts of alcohol than a well person, so even one drink or one beer can significantly reduce their ability to function. They may be unable to tolerate the same amount of alcohol that they used to be able to handle.

It helps to recognize that the brain impairment may make it impossible for the person to control their drinking or other behaviors and that you may have to provide this control for them. Doing so will include taking steps to make alcohol unavailable to them. Do so quietly but firmly. Try not to feel that their unpleasant behavior is aimed at you personally. Avoid saying things that put the blame for the situation on anybody. Do what needs to be done, but try to find ways for the person to retain their self-esteem and dignity. There should be no alcohol in the house unless it is locked away. One family was able to arrange with the local liquor store to stop selling to the person who had dementia.

You may need help from a counselor or physician to manage the behavior of a person with a memory problem who also abuses alcohol or drugs.

Apathy and Listlessness

Many people who have dementia become apathetic and listless. They just sit and don't want to do anything. Such people may be easier to care for than people who are upset, but it is important not to overlook their needs.

Apathy and listlessness are evidence that the parts of the brain that control initiative and energy are not working properly. It is important to keep people who have dementia as active as possible. They need to move around and to use their minds and bodies as much as possible.

Withdrawing may be a person's way of coping when things get too complicated. If you insist on their participation, they may have a catastrophic reaction. Try to reinvolve them at a level at which they can feel comfortable, can succeed, and can feel useful. Ask them to do a simple task, go for a walk with them and point out interesting things, play some music, or go for a car ride.

It often seems that getting the body moving helps cheer a person up. Once a person starts doing something, they may begin to feel less apathetic. Perhaps they can peel only one potato today. Tomorrow they may feel like doing two. Perhaps they can weed the garden. Even if they spade for only a few minutes, it may have helped for them to get moving. If they stop a task after a few minutes, instead of urging them to go on, focus your attention on what they have accomplished and compliment them on that.

Occasionally, when you try to get a person active, they may become upset or agitated. If this happens, you will need to weigh the importance of their being active against their being upset.

Remembering Feelings

People who have dementia may remember their feelings far longer than they remember the situation that caused the feelings.

•

Mrs. Bishop stayed angry with her daughter for days, but she forgot that there was a good reason why her daughter had acted as she did.

•

Likewise, some people constantly restate the same suspicious ideas. Their families understandably wonder why they can't remember other things as well as they remember these suspicions. Our brain probably processes and stores the memory of feelings in different places and ways than it does memories of facts. For reasons we don't understand, emotional memories seem to be less vulnerable to the devastations of the illnesses that cause dementia. This can have a good side, because people often remember good feelings longer than the facts surrounding them.

•

One woman insisted that she had been dancing at the day care center, although she was confined to a wheelchair. She meant that she had had a good time there.

•

One man always stayed happy for hours after a visit from his grandchildren, even though he forgot their visit itself soon after they had left.

•

Anger and Irritability

Sometimes people who have illnesses that cause dementia become angry. They may lash out at you as you try to help them. They may slam things around, hit you, refuse to be cared for, throw food, yell, or make accusations. This behavior can be upsetting for you and may cause problems in the household. It can seem as if all this hostility is aimed at you despite your best efforts to take care of the person, and you may be afraid that they will hurt themselves or someone else when they lash out in anger. This is certainly a concern. However, our experience has been that it occurs rarely and can usually be controlled.

Exaggerated or misdirected anger is common in people with brain damage, such as in dementia

---

Angry or violent behavior is usually a catastrophic reaction and should be handled as you would any other catastrophic reaction (see Chapter 3). Respond calmly—do not respond with anger. Remove the person from the situation or remove the upsetting stimulus. Look for the event that triggered the reaction so that you can prevent or minimize a recurrence.

Try not to interpret anger in the same way as you would if it came from a well person. Anger from a person who has dementia is often exaggerated or misdirected. The person may not really be angry at you at all. The anger could likely be the result of misunderstanding what is happening or of frustration at not being able to do something they always did well. For example:

•

Mr. Jones adored his small grandson. One day the grandchild tripped and fell and began to cry. Mr. Jones grabbed a knife, began to yell, and would allow no one near the child. Mr. Jones had misinterpreted the cause of the child's crying and overreacted. He thought someone was attacking the child. Fortunately, the child's mother understood what was happening. "I will help you protect the baby," she said to Mr. Jones. She gave Mr. Jones a job to do: "Here, you hold the door for me." Then she was able to pick up and quiet the child.

•

Ironically, forgetfulness can be an advantage because the person may quickly forget the episode. Often you can distract a person who is behaving this way by changing the topic of discussion to something you know they like.

•

Mrs. Williams's mother-in-law often got angry and nasty when Mrs. Williams tried to prepare supper. Mr. Williams began distracting his mother by spending that time each day visiting with just her in another part of the house.

•

Once in a while, a person experiencing a catastrophic reaction will hit someone who is trying to help them. Respond to this as you would to a catastrophic reaction. Try to remain calm and not react in anger. When at all possible, avoid restraining the person.

If angry outbursts occur frequently, you may need to ask a clinician to help you review what is upsetting the person. In rare instances medication might be necessary.

> **Try distracting a person who is behaving angrily or irritably by suggesting that you both do something you know they like**

If you are frequently angry or irritable or are hitting or yelling a lot, you must seek help for yourself and the person who has dementia. These are signs that the burden of the situation is overwhelming for you. Find a way to have time for yourself away from the person who has dementia so that you can keep your emotional "balance."

Anxiety, Nervousness, and Restlessness

People who have dementia may become worried, anxious, agitated, and upset. They may pace or fidget. Their constant restlessness can get on your nerves. The person may not be able to tell you why they are upset. Or they may give you an unreasonable explanation for their anxiety. For example:

•

Mr. Berger was obviously upset over something, but whenever his wife tried to find out what it was, he would say that his father was coming to get him. Telling him that his father had been dead for years only caused him to cry and pace.

•

Some anxiety and nervousness may be caused by the changes within the brain. Other nervousness may come from real feelings of loss or tension. The emotional distress that arises from not knowing where one is, what one is expected to do, and where one's familiar possessions are can lead to almost constant feelings of anxiety. Some people sense that they often do things incorrectly and become anxious about "messing up." Longing for a familiar environment ("I want to go home") or worrying about people from the past ("Where are my children?") can create even more anxiety. Reassurance, affection, and distraction may be all you can offer. Medication only occasionally helps relieve these feelings and should be tried only if other options have failed and if the anxiety is very severe and occurs frequently.

Even people who have a severe dementia remain sensitive to the moods of the people around them. If there is tension in the household, no matter how well you try to conceal it, the person may respond to it. For example, Mrs. Powell argued with her son over something minor, and just when that was solved, her confused mother began to cry because she "felt like something dreadful was going to happen." Her feeling was a real response to the mood in the house, but because she was cognitively impaired, her interpretation of the cause of the feeling was incorrect.

The person may be sad and worried over losing some specific item, like a watch. Reassuring them that you have the watch may not seem to help. Again, they have an accurate *feeling* (something is lost: the memory is lost, time is lost, many things are lost), but the *explanation* of the feeling is inaccurate. Respond with affection and reassurance to their emotions, which are an accurate reflection of what they are experiencing, and avoid trying to convince them that what they are expressing is unreasonable.

Trying to get the person to explain what is troubling them or arguing with them ("There is no reason to get upset") may only make them more upset. For example:

•

Every afternoon at 2:00, Mrs. Novak began to pace and wring her hands at the day

care center. She told the staff that she was going to miss the train to Baltimore. Telling her she lives in Denver and was not going to Baltimore only upset her more. The staff realized that she was probably worried about going home, and they reassured her that they would see that she got home safely. This always calmed her down. (They had responded appropriately to her feelings.)

•

Not all anxiety and nervousness go away so easily. Sometimes these feelings are inexplicable. Offering the person comfort and reassurance and trying to simplify their environment may be all that you can do to counteract the effects of the brain disease.

When people who have dementia pace, fiddle with things, resist care, shove the furniture around, run away from home or from the day care center, or turn on the stove and all the water faucets, they may make others around them nervous. Their restless, irritable behavior is hard for families to manage without help.

Among the causes of agitation are pain, medications, a distressing environment, and disease

---

Agitation may reflect the fact that people are feeling depressed, angry, or anxious. It may be a manifestation of restlessness or boredom, a symptom of pain, a side effect of medication, or an inexplicable part of the illness that is causing their dementia. Respond calmly and gently. Try to simplify what is going on around the person and avoid "overloading their mental circuits." Your calmness and gentleness will be communicated to them.

You may find it helpful to give the person who is mildly restless something to fiddle with. Giving the person something constructive to do with their energy, such as walking to the mailbox to get the mail, may help. If the person is drinking caffeinated beverages (coffee, cola, tea), switching to noncaffeinated drinks might help.

•

One woman was restless much of the time. She paced, fidgeted, and wandered. Her husband stopped telling her to sit down and instead began handing her a deck of cards, saying, "Here, Helen, play some solitaire." He took advantage of her lifelong enjoyment of this card game, even though she no longer played it correctly.

•

Sometimes physical overactivity is the result of frequent or almost continuous catastrophic reactions. Try to find ways to reduce the confusion, extra stimulation, noise, and change around the person. (Read the sections on catastrophic reactions in Chapter 3 and on wandering in Chapter 7.)

False Ideas, Suspiciousness, Paranoia, and Hallucinations

Forgetful people may become unreasonably suspicious. They may suspect or accuse others of stealing their money or their possessions, even things nobody would take, like an old toothbrush. They may hoard or hide things. They may shout for help or call the police. A person who has dementia may begin accusing their spouse of infidelity.

People who have dementia may develop unshakable ideas that things have been stolen from them or that people are going to harm them. Carried to an extreme, these ideas can make the person fearful and resistant to all attempts at care and help. Occasionally, people who have dementia develop distressing and strange ideas that they seem to remember and insist on. They may insist that this is not where they live, that people who are dead are alive

and are coming for them, or that someone who lives in the house is a stranger and perhaps dangerous. Occasionally a person will insist that their spouse is not their spouse—that they are someone who looks like their spouse but is an impostor.

People who have dementia may hear, see, feel, or smell things that are not there. Such hallucinations may terrify them (if they see a strange person in the bedroom) or amuse them (if they see a puppy on the bed).

These behaviors are upsetting for families because they are strange and frightening and because we associate them with insanity. They may never happen to your family member, but you should be aware of them in case you have to respond to such an experience. When they occur in the presence of an illness that causes dementia, they are usually the result of the brain injury or a superimposed delirium (see page 305) and are not symptoms of other mental illness.

Misinterpretation

Sometimes these problems are due to people misinterpreting what they see and hear. If they see poorly in the dark, they may misinterpret the moving curtains as a stranger. If they hear poorly, they may suspect conversations to be people talking about them. If they misplace their shoes, they may misinterpret the loss as a theft.

> **If the person is misinterpreting things, avoid directly disagreeing with them since this may trigger a catastrophic reaction. Instead, explain what they are seeing or hearing.**

Is the person seeing accurately in the dark, and are they hearing as well as they should? You will need to help the person with cognitive impairment see and hear as well as possible because they may not realize their sensory limitations. Be sure that glasses and hearing aids are working well. If the room is dimly lit, see if improving the lighting helps. If the room is noisy or if sounds are muted, help the person identify sounds (see "Hearing Problems" in Chapter 6). Closing the curtains may help if they are seeing someone outside at night.

If you think the person is misinterpreting things, you may be able to help by explaining what they see or hear.

Say, for example, "That movement is the curtains" or "That tapping noise is the bush outside your window." This is different from directly disagreeing with them, which may cause a catastrophic reaction. Avoid saying, "There is no man in the bedroom" or "Nobody is trying to sneak in. Now go to sleep."

If the person does not hear well, it may help to include them in the conversation by addressing them directly rather than talking about them. Look directly at the person. Some people who have dementia can gain understanding from nonverbal aspects of communication such as facial expression, tone of voice, and body language even when their hearing is poor. Include the person in the conversation. You might say, "Mom, John says the weather has been terrible lately," or "Mom, John says your new grandchild is sitting up now." Never talk about someone in the third person, as if they weren't there, no matter how "out of it" you think the person is. This is dehumanizing and can understandably make a person angry. Ask other people to avoid doing it too.

Sometimes the person's brain incorrectly interprets what their senses see or hear. This is often what happens when a person becomes unrealistically suspicious. Sometimes you can help by giving the person accurate information or writing down reminders. You may have to repeat the same information frequently because the person will tend to quickly forget what you say.

Failure to Recognize People or Things (Agnosia)

People who have illnesses that cause dementia may lose the ability to recognize familiar things or people, not because they have forgotten them or because their eyes are not working, but because the brain is not able to correctly put together the information it is receiving. This can cause them to insist that their spouse is not their spouse or that their home is not their real home. This is called *agnosia*, from the Greek meaning "to not know or recognize." It can be a baffling symptom. For example:

Mrs. Kravitz said to her husband, "Who are you? What are you doing in my house?"

This is not a problem of memory. Mrs. Kravitz had not forgotten her husband. In fact, she recognized him immediately from his voice, but her brain could not figure out who he was from what her eyes saw. If the person does not recognize you as their spouse, reassure them. Try saying, "I know I look old, but I am your husband," but avoid arguing. Although this is heartbreaking, it is important for you to reassure yourself that it is not a rejection of you (the person does remember you). It is just an inexplicable misperception by the damaged brain.

Mr. Clark insisted that this was not his house, although he had lived there many years. When asked to describe his house he did so accurately, but when it was pointed out that his description matched the house he was in, he accused his daughter of lying to him.

Mr. Clark had not forgotten his home, but because his brain could not connect what he was accurately seeing with what it remembered about the appearance of his house, the place did not look familiar.

Some people do not recognize themselves in a mirror. They may interpret what they see as meaning a stranger is in the house. This is likely an agnosia for self.

If the person cannot recognize familiar faces but still recognizes voices, they may recognize you when you speak to them

---

You can help by giving the person other information. It may help to say, "I guess it doesn't look familiar, but this is your house." Hearing your voice may help them recognize who you are if their voice recognition is still accurate. It may be necessary to remove mirrors or cover them if they repeatedly upset the person.

"My Mother Is Coming for Me"

Someone who has an illness that causes dementia may forget that a person they once knew has died. They may say, "My mother is coming for me," or they may say that they have been visiting with a long-deceased grandmother. Perhaps their memory of the person is stronger than their memory of the death. Perhaps in their mind the past has become the present. In Alzheimer disease, older memories are better retained than newer memories. Therefore, the person may not be able to recall a more recent death but may retain childhood memories of being with the person.

Instead of either contradicting the person or playing along with them, try responding to their general feelings of loss if you feel that this is what they are expressing.

Telling the person who has dementia outright that their mother has been dead for years may upset them terribly. Most of us want to tell "the truth," and it is reasonable to see how the person reacts to the truth. Most of the time, unfortunately, the person who has dementia cannot remember this very important piece of information even after being told several times. Their focus on these memories probably means that they are important to them. Ask the person to tell you about their mother, look through a photo album from those years, or retell some old family stories. This responds to their feelings without hurting them again and again.

Sometimes people feel that this idea is "spooky" or that the person is "seeing the dead." It is much more likely to be another symptom, like forgetfulness, wandering, or catastrophic reactions.

Perhaps you will decide that this issue is not worth the argument.

Suspiciousness

If a person is suspicious or "paranoid," one must consider the possibility that their suspicions are founded on fact. Sometimes when a person is known to be unusually suspicious, real causes for their suspiciousness are overlooked. In fact, they might be being victimized, robbed, physically abused, or harassed. However, some people who have dementia do develop a suspiciousness that is inappropriate to the situation.

Paranoia and suspiciousness are not difficult to understand. We are all suspicious—a certain amount of suspicion is probably necessary to our survival. The innate naivete of the child is carefully replaced by a healthy suspiciousness as we grow up. We are taught to be suspicious of strangers who offer us candy, overly friendly salespeople, and people making offers "too good to be true." Some of us were taught as children to be suspicious of people of other races or religions. Some people have always been suspicious and others, always trusting. An illness that causes dementia may exaggerate these beliefs.

•

Ms. Henderson returns to her office to find her purse missing. Two other purses have disappeared this week. She suspects that the new file clerk has stolen it.

•

As Mr. Starr comes out of a restaurant at night, three teenagers approach him and ask for change for the bus. His heart pounds. He suspects that they plan to mug him.

•

Mrs. Bellotti called her friend three times to meet for lunch, and each time the friend refused, giving the excuse that she had extra work. Mrs. Bellotti worries that her friend is avoiding her.

•

Situations like these occur frequently. One difference between the response of a well person and that of a person who has dementia is that the latter's ability to reason may become overwhelmed by the emotions the suspiciousness raises or the inability to make sense out of their world.

•

Ms. Henderson searched for her purse and eventually remembered that she had left it in the cafeteria, where she found it being held for her at the cash register.

•

The person who has dementia lacks the ability to remember and to reason out complex problems. Therefore, Ms. Henderson will never find her purse and will continue to suspect the file clerk.

•

Knowing that he is in a well-lit, high-traffic area, Mr. Starr suppresses his panic and hands over some change to the three teenagers. They thank him and run to the bus stop.

•

The person who has dementia lacks the ability to assess their situation realistically and to control their panic. They often overreact. In this situation, Mr. Starr might have screamed, the teenagers would have run, the police would have been called, and so on.

•

Mrs. Bellotti discussed her concerns with a mutual friend and learned that her friend had been sick, had gotten behind in her work, and was eating lunch at her desk.

•

The person who has dementia lacks the ability to test out their suspicions against the opinions of others and then evaluate them.

People with dementia live in a world in which each moment is starting over with no memory of the moments that went before

---

The person who has dementia and becomes "paranoid" has not gone crazy. They live in a world in which each moment is starting over with no memory of the moments that went before. For them, things disappear, explanations are forgotten, and con-versations make no sense. In such a world it is easy to see how healthy suspiciousness can get out of hand. For example, the person who has dementia forgets that you carefully explained that you have hired a housekeeper. Lacking the information they need to assess accurately what is going on, they make exactly the same assumption we would if we found a strange person in the house—that the person is a thief. Home care workers are often of a different ethnicity from the person who has dementia. It may help the person who has dementia become comfortable with a new care worker if you stay at home the first few times. The person who has dementia may treat the home care worker as a "maid." Be sure that the home care worker knows that they are accountable to you, not anyone else.

When a person who has dementia hides something, they often forget where they put it and conclude that it has been stolen

---

The first step in coping with excessive suspiciousness is to understand that this is not behavior that the person can control. Second, it only makes things worse to confront the person or to argue about the truthfulness of the complaint. Avoid saying, "I told you twenty times, I put your things in the attic. Nobody stole them." Perhaps you can make a list of where things are: "Love seat given to cousin Mary. Cedar chest in Ann's attic."

When the person says, "You stole my dentures," don't say, "Nobody stole your teeth, you lost them again." Instead say,

"I'll help you find them." Locating the lost article will often solve the problem. Even if you don't find them, trying to do so can make the person feel acknowledged. Articles that are mislaid seem stolen to the person who cannot remember where they put them and who cannot reason that nobody would want their dentures.

•

One son securely fastened a key to the bulletin board (so his mother could not remove and hide it). Every time she accused him of stealing her furniture, he replied gently, "All your things are locked in the attic. Here is your key to the attic, where they all are."

•

Sometimes you can distract a person from their suspiciousness. Look for the lost articles or try going for a ride or getting them involved in a task. Sometimes you can look for the real cause of their complaints and respond with empathy and reassurance to their feelings of loss and confusion.

When many of a person's possessions must be disposed of so they can move into someone's home, residential care, or a nursing home, they may insist that their possessions have been stolen. When you have assumed control over a person's finances, they may accuse you of stealing from them. Repeated explanations or lists sometimes help. Often they do not because the person cannot make sense of the explanation or forgets it. Such accusations can be discouraging when you are doing the best you can for someone. The accusations are often, at least in part, an expression of the person's overwhelming feelings of loss, confusion, and distress. They are not really harmful to anyone, even though they are very distressing to you. When you understand that they occur because of the brain damage, you will be less upset by them.

Few things make us angrier than being falsely accused. Consequently, a person's accusations can alienate sitters, other family members, neighbors, and friends, causing you to lose needed sources of friendship and help. Once you are sure that the accusations are false, make it clear to people that you do not suspect them of anything and explain to them that the accusatory behavior results from the person's inability to assess reality accurately. Your trust in them must be obvious and strong enough to override the accusations made by the person who has dementia. Sometimes it is helpful to share with others written materials such as this book, which explain how the brain impairment affects behavior. Part of the problem is that the person who has dementia may look and sound reasonable. Because they may not look and sound as if this behavior were beyond their control, others may not realize what is happening.

When a person makes untrue accusations, make it clear to the person being accused that the suspicious ideas are part of the person's illness and that you do not suspect them

---

Some suspiciousness goes beyond this explanation—it cannot be explained by the forgetfulness and loss of the ability to correctly assess reality. Such suspiciousness may be caused by the disease process itself. Low doses of medication are occasionally necessary when the untrue beliefs lead to threats to harm others or to severe distress in the person who has dementia that cannot be relieved by reassurance, activity, and empathy. Treatment not only makes life easier for you but also relieves the person of the anxiety and fear that arise from their suspicions.

Hiding Things

In a world that is confusing and in which things inexplicably disappear, it is understandable that a person would put things of importance in a safe place. The difference between being well and being impaired is that the person with dementia forgets where that safe place is more often than the well person. Hiding behaviors often accompany suspiciousness. Because these behaviors cause so many problems of their own, we have discussed them separately in Chapter 7.

Delusions and Hallucinations

Delusions are untrue ideas unshakably held by one person. They may be suspicious in nature ("The mafia are after me," or "You have stolen my money") or self-blaming ("I am a bad person," or "I am rotting inside and spreading a terrible disease"). The nature of the delusion can help doctors diagnose the person's problem. Self-blaming ideas, for example, are often seen in people who are depressed. However, when delusions occur in a person who is known to have a brain impairment from stroke, Alzheimer disease, or certain other conditions, the delusion is believed to arise out of the injury to brain tissue. It can be frustrating to have a person seem able to remember a false idea but be unable to remember real information.

Sometimes delusions appear to come from misinterpreting reality. Sometimes they are tied to the person's past experiences. (A note of caution: not every odd thing that a person says is a delusion.)

Hallucinations are sensory experiences that are real to the person having them but that others do not experience. Hearing voices and seeing things are most common, although occasionally people feel, smell, or taste things that others do not.

·

Mrs. Singer sometimes saw a dog asleep in her bed. She would call her daughter to "come and get the dog out of my bed."

·

Mr. Davis saw tiny little men on the floor. They distracted him, and often he sat watching them instead of taking part in activities at the senior center.

·

Mrs. Eckman heard burglars outside her window trying to break in and discussing how they would hurt her. She called the police several times and earned herself the reputation of being a "nut."

·

Mr. Vaughan tasted poison in all his food. He refused to eat and lost so much weight that he had to be hospitalized.

·

Hallucinations are a symptom, like a fever or sore throat, that can arise from many causes. Certain drugs can induce hallucinations, even in otherwise well people, and so can several disease processes. As with a fever or sore throat, the first step is to identify the cause of the hallucination. In an elderly person, hallucinations are not necessarily an indication of an illness that causes dementia. They may result from several other causes, many of which are treatable. Delirium is one example. If hallucinations or delusions suddenly occur in a person who has previously been functioning well, they are probably not associated with dementia. Do not let a doctor dismiss this symptom. The examples we have given are not all examples of people in whom the hallucination is a symptom of dementia.

If delusions or hallucinations occur, react calmly so that you do not further upset the person. Reassure the person that you are taking care of things and that you will see that things are all right. Although this is not an emergency situation, you will want to check with the doctor as soon as convenient. If these symptoms distress the person who has dementia, medication may make them more comfortable and make life easier for you. However, the drugs used to treat these symptoms have powerful side effects and should be used only when non-medication interventions have failed and the person with dementia is either very distressed or is causing harm to others.

Avoid denying the person's experience or directly confronting them or arguing with them. This will only further upset them. Remember, the experience is real for them. You don't have to agree or disagree, just listen or give a non-committal answer. You can say, "I don't hear the voices you hear, but it must be frightening for you." This is not the same as agreeing with the person. Sometimes you can distract the person so that they forget about their hallucinations. Say, "Let's go in the kitchen and have a cup of warm milk." When they return to their bedroom, they may no longer see a dog on the bed and you will have avoided an upsetting confrontation.

Hallucinations are a symptom, like a fever or sore throat, and can happen for many reasons

---

It is often comforting to touch the person physically as long as they do not misinterpret your touch as an effort to restrain or harm them. Say, "I know you are so upset. Would it help if I held your hand (or gave you a hug)?"

One woman insisted that there was a snake in her bed. The staff took a bag to her bedroom and told her they had caught the snake. This may seem like lying to the person, but it made her comfortable and avoided an argument.

Having Nothing to Do

As they progress, illnesses that cause dementia greatly limit the things the person can do. It becomes impossible to remember the past or to anticipate the future. The person cannot plan ahead or organize a simple activity like taking a shower. Many people who have dementia cannot follow the action on television. While you or the nursing home staff are getting work done, the person may have nothing to do but sit with vacant time and empty thoughts.

> **Restlessness, wandering, trying to go "home," repetitive motions, asking the same question over and over, scratching, masturbating, and many other behaviors can begin as an effort to fill empty hours**

For the person who has dementia, restlessness, wandering, trying to go "home," repetitive motions, asking the same question over and over, scratching, masturbating, and many other behaviors begin as an effort to fill this emptiness. But for the family caregiver, the hours are full. We do not think that family caregivers, with all the burdens they face, should be expected to take on the additional responsibility of planning recreation. We do think that activity is important and urge the use of a day care center, other family, friends, or paid help, if possible.

Whenever you or someone else initiates an activity for a person who has dementia, you must walk a fine line between providing meaningful activity and overstressing the person. Move at the confused person's pace. Never let an activity become a test of their abilities—arrange things so that they will succeed. Having fun should be more important than doing something correctly. Stop when the person becomes restless or irritable.

CHAPTER 9

Special Arrangements If You Become Ill

Anyone can become ill or have an accident. If you are tired and under stress from caring for a chronically ill person, your risk of illness or accident *increases*. The spouse of a person who has dementia, themselves no longer young, is at risk of developing other illnesses.

What happens to the confused, forgetful person if you, the caregiver, are injured or become ill? It is important to have a plan ready. Perhaps you will never need to put your plan into effect, but because dementia disables a person in such a way that they cannot act in their best interests, you must have plans in place that protect both you and the person who has dementia. You need a physician familiar with your health to whom you can turn if you become ill, one who is available quickly in a crisis. In addition, you need to plan in advance for several kinds of possible problems: the sudden, severe problems that would arise if you had a heart attack or a stroke or if you fell and broke a bone, the less sudden problems that would arise if you had an illness and required hospitalization or surgery, and the

problems that would arise if you got the flu or for some other reason were at home sick for a few days.

What happens to the confused, forgetful person if you, the caregiver, are injured or become ill?

•

Mrs. Brady suddenly began having chest pains and knew she should lie quietly. She told her husband, who had dementia, to go get their neighbor, but he kept pulling at her arm and shouting. When she finally was able to reach her phone and call 911, he refused to let the ambulance attendants into the house.

•

People who have dementia, even if they appear to function well, may, when upset, become unable to do things they can usually do. Should you suddenly become ill and unable to summon help yourself, the upset and confused person may not be able to summon help for you. They may misinterpret what is happening and impede efforts to get help.

Ways to Get Help

There are several possible ways you can plan to get help. Post "Emergency. Call 911" by all landline phones. However, you cannot depend on the person who has dementia, especially when they are under additional stress, to be able to respond to an emergency.

Invest in a personal security alarm. This is a small device that you wear on your wrist or around your neck. When you press a button on it, you are connected with someone at the security service. You can talk to that person as they call for help for you. There are several manufacturers of these devices. You pay a purchase fee, plus a monthly service fee. The fees are reasonable and can save both your life and the life of the person who has dementia. Select a device that will work in the shower.

Carry a card in your wallet that states that the person you are with has dementia. Briefly list their immediate needs and give the phone number and name of a person who can assume care on an emergency basis. Carry with you a card that gives diagnoses and current medications for both yourself and the person who has dementia. Securely tape a copy of this to the refrigerator for emergency personnel as well. Keep it current (even marking up the copy in ink is better than letting it slide until you have time to redo it).

Keep your cell phone with you at all times. Keep your contacts list up to date so that you can get in touch with help immediately.

Many communities have programs for senior citizens in which someone will call once a day to see if the senior is alright. This may mean a long delay in getting help, but it is better than nothing.

> **The ideal substitute caregiver is someone the person with dementia knows and someone who knows the person's daily routines**

Be sure that the person who would respond in a crisis has a key to your house. The upset, confused person with dementia may refuse to let anyone in.

In case you must go into the hospital or if you are sick at home, you will want to carefully plan ahead for the care of the person who has dementia. Changes will be upsetting for them, so you should minimize change as much as possible. The substitute caregiver should be someone the person knows and someone who knows your care routines. See Chapter 10 for possible sources of temporary help. Be sure that the names and phone numbers of your doctor, the person's doctor, the pharmacist, your lawyer, and close family members are written down where the person helping out in an emergency can find them.

Some families make a "cope notebook" in which they jot down the things another person would need to know, for example, "Dr. Khan (773-555-8787). George gets a pink pill one hour before lunch. He will take it best with orange juice. The stove won't work unless you turn on the switch that is hidden behind the toaster. George starts to wander around suppertime. You need to watch him then." Some families give a "care sheet" of instructions to all family members or friends who may be called on to help. This care sheet covers all the important aspects of the person's care, from meals to medications and activities, and it includes essential phone numbers of responsible people and professional caregivers.

In the Event of Your Death

When someone close to you has an illness that causes dementia, you have a special responsibility to provide for them if you should die. While there is a good chance your plans will never have to be put into action, they must, for the sake of the person who has dementia, be made.

When a family member is unable to take care of themselves, it is important that you have a will that provides for their care. Find a lawyer whom you trust, and have them draw up a will and any other necessary legal papers. Every state has a law that determines how property will be divided among your heirs if you do not make a will or if your will is not valid. However, this may not be the way you want your estate to be distributed. In addition to the usual matters of dividing your estate among your beneficiaries, the following questions must be addressed and appropriate arrangements made. (Also see Chapter 14.)

What arrangements have been made for your funeral, and who will carry these out? You can select a funeral director in advance and specify, in writing, what kind of funeral you will have and how much it will cost. You can usually pay in advance for the arrangements and obtain a certificate specifying what services will be provided for the advance payment. (Be sure to provide a copy to trusted family members, a legal representative, or friends so there are no questions when the time comes.) Far from being macabre, this is a considerate and responsible act that ensures that things will be done as you wish and that saves your distraught family from having to make these arrangements in the midst of their grief. Funerals can be expensive, and advance plans make it possible for you to see that your money is spent as you wish.

All members of the family should know what is wrong with the person and what plans have been made

What immediate arrangements have been made for care of the person who has dementia, and who will be responsible for seeing that they are carried out? Someone must be available immediately who will be kind and caring.

Does the person who will be caring for the person who has dementia know their diagnosis and doctor? Do they know as much as possible about how to make them comfortable?

What financial provisions have been made for the person who has dementia, and who will administer them? If they can no longer manage their own affairs, someone must be available with the authority to care for them. You will want to select a person whom you trust to do this rather than leave such an important decision to a court or judge. When such decisions are made by a court, they involve long delays and considerable expense.

Sometimes a husband or wife cares for years for a spouse with an illness that causes dementia and does not want to burden their children with the knowledge of this illness.

•

Said a daughter, "I had no idea anything was wrong with Mom, because Dad covered for her so well. Then he had a heart attack and we found her like this. Now I have the shock of his death and her illness all at one time. It would have been so much easier if he had told us about it long ago. And we didn't know anything about dementia. We had to find out all the things he had already learned, and at such a difficult time for us."

•

An experience like this is one example of the disservice of "protecting" other members of the family. All members of the family need to know what is wrong with the person and what plans have been made.

You should have a brief summary of your assets available for the person who will take over. This should include information on the location of wills, deeds, stocks, cemetery plot deeds, and information about the care of the person who has dementia. Tell someone you trust where it is.

CHAPTER 10

Getting Outside Help

Throughout this book we have emphasized the importance of finding time for yourself away from the responsibilities of caring for the person who has dementia. You may also need other kinds of help: someone to see that a person with dementia who is alone during the day gets their meals; someone to help give them a bath; someone to watch them while you shop, rest, or take a break; someone to help with the housework; or someone with whom you can talk things over.

You may want someone to stay with the person part of the day, or you may need a place where they can stay for several days while you take a vacation or get medical care. At some point you may need to find a place where the person with dementia can spend time away from you and where they can make friends of their own. Such outside help is called *respite* because it gives you a break from caregiving. This chapter describes the kinds of services that may be available. The second part of the chapter discusses some of the problems you may encounter.

Help from Friends and Neighbors

Usually, caregivers who feel that they have the support of others manage the burdens of care more successfully. It is important that you not feel alone with your burden. Most people first turn to family members, friends, or neighbors for support and help. Often people will offer to help, but sometimes you have to ask.

Family members sometimes disagree or don't help out. You may be reluctant to ask them for the help you need. In Chapter 11 we discuss some ways to handle family disagreement and to ask for help.

Others are frequently willing to help. Sometimes a neighbor will look in on the person who has dementia; the pharmacist will keep track of prescriptions for you; the minister, priest, imam, or rabbi will listen when you are discouraged; a friend will sit with the person in an emergency; and so forth. As you plan, you should consider these resources, because they are important to you.

How much help should you accept or ask for from friends and neighbors? Most people like to help, yet making too many demands on them may eventually cause them to pull away.

When you turn to friends and neighbors for help, there are several things you can do to make them feel comfortable helping you. Some people are uncomfortable around those who are visibly upset. You may not want to express all your distress to such people. Close friends may be more willing to share some of the emotional burden with you than people who do not know you well.

Although most people have heard of Alzheimer disease, many need more information to understand why the person acts as they do. Explain that the behaviors are the result of damage to the brain, that they are not deliberate or dangerous.

People may be reluctant to "sit with" or visit with the person because they feel uncomfortable and do not know what to do. You can help by suggesting specific things that the visitor might do with the person. For example, mention that going for a walk might be more fun than a conversation or that reminiscing about old times might be fun for both of them. Tell the visitor what you do when the person who has dementia becomes irritable or restless.

Some Area Agencies on Aging and local chapters of the Alzheimer's Association have programs to train family members or friends to be special visitors. Such visitors bring pleasure to the person who has dementia, as well as giving you time away from caregiving.

When you ask people to help you, give them enough advance notice, if possible, so they can make time in their schedule. Remember to thank them, and avoid criticizing what they have done.

Look for things others can do that they will not consider inconvenient. For example, neighbors may not mind "looking in" on the person with dementia because they live close by, while more distant friends might resent being asked to make a long drive.

Finding Information and Services

At some point, most families look for outside help in obtaining information, making decisions, and planning for the long-term care of their afflicted family member. Most families also need some time for themselves away from caregiving. Many families find the help they need and manage effectively without extensive professional assistance. However, the burdens of caring for a person who has dementia can be enormous, and many people have difficulty finding the services that might make caregiving easier.

> **Caring for a person with dementia can be overwhelming. Many families will need help from friends, family, or someone outside the family.**

Kinds of Services

People who have dementia and their families may need several kinds of services. Most are available for a fee, but a few are available without charge. See Chapter 14 for a discussion of financial resources.

An increasing number of people who develop dementia are under age 60. The Alzheimer's Association can direct them and their family to community resources with expertise in the unique problems they are likely to face.

There are additional resources for people 60 years and older. Most local offices on aging and senior centers have a list of free or reduced-fee programs for people over age 60 or 65. AARP is also a good source of information about such resources.

Some programs offer services such as dental care, discounted dentures, relatively low-cost eyeglasses, legal counseling, social work help, referral services, and free tax assistance to people over age 60, their spouses, and people who are disabled. Some programs provide prescription medications or medical appliances at reduced cost. Some provide transportation.

There are a few programs that repair older people's homes at reduced rates. You may be able to use such a program to install wheelchair ramps, locks, grab bars, and other safety features.

In some areas, programs such as Meals on Wheels will bring a daily hot meal to people who cannot get out. These meals are often delivered by friendly, dedicated volunteers who will also check to see how a person living alone is doing, but they provide limited help for a person who is becoming confused and are not a substitute for supervision.

Expanded nutrition programs offer a hot lunch and a recreation program in a sheltered group setting for several hours each weekday. They usually do not provide medical care, give medicines, or accept wandering, disruptive, or incontinent people. They are often staffed by lay or paraprofessional people. People who have a mild or moderate dementia may enjoy the group setting.

Nutrition programs funded through the Older Americans Act serve people over age 60 and their spouses. You can find them by calling your local senior center or commission on aging. Some hot lunch programs are intended for well older people, and a person who has dementia would not fit in. Other programs under the same or similar funding offer services to "frail" elderly people. You may be able to attend with your spouse if you wish. *Such programs do not provide adequate supervision for a person living alone.*

Mr. Williams was confused and often became restless. His wife arranged for a senior volunteer to visit and play checkers with him. He loved checkers, and the volunteer understood and did not mind that Mr. Williams often forgot the rules. The volunteer became his "checkers pal" and made it possible for Mr. Williams to have a friendship and an enjoyable activity. At the same time, Mrs. Williams got a break.

•

Two online sources of information are the Eldercare Locator (https://eldercare.acl.gov) and the National Adult Day Services Association (www.nadsa.org).

There are many other programs; we have referred to some of them in other parts of this book. You should find out what is available in your area even if you don't feel you need the service now.

Having Someone Come into Your Home

Many families arrange for someone to come into their home to help with the person's care. A *homemaker* will help you with tasks such as housework, cooking, laundry, or shopping. A *home health aide* or a *personal care aide* will help the person who has dementia dress, bathe, eat, and use the bathroom. Families of people who have dementia most commonly turn to a *paid companion* or *sitter*. Sitters provide supervision and may help the person with meals. Some will give baths. Some have had special training to provide the person who has dementia with socialization and meaningful activities.

Visiting nurse and home health agencies send professionals—nurses, social workers, and other therapists—into homes to provide evaluation and care. A nurse, for example, may monitor the person's status, change a catheter, and give injections. A speech therapist can help a person who has had a stroke regain language skills, while a physical therapist can help the person exercise. Because a nurse is expensive

and because Medicare will pay for this care only under strict guidelines, most families employ a nurse only when the person who has dementia has an acute illness that is difficult to manage at home. Hospice team members can teach you how to care for a dying person at home.

Home care provides supervision and personal care

Home Care

Home care is the first choice for many families. It is helpful when the person with dementia is ill or cannot get out of the house. It can be painful to realize that you need outside care, and you may not want another person in your home. However, in-home care gives you much needed respite, and often the person with dementia will feel that the home care worker is a visiting friend and enjoy spending time with them.

There is little state and federal regulation or licensing for home care (also see pages 187–88). You are on your own. The quality of care you receive often depends on the agency and the individual caregiver. Interview more than one agency and compare costs. But the cheapest agency may not be the best. Ask what training the aides are given about dementia. Is the agency bonded? What are your state's regulations and licensing requirements?

Most care workers are honest, but do not leave pain medications and money out, and do not give the person access to a credit card or checkbook.

It is important that the caregiver be consistent. Under what circumstances does the agency substitute a new caregiver? How much warning will the agency give you if the caregiver is not coming? Care workers may not show up at the last minute. You need to have a "back up" plan if the care worker does not show up or if a stranger arrives. Can a family member or neighbor fill in on short notice?

Will the caregiver be driving the person with dementia to doctor appointments or other places? Are they qualified? Can the care worker manage with the person with dementia in the car? If you can't, the aide may not either. If you take the person to the doctor, take the caregiver along to help you manage.

Teach the caregiver about dementia and give them detailed information about the person's needs. The paid caregiver will be more successful if you inform them about triggers that upset the person and instruct them on how to calm the person down. Try leaving a note for the person with dementia telling them that you have asked "Alice" to visit and that you will return. Make sure the caregiver knows that only you make decisions, give orders, and make plans for the day. Make sure the caregiver knows that only you can fire them—never the person with dementia (if the person with dementia "fires" the caregiver, the caregiver should check with you).

If possible, stay with the caregiver and person with dementia the first few times to show the caregiver what you do. This also helps if the person with dementia rejects the care worker. You can gently reassure them.

Do not expect the care worker to also do housework in addition to their caregiving tasks. They should be fully occupied in caring and socializing with the person with dementia. You may hire the caregiver under the guise of being a housekeeper, but make sure the caregiver knows that their primary responsibility is to care for the person with dementia.

Be sure to inform the caregiver that only you have the authority to hire and fire

---

Talk to the care worker when they arrive and before they leave to share information about how the day went. This is especially important when the confused person gives a muddled account of what happened.

Some families have used a baby monitor, remote video camera, or similar devices to keep track of what is going on. Caregivers prefer to know that they are being monitored.

Home care workers often do not earn a lot from home caregiving. Treating them with courtesy and correcting them kindly works best. Talking to the agency about any problems is usually helpful.

Adult Day Care

Adult day care offers several hours a day of structured recreation in a group setting. Lunch and activities such as exercise, crafts, discussion, and music are offered. Programs may be open from one to five days a week; a few offer weekend or evening care.

Some day care programs accept both people with a range of physical impairments and people who have dementia, but others specialize in the care of people who have dementia. Those that do may take people with severe impairments and may offer more activities designed for people who have dementia. Many programs that mix people who have dementia and those with other conditions provide good care to both groups. The skill of the staff and the philosophy of the program are most important in determining the quality of a program's care.

> **The skill of the staff and the philosophy of the program determine the quality of adult day care programs**

Adult day care is one of the most important resources for families. It provides urgently needed respite for the caregiver and *often benefits the person who has dementia*. For most of us, the pressures of daily life can be relieved by getting away sometimes to be with friends or to be alone. The person who has dementia does not have this opportunity. They must be with their caregiver day after day, but their impairment does not take away the need to have their own friends and time apart. The burden of this enforced togetherness may be as difficult for the person who has dementia as it is for the family caregiver.

People who have dementia experience failures and reminders of their inadequacies at every turn. But even when they cannot feed or dress themselves, they often retain their ability to enjoy music, laughter, friends, and the pleasures of doing some simple activity. People who have dementia may make friends with other people at the center, even when their impairment means that they may not be able to tell you about their friend. Day care staff observe that participants regain a sense of humor, appear more relaxed, and enjoy the activities. Good day care programs find ways for people to succeed at little things and thereby feel better about themselves. Day care programs fill empty time with activities the person can do well. Some programs do not offer much stimulation or socialization for the person who has dementia, but they remain a valuable source of time away for you.

Some programs offer both day care and in-home care. They are flexible so that you can shift from one to the other as your needs change.

> **People who have dementia can still enjoy music, laughter, friends, and doing activities even when their impairment is severe**

Day care programs sometimes will not take clients with severe behavior problems. They may not take those who are incontinent or those who cannot walk independently, although some dementia-specific programs accept individuals with these very severe impairments. Some day care centers specialize in people who have a mental illness or who are developmentally disabled. Some accept only frail people who are not cognitively impaired. Some offer few activities. Check out the program to be sure it will meet the needs of the person you are caring for.

A major barrier to day care is transportation. Transporting people to and from day care is time-consuming and expensive. Some programs pick people up, some contract with local transportation or taxi services, and some require that you transport the person yourself. Be sure that the person will be given enough supervision while en route to the program.

Many families turn to day care or home care as a last resort, when residential care or nursing home care is what the person needs. We think this is a mistake. The person's ability to adjust to and benefit from the respite care program is usually greater if you seek respite care *early*, when the person still has the capacity to adjust to and enjoy the new program. Your continued ability to provide care also depends on getting relief for yourself early.

> **Even if you think the home care worker is not doing much, the respite is still important for you**

While you cannot expect home care or day care to be the same as what you yourself provide, you will want to be sure that the care is adequate. If you have real concerns about the quality of care, talk to the local office on aging about the program. You can "drop in" unexpectedly at a day care center. However, even if the person spends time sitting and looking at the television, the respite is still important for you.

Short-Stay Residential Care

In short-stay respite settings, the person who has dementia lives in a nursing home, an assisted living facility, or a boarding home for a short period—a weekend, a week, or a few weeks—while the caregiver takes a vacation, receives needed medical care, or just rests. The concept of short-stay respite care may be unfamiliar to you, but you should consider trying it. Caregivers who use it are enthusiastic about it.

> **As with all support programs, respite care is more effective when families use it *before* they reach the breaking point**

There is little government funding or insurance coverage for short-stay care. Some caregivers are reluctant to use short-stay respite because they fear that once they give up the demands of care, even temporarily, they will be unable to shoulder them again. There must be a clear understanding between the provider and the family about the duration of the stay. As with all support programs, respite care is more effective when families use it *before* they reach the breaking point.

You may negotiate for this service yourself with a facility or an individual who will take in one or two clients. Because there is often little government oversight of such care, you must make sure that the provider understands how to care for your family member and is a kind and gentle person. New surroundings may stress people who have dementia, so short-stay respite programs need enough skilled staff to give individual attention to their guests.

A range of combinations of respite programs has been developed for people who have dementia and their families. Some respite programs offer resources for the caregiver as well as the person who has dementia. Some programs designed for people who have dementia create positive experiences that go far beyond being merely a "sitter" service. A local dementia-support program or the local chapter of the Alzheimer's Association may be able to help you find resources.

Planning in Advance for Home Care, Day Care, and Respite Care

Once you have found a good program, there are a few things you must do to make the visits go smoothly. Be sure that the provider understands the nature of the dementia and knows how to handle problem behaviors. Write out special information for the provider. How much help will the person need in the bathroom or with meals? What do they like for lunch? What cues do they give that they are becoming irritable, and how do you respond? What special needs do they have?

Be sure the care provider knows how to reach you, another family member, and the doctor. Be sure that the provider is informed by you that only you have the authority to hire and fire.

> **Be sure that the care provider understands the nature of the person's dementia and knows how to handle problem behaviors. Be sure the care provider knows how to reach you, another family member, and the doctor.**

If the person with dementia has complicating health problems, such as a heart or respiratory condition, a tendency to choke or fall, or seizures, you must carefully consider the skills of the person with whom you leave them.

When the Person Who Has Dementia Rejects the Care

Families often think their family member who has dementia would never go to day care or accept a home visitor. People who have dementia often surprise everyone by enjoying day care or a home visitor. Avoid asking the person with dementia if they would like to go to day care. They are likely to answer "no" because they do not understand what you are suggesting. Some people continue to say they don't want to go even when they are clearly enjoying themselves. This usually means that they do not understand or do not remember their enjoyment. Continue to cheerfully take the person to day care.

When a family is able to arrange for someone to stay at home with the person who has dementia, the person may fire the sitter or housekeeper, may get angry or suspicious, may insult them, may refuse to let them in, or may accuse them of stealing. People who have dementia may refuse to go to day care or put up such a fuss getting ready that the caregiver gives up.

To the person who has dementia, the new person in the house may seem like an intruder. The person entering day care may feel lost or abandoned. What she says may reflect these *feelings* more than fact.

People who have dementia often surprise everyone by enjoying day care or a home visitor

---

Be prepared for a period of adjustment. People who have dementia adjust to change slowly: it may take weeks for such a person to accept a new program. When you are already exhausted, arguments over respite care may seem overwhelming. You may feel guilty about forcing your loved one to do this so that you can get a break. Make a commitment to yourself to give the program a good trial. Often the person who has

dementia will accept the new plan if you can weather the initial storm.

What you say will make a difference. Refer to the respite plan as an activity the person will like. Present the home care provider as a friend who has come to visit. Find things the person who has dementia likes to do that the two of them can do together: take a walk, groom the dog, play a game of checkers (even if not by the rules), or make brownies. Call day care anything the person will accept, for example, "the club."

Make a commitment to yourself to give the day care program or home care worker a good trial

---

Often people who have a mild impairment prefer to "volunteer" at the day care center. Most day care programs will support this. "Helping" people who are more impaired allows the person to feel successful while reducing the pressure on them to perform or adapt to a new place.

Write the person who has dementia a note—explain why they are there (or why the home care provider is there), when you will return, and that they are to stay there and wait for you. Sign the note and give it to them or to the provider. If this does not work, have your doctor write and sign a "prescription." The provider can read it with the person with dementia each time they become restless.

Some families make a short video on a smartphone, tablet, or computer about the care of the person. This is particularly helpful when the provider will be assisting in personal care such as dressing or eating. You can demonstrate the order in which you do things, like which arm goes into its sleeve first. You might leave written instructions as well.

Day care and home care providers have found that people with dementia adjust better when the family does the following:

- The first visits by the in-home provider or to day care are short enough that the person who has dementia does not get tired from being in an unfamiliar situation.

- The primary caregiver stays with the person who has dementia the first few times an in-home visitor is used. This may help the person begin to feel that they know this visitor. Although many day care programs ask caregivers to stay with the person the first time or two, a few prefer that they not remain. For most people who have dementia, the presence of the caregiver is reassuring. However, a few do better on their own away from the caregiver's tension and uncertainty.

- Someone from the day care program visits the person who has dementia at home before their first visit to the day care center.

Remember, for the person who has dementia, each visit is like starting over. However, most people gradually accept the new routine. More frequent visits to day care or from the home care provider may help the person experience a sense of continuity.

Some caregivers find that the hassle of getting the person ready is so great that day care is not worth it. Perhaps you can arrange for a friend, neighbor, or aide to come in to help with this chore. Allow plenty of time. Feeling rushed will upset the person who has dementia even more.

Occasionally a person in day care will come home and say to their spouse, "My husband (or wife) is at the center." Of course, this is distressing for the caregiving spouse. The person with dementia usually does not mean "husband" or "wife" in such a situation. Perhaps they are trying to say "friend" but cannot find the word. Perhaps "husband" or "wife" is the closest word they can find to mean companion. It does not necessarily imply a romance.

Sometimes the person will say, "She hit me," or "They wouldn't give me anything to eat," or "The fat one took my purse." Ask the program staff about the incident, but keep in mind that people who have dementia can misperceive, misremember, and express themselves inaccurately. Perhaps they can't remember having lunch or misplacing their purse.

You may ask the person, "What did you do today?" and they may reply, "Nothing." "Well, did you have a good time?" "No." Answers like this may indicate that they can't remember what went on. Don't embarrass them by continuing to ask. Ask a staff member what they enjoyed today.

When people who have dementia say that they do not want to go to day care (or have the home care provider visit them), you do not have to take this literally. They may mean that they do not understand what you are suggesting. They may not remember earlier visits at all. Avoid getting into arguments. Reassure them that this is something they can handle and enjoy, that you will come back for them, and that the people there are nice and will help them.

A few people who have dementia cannot adjust to home care or day care. Try several different providers. Some people have a way with those who have dementia. Ask yourself whether your attitude is affecting their adjustment (see below). If you cannot use a respite program now, try again in a few weeks or months. Often changes in the person's condition will make it easier for them to accept the program later.

Your Own Feelings about Getting Respite for Yourself

It is not unusual for a family to be discouraged by their first visit to a day care center.

·

Mr. Wilson said, "I went to see the day care center. The hospital told me this was an excellent center. But I can't put Alice in there. Those people are old and sick. One of them was dragging a shopping bag around and mumbling. One was drooling. Some of them were sleeping in these chairs with a tray across them."

·

The sight of other disabled or elderly people can be distressing. Our perception of the person we live with is colored by our memory of how they used to be. You may feel that such a program does not offer the individual care that you can give at home, or you may feel that no one else can manage the person.

Some families are reluctant to bring caregivers into their home. You may not like strangers in your home, or you may worry about their honesty. You may not want anyone to see your house in a mess. And many people may feel that

"My family and I are private people. We take care of our own. We just aren't the kind of people who use public help."

Like you, American families provide almost all the care of frail elderly people; 75 to 85 percent of all such care comes from family members. Illnesses that cause dementia create particularly devastating burdens for family members.

Seventy-five to 85 percent of all care is provided by family members

Because dementias are diseases of the brain and mind, you are faced with the grief of losing companionship and communication; with the tasks of dressing, feeding, and toileting the person; and with difficult behavior. These diseases last many years, and caregivers usually cannot leave the person who has dementia alone for even a few minutes. Many caregivers are doing little more than surviving—just barely hanging on.

If you become ill, as many caregivers do, others will have to assume responsibility for the person you care for. Good care means caring for yourself too. If you are tired and depressed, you may snap at the person. They will usually sense your distress and may respond (they can't help it) by whining or wandering or arguing even more. Many caregivers wonder whether medications would control these behaviors. As we noted earlier, such medications can have serious side effects and are not particularly effective. They may even make the person more confused. Ask yourself, Am I rushing them? snapping at them? slapping them?

Coming back rested and in better humor after having time for yourself will help you keep the person at home for as long as possible

The best prescriptions we know are to talk with other families and to take some time to be away from the person who has dementia. Arranging a little time for yourself and coming back rested and in better humor can enable you to continue caring.

If the other participants at the day care center seem more impaired than your family member, it is likely that your loved one will feel comfortable in a place where their difficulties will not be noticed and where they can be the helper. If you have checked references, it is likely that the person coming into your home is honest. If you have hired them through an agency, they should be bonded. Home care workers say they rarely notice how messy the house is. Talk with other families: often they too were reluctant but will tell you that the time apart helps the person who has dementia as well as themselves. Caregivers have told us that knowing that a professional provider is also having difficulty with the person makes them feel better about their own efforts to manage.

Even if the respite situation is not perfect—if the home sitter watches videos on their phone, or the participants in day care seem to just sit a lot of the time—you may want to continue with it. Your continued strength and your ability to keep providing care may depend on your getting regular breaks from caregiving.

Some in-home providers urge you to leave the house while they provide care. This is because they think caregivers need the time away. It is tempting to stay and talk with the respite worker or help with the person who has dementia, but you may manage better in the long run if you get away, even if all you do is take a walk, play bridge, or visit with a neighbor. If you stay at home, go into another room, away from the person who has dementia.

Locating Resources

Some towns and cities have a central information source that can tell you what services are offered and how to get them. Even when this is available, their information may not be complete or current. Therefore, you will need to be persistent and may have to contact several individuals or agencies. The process of locating resources can be long and tedious. If you are providing most of the supervision and care of a person who has dementia, you may feel too overwhelmed to do this. It may be difficult to make phone calls in their presence. If you are overwhelmed, ask another family member or a close friend to take on the job of locating outside help. If you are not the person with daily responsibility for care, offer to help the caregiver locate outside services.

Before you begin, think about what kinds of help would be right for you and the person who has dementia:

- Do you need help with financial planning?

- Do you need more information about the disease or about diagnosis?

- Should you try day care or a sitter at home?

- If you use day care, will you need transportation for the person?

- Do you need help for specific tasks, such as giving baths?

- Do you want to get out one night a week? Or do you need to get out during the day when you can drive?

- Do you need someone to talk to?

- What kind of help will the person need? (If they become agitated, wander, or are incontinent, be sure that the provider can manage this.)

- Do they need help walking, or do they need bed care?

Write down your questions before you begin making calls. Keep notes of your conversations. Write down the names of the people you talk to. If you call back later for additional information, this record will be helpful. If the person you speak to does not have the answers to your questions, ask to speak to someone who does. If a person brushes you off, ask to speak to someone else.

Begin by contacting the local chapter of a dementia support agency or the Alzheimer's Association. Their phone number should be listed on their website. Most chapters have paid, professional staff and will be able to tell you about good programs in your area that accept people who have dementia. A concerned person—often someone who also has a family member who has dementia—will listen to your needs and make suggestions. Chapters usually do not make formal evaluations of the quality of programs, but they can often tell you what other families have thought of a service.

Also call the local office on aging. The name of this state and federally funded organization varies from place to place, but you can usually find it online under local government listings or by searching "senior citizens" or "older adults." Some of these agencies have professionals who will help you locate resources. Some have special programs for people who have dementia, including in-home sitters or day care. Some will provide transportation to day care. Some fund limited amounts of day care or in-home care. Most offices on aging are knowledgeable about dementia and have an effective referral system. However, they may know little about the quality of the services they refer people to.

Adult day care staff often know about other services available in your area. It is worth calling them even if you don't want adult day care. If there is a regional Alzheimer disease center or resource center near you, its staff members probably know what resources are available for people who have dementia. Other potential resources include community health centers, geriatric assessment programs, senior centers, social service agencies, family services (such as Catholic Family Services, Lutheran Family Services, and Jewish Family Services), and nursing home ombudsperson programs. They often have information and referral services. Some will be helpful; others will not. The staff of an agency may not know about local services. In a few places, each of these agencies provides outstanding day care or in-home care to people who have dementia, but in other areas they do not serve people who have dementia or their families.

You may not find what you need. Unfortunately, the resources needed by the families of people who have dementia are often not available. Don't blame yourself if you can't find the resources you need. Some agencies have a waiting list or will only take people with certain diseases or disabilities, while other agencies may be too expensive.

Perhaps you will want to accept what resources are available, even if they are not ideal, because you may find that having some help is better than trying to cope alone.

Occasionally families are able to exchange services. Such plans can be simple or elaborate. Basically, two or three families agree to take turns sitting. You may sit with two people in your home for one afternoon a week. Then the next week someone else will sit while you have an afternoon out. This works best when the people who have dementia are not agitated and do not wander. They will enjoy the contact with others. The "rules" of such exchange services should be clearly spelled out.

> Dementia support programs such as the Alzheimer's Association seldom make formal evaluations of the quality of programs, but they can often tell you what other families have thought of a service

An organization of families might want to train one or two people in the management of people who have dementia. Such a person would have a full-time job dividing their time among several families.

The person who helps you may be a family member, a friend, a neighbor, or a member of your place of worship. Alzheimer's Association chapters often provide training for such people so that they will feel more secure in helping care for the person who has dementia while you have some time away. Some families locate a respite care worker by advertising or through word of mouth. Older people who need work but lack formal skills are a good source of help. Also consider college students. Some students are gentle and kind and have had experience with their own grandparents.

Paying for Care

Check to see if the person has long-term care insurance. Some policies cover only nursing home care, while others cover home care, day care, hospice, and residential care.

Fees for day care and in-home care vary, often depending on the sources of government or private funding the program has access to. There is no national resource for assisting middle-class families with the costs of day care or in-home care. Medicare does not pay for long-term care. If a person is hospitalized and needs rehabilitation services, these might be covered as long as the person is improving as a result of the rehabilitation therapy. Medicare rarely pays for home care unless the person is unable to leave the home. Medicaid may pay for day care that it deems "medical day care," but it will not pay for day care that provides only social enrichment. Find an experienced home health agency and discuss whether it will be able to help you get Medicaid coverage for its services.

Medicare regulations change with changes in federal policy and can be confusing to interpret. Ask a social worker or service agency staff to help you find out whether their services to you are reimbursable. It may be worthwhile to request that a decision be reviewed by Medicare. In general, except for a few demonstration projects, Medicare does not pay for respite for caregivers of people who have dementia.

Home nursing and home health aides can also be hired from nursing agencies. If you use an agency, be sure the person is bonded and that you know whether it will replace aides who do not show up. You should ask how much training or experience the aide has had in caring for people who have dementia. Emphasize that you will need someone the person who has dementia can communicate with.

Home health aides and companions that you locate and contract with are usually less expensive than agency staff members, but you can spend considerable time locating them, and some are unpredictable. Some people advertise for help online or in local newspapers, and some home health aides advertise their availability online, in newspapers, or on bulletin boards in local stores. Families suggest that you seek advice from a home aide who is working with someone you know since they may have friends who are looking for work.

If you hire someone, recognize that it is unreasonable to ask a person to both clean the house and watch a person who has dementia. It is challenging for *you* to do both and often impossible for someone unfamiliar with your house and with the person who has dementia. You may have to settle for a sitter and a house that is not very well kept. Discuss fees, hours, and exact responsibilities before you hire the aide. Fees may be surprisingly high, particularly in metropolitan areas.

In some states, Medicaid pays for home care and day care for some people with low incomes, but eligibility is limited, and even this is not available in most areas. Some states have limited funds to pay for in-home or day care through the office on aging. Federal and state governments and some foundations are funding respite care demonstration programs, but these serve only a few people for limited periods of time.

Some programs provide trained volunteers as in-home or day care workers. These programs work well, but there are costs: for supervisory and training personnel, transportation, and insurance. A fee may be charged to cover these costs.

In some states, low-income people with a disability are eligible for a paid personal assistant to help with household chores and personal care. People eligible for Medicaid or Supplemental Security Income (SSI) may automatically qualify for this help, and in some states, families with somewhat higher incomes can obtain these services if they pay a share of the cost. An increasing number of states will pay a family member or a relative to provide this care. People who have dementia often are eligible for help in the home even when they are able to carry out tasks like dressing, because they need supervision to do so.

A few local dementia support programs such as Alzheimer's Association chapters have funds to assist families who need home care or day care. Some programs have sliding fee scales, and some can provide financial aid.

All these resources are extremely limited, however. Most families can expect to pay at least part of the cost of respite care. Many families fear the enormous costs of residential or nursing home care. While they hope never to need such care, they feel they must conserve their resources rather than spend money on respite. However, because Medicaid pays for nursing home care only after the person has exhausted their own resources, the family may decide to spend part of the person's (*not the spouse's*) resources on respite care, keeping detailed records to prove that the money was spent on their care. Keep sufficient funds to pay privately for the first few months of nursing home care (to ensure access to a nursing home). When this money is spent, you can apply for Medicaid funds. Because Medicaid rules change frequently, vary from state to state, and are extraordinarily complex, you must evaluate the person's resources carefully and *consult someone knowledgeable about Medicaid law in your state before taking this step.*

Should Respite Programs Mix People Who Have Different Problems?

You may have heard that respite programs that specialize in the care of people who have dementia are supposed to be better than programs that mix people with different kinds of health problems. Families sometimes worry about what might happen if a frail, elderly person who has Alzheimer disease is in the same program with a younger, stronger person who has had a head injury or similar trauma.

Staff skill is more important than the diagnoses of attendees in determining the quality of a day care program

Programs that serve a group of people whose needs and levels of functioning are similar can more easily provide specialized programming that meets their needs. However, many programs have successfully mixed people who have dementia with people who have head trauma or physical disabilities. In some areas there are programs that serve both frail individuals and people who have dementia. These can be successful because diagnosis does not describe a person's needs and level of function well: the care of an active younger individual with Alzheimer disease may be more like that of a person with a head trauma than like the care of a frail older person with Alzheimer disease. Finally, staff skill is more important than diagnosis in most cases.

It is best to judge a program on how well it provides individual care and how well you think your family member will fit in with the group. A person who has dementia can take great satisfaction from pushing a wheelchair or handing a dish of cookies to a physically impaired person. On the other hand, a program that offers primarily discussion groups, reading, and movies focuses on activities that will leave out most people who have dementia. If you are concerned that your family member will not fit in or is too frail, discuss your concerns with the program director. Some programs are flexible and try to match activities to a person's current abilities. A trial period in the program is often the best idea. People who have dementia often surprise us by how well they adapt to what is offered.

Determining the Quality of Services

Because the person may not be able to tell you about the care they receive, you must know about the quality of care the program provides. *Many of the agencies that refer you will not have reliable information about the quality of the services they refer you to.* This is true even of government agencies, which may never have visited the program. To prevent discrimination, some referral programs are required to recommend all programs equally, without regard to quality. To complicate matters even further, hospital social workers are often under pressure from the hospital to place people quickly.

Many people assume that some government agency is responsible for safeguarding the quality of programs such as adult day care and in-home care. In fact, the federal government has almost no control over such programs. Many states license programs of these kinds or have standards and enforce them, but others have no or minimal standards. Existing standards may not take into account the special limitations of people who have dementia (for example, that they need more supervision or that they cannot respond to fire alarms).

Never assume that because you were given the name of a service by an authority it is a good-quality program, meets industry or state standards, or has been recently inspected.

In most of the programs we have seen, providers work because they love the job, and they give good care. However, there is an occasional bad apple. Checking on the quality of a service is up to you. Always ask if the program is licensed and by what agency and whether it meets existing voluntary or required standards. Ask when it was last inspected and ask to see the findings.

At a minimum, a day care center should be bonded. Workers should be supervised by a professional (usually a nurse or social worker) and should be trained in the safe care of elderly people and in the special care of people who have dementia. Ask the providing agency whether your state certifies this level of worker and whether the day care center staff or the in-home caregiver is certified. Ask questions, check references,

and monitor the care given, particularly in the beginning. In a day care center, ask about meal preparation, supervision of wandering, fire emergency plans, and the kinds of activities provided.

People who have dementia often misunderstand or misinterpret things. As a result, they may report neglect or poor care that did not really happen. Carefully investigate complaints such as "They didn't give me any lunch" or "She is spying on us."

•

When her mother was sick, Mary had a woman stay with her in their home. On one occasion Mary came home earlier than expected and found that the aide had been watching soap operas all afternoon instead of spending time with her mother.

•

It can be difficult to know how well another person is caring for your family member. Caregivers are almost always honest and caring, and it is important that you have some respite time. Do not avoid getting help because you worry about the quality of care. At the same time, be alert to potential problems. If you have real concerns about the quality of care, talk to the local office on aging or ombudsperson about the program. Many will look into complaints and concerns.

Research and Demonstration Programs

The federal government, a few state governments, and some universities have established Alzheimer research centers and Alzheimer disease clinics. Some fund demonstration programs to determine if new approaches to care

are feasible. Some centers carry out research into potential treatments, prevention, or possible cures. Others focus on diagnosis, medical care, and educational services for families. Some centers are closely allied with Alzheimer's Association chapters. Others have no such affiliation or are affiliated with a different dementia support program. Some provide information about respite only to families they serve; others provide information to anyone who requests it. Such centers are a great resource to the families near them. The scope and budget of these centers vary. The Alzheimer's Association can guide you.

CHAPTER 11

You and the Person Who Has Dementia

A chronic illness that causes dementia places a heavy burden on the whole family: it may mean a lot of work and financial sacrifices; it may mean accepting the reality that someone you love will never be the same again; it may mean that responsibilities and relationships within the family will change; it may mean disagreements within the family; it may mean that you feel overwhelmed, discouraged, isolated, angry, or depressed. And, it continues on and on. You and the person who has dementia, as well as the other people close to them, all interact as part of a family system. This system can be severely stressed by an illness that causes dementia. It is helpful to consider the changes that may occur in families facing a chronic illness and to identify the feelings you may experience. Sometimes just knowing that what is happening to you has also happened to others can make life easier. In addition, knowing what is happening can help you identify ways to improve things.

Almost all families care for their elderly and sick members as long as possible. It is simply not true that most Americans abandon their elderly or "dump" them into nursing homes. Studies have shown that grown children usually keep close tabs on or directly provide care for their parents and other elderly relatives even though many older people do not live with their children. Families usually do all they can, often at great personal sacrifice, to care for ill elderly family members before seeking help. Of course, there are families who do not provide care for ill family members. There are some who, because of illness or other problems, are unable to give the care; there are a few who do not wish to. There are some elderly people who have no family to help them. But in the majority of cases, families are struggling to do the best they can for their ill elderly members.

Almost all families care for their elderly and sick members as long as possible

---

Most family members discover a closeness and cooperation as they work together to care for someone who has dementia. Sometimes, however, the pressures of caring for a person create conflicts in families or cause old disagreements to flare up. For example:

Mr. Higgins said, "We can't agree on what to do. I want to keep Mother at home. My sister wants her in a nursing home. We don't even agree on what is wrong with Mother."

Mrs. Tate said, "My brother doesn't call and he refuses even to talk about it. I have to take care of Mother alone."

In addition, the burden of caring for a person who has dementia can be exhausting and distressing for you.

Mrs. Fried said, "I get so depressed. I cry. Then I lie awake at night and worry. I feel so helpless."

Watching someone close to you decline can be a painful experience. This chapter discusses some of the problems that arise in families, and Chapter 12 covers some of the feelings you may experience individually.

We have observed that sometimes the caregiver, family, and friends fail to recognize the severity of the person's impairment. They may let them live alone or continue to drive past the time when doing so is safe. A clear evaluation of the person's impairment from a physician who is familiar with dementia will help you cope with the challenges of caregiving.

Try not to lose sight of the fact that not all of your experiences will be unhappy. Many people feel a sense of pride in learning to cope with difficult situations. Many family members rediscover one another as they work together to care for the person who has dementia. As you help a forgetful person enjoy the world around them, you may experience a renewed delight in sharing little things—playing with a cat or enjoying flowers. You may discover a new faith in yourself, in others, or in God. Most illnesses that cause dementia progress slowly, so you and your family member can look forward to many good years.

Mrs. Morales said, "Although it has been hard, it's been good for me in a lot of ways. It's given me confidence to know that I can manage things my husband always took care of, and in some ways my children and I have grown closer as he has gotten sick."

Because this book is designed to help you with problems, most of what we discuss are unhappy feelings and difficulties. We know that this is a one-sided view that reflects only part of what life is like for you.

The feelings and problems you and your family experience interact and influence one another. However, for simplicity, we discuss them separately.

Changes in Roles

Roles, responsibilities, and expectations within the family change when one person becomes ill. For example:

•

A spouse said, "The worst part is managing the finances. We've been married thirty-five years, and now I have to learn to manage the accounts and pay the bills."

•

A husband said, "I feel like a fool washing ladies' underwear in the laundromat."

•

A son said, "My father has always been the boss. How can I tell him he can't drive?"

•

A daughter said, "Why can't my brother help out and take his turn keeping Mother?"

•

Roles are different from responsibilities, and it is helpful to recognize what roles mean to you and to others in the family. Responsibilities are the jobs each person has in the family. Roles include who you are, how you are seen, and what is expected of you. By *role*, we mean a person's place in their family (for example, head of the household, peacemaker, or "the person everyone turns to"). Roles are established over many years and are not always easy to describe. Tasks often symbolize our roles. In the examples above, family members describe both having to learn new tasks (doing the wash or balancing the checkbook) and changes in roles (money manager, homemaker, head of the household).

Learning a new responsibility, such as managing the finances or washing clothes, can be difficult when you are also faced with the many day-to-day needs of the person who has dementia, yourself, and your family. However, changes in roles are often more difficult to accept or adjust to. Understanding that each person's responsibilities change and that roles and expectations of others change also will help you to understand the personal feelings and problems that may arise in families. It is helpful to remember that you have coped with changes in roles at other times in your life and that this experience will help you adjust to new responsibilities.

> **Changes in roles are often more difficult to adjust to or accept than changes in responsibility. Recognizing this can help you understand the personal feelings and problems that arise in your family.**

There are many relationships in which role changes occur as the person's dementia worsens. Here are four examples.

1. *The relationship between a husband and wife changes when one of them becomes ill.* Some of these changes may be sad and painful; others can be enriching experiences.

John and Mary Douglas had been married forty-one years when Mary developed dementia. She had always been the principal breadwinner: her salary paid the majority of the bills, and she was seen as having more input into big decisions. John was a writer and saw himself as a person who always leaned on his wife. When she developed dementia, John realized that he did not know how much money they had, what insurance they had, or even how to balance a checkbook. Bills were going unpaid, yet when he asked Mary about it, she yelled at him.

For their anniversary John fixed a small turkey and planned a quiet time together when they could forget what was happening. When he lit some candles, she became frightened and began yelling that he was trying to burn down the house. Trying to keep the peace, John blew out the candles and took them into the kitchen. Mary cried that he was abandoning her. John stormed out. Neither of them felt like eating supper that night.

Failing to celebrate the anniversary as they had always done seemed like the last straw for John. He realized that Mary could not contribute actively to celebrations, nor could she manage their finances. He suddenly felt overwhelmed and lost. Throughout their marriage, John had looked to Mary to solve problems. Now he had to learn to do the things she had always done at the same time that he had to face her illness.

Learning new skills and responsibilities involves energy and effort and means more work on top of what you already have to do. You may not want to take on new tasks. Few people who have never done laundry want to learn how, and more than one has had a load of shrunken sweaters and newly pink towels before finding out that one can't wash red sweaters with white towels. A spouse who has never managed the finances may feel unable to manage money and be afraid of making serious errors.

In addition to having to do the job itself, the realization that you must take this job away from your spouse may symbolize all the sad changes that have taken place. For John, the inability to celebrate his and Mary's anniversary as they always had symbolized the loss of his role in their relationship.

Having to learn new skills when you are upset and tired is difficult. If possible, do so when you are rested and not under pressure.

Spouses may gradually realize that they are alone with their problems, having lost the partner with whom they shared things. John could no longer see himself relying on Mary's decisiveness in her role as the decision maker of the family. He suddenly found himself, at age 60, on his own, forced to be independent with no one to help him. No wonder he felt overwhelmed by all the tasks he had always deferred to her. But at the same time, learning new skills gradually gave John a sense of accomplishment. He said, "I really surprised myself that I could handle things I had always avoided. Even though it was upsetting, it was good for me to learn that I could take on these new tasks and do them well."

Sometimes problems seem insurmountable because they involve both changes in roles and the need for you to learn new tasks. Having to learn new skills when you are upset and tired can be difficult. As well as recognizing the distress that may be caused by changing roles, you may need some practical suggestions for getting started with new responsibilities.

If you must take over the housework, often you can do it gradually and learn as you go. But you can save yourself the frustration of burned suppers and ruined laundry by getting some advice. Most people who cook for themselves and work full-time have many tricks for preparing tasty, quick meals. You may find useful recipes online or in cookbooks written for single people.

·

Mrs. Stearns says, "I know my husband can't manage his money anymore, but it seems like it is taking away the last of his manhood to take away the credit and debit cards. I know I have to, but I just can't seem to do it."

·

Having to take this symbol of independence away from someone you love can be difficult. It can be worse when you are not accustomed to managing money.

If you have never managed bank accounts or paid the bills, you may find it hard to learn this new responsibility. Actually, managing household finances is not difficult, even for people who dislike math. Some banks and retirement programs have staff who will advise you, without charge, and there are many websites that can teach you how to budget and keep up with expenses. If the person who has dementia paid bills online, ask a family member or friend to help you learn how. Sometimes, what is hard is not the task itself, but the fact that this means your loved one is no longer able to do it.

The bank or a lawyer can also help you draw up a list of your or the person's assets and debts. Sometimes a person has been private about financial affairs, has told no one about them, and now cannot remember them. Chapter 14 lists some of the potential resources you should look for.

If you don't drive or do not like to drive and must take over the driving responsibilities, look for a driver's education course designed for adults. Inquire through the police or the AARP for driver's education courses and defensive driving programs for older adults. Life will be much easier if you are comfortable behind the wheel.

2. *The relationship between a parent who has dementia and their adult children often changes.* The changes that occur when an adult child must assume responsibility for and care of a parent are sometimes called "role reversal." We think it is better to describe the needed changes as *shifts* in roles and responsibilities, in which the adult son or daughter gradually assumes increasing responsibility for a parent while the roles remain much like they always have been, those of parent and adult child. These changes can be difficult. You, the adult son or daughter, may feel sadness and grief at the losses you see in someone you love and look

up to. You may feel guilty about "taking over."

•

"I can't tell my mother she shouldn't live alone anymore," Mrs. Russo says. "I know I have to, but every time I try to talk to her, she manages to make me feel like a disrespectful child who has been bad."

•

To varying degrees, many of us as adults still feel that our parents are parents and that we are the children, even if we have lived independently and have families of our own. In some families the parents seem to maintain this kind of relationship with their adult children past the time when adult sons and daughters usually come to feel mature in their own right.

Not everyone has had a good relationship with their parents. If a parent has not been able to let their grown children feel grown up, a lot of unhappiness and conflict may develop. Then as the parent develops dementia, they can seem to be demanding and manipulative of you. You may find yourself feeling trapped. You may feel used, angry, and guilty at the same time.

Show by your actions that you still respect the person who has dementia: consult them, talk with them, listen to them

---

What seems demanding to you may feel different to the person who has dementia. They may be feeling that with "just a little help" they can hold on to their independence, perhaps continue to live alone. As they sense their de-

cline, this may seem the only way they can respond to their losses.

Adult children often feel embarrassed by the tasks of physically caring for a parent—for example, giving their mother a bath or changing their father's underwear. Look for ways to help your parent retain their dignity at the same time that you give needed care.

3. *People who have dementia must adjust to their changing roles in the family.* This often means giving up some of their independence, responsibilities, or leadership—changes that can be difficult for anyone. They may become discouraged or depressed as they realize that their abilities are waning. Sometimes they are unable to change or to recognize their decline.

The roles people have held within the family in the past, and the kind of people they are, will influence how family members approach them as the dementia develops. You can help them maintain their position as important members of the family even when they can no longer do the tasks they once did. You can still consult them, talk to them, listen to them (even if what they say seems confused). Let them know by these actions that they are still respected.

4. *As the responsibilities of people who have dementia change, the expectations and roles of family members in relationship to other family members often change.* Your relationships and expectations of members of the family are based on family roles that have been established for years. Changes often lead

to conflicts, misunderstandings, and differing expectations of each other. At the same time, adjusting to changes and facing problems can bring families closer together even if they have not been close for years.

Understanding Family Conflicts

Mrs. Eaton says, "My brother doesn't have anything to do with Mom now—and he was always her favorite. He won't even come to see her. All the burden is on my sister and me. Because my sister's marriage is shaky, I hate to leave Mom with her for long. So I end up taking care of Mom pretty much alone."

•

Mr. Patel says, "My son wants me to put my wife in a nursing home. He doesn't understand that, after thirty years of marriage, I can't do that to her." His son says, "Dad isn't being realistic. He can't manage Mother in that big two-story house. She's going to fall one of these days. And Dad has a heart condition that he refuses to discuss."

•

Mr. Vane says, "My wife's brother says if I kept my wife more active, she would get better. He says I should answer her back when she gets nasty, but I know that only makes things worse. He doesn't live with her. He just stays in his own apartment and criticizes."

•

Mr. Wilson says, "John has an early onset dementia. He and I have been together thirteen years and we got married when they changed the law. I love him more than life itself. I think we can manage ok except for his parents. They disowned him when we first started to live together, but *now they visit all the time. They deny he has dementia and they say that he isn't gay. It upsets him terribly and he screams and sobs."*

•

Division of Responsibility
The responsibility of caring for a person who has dementia often is not evenly shared by the family. Like Mrs. Eaton, you may find that you are carrying most of the responsibility of taking care of the person who has dementia. There are many reasons why it is difficult to divide care evenly. Some members of the family may live far away, may be in poor health, may be financially unable to help, or may have problems with their children or their marriage.

Sometimes families accept stereotypes about who should help without really considering what is best. One such stereotype is that daughters (and daughters-in-law) are "supposed" to take care of the sick. But the daughter or the daughter-in-law may already be heavily burdened and not able to take on this task. Perhaps she has young children or a full-time job. Perhaps she is a single parent.

Long-established roles, responsibilities, and mutual expectations within the family, even when we are unaware of them, can play an important part in determining who has what responsibility for the person with dementia. For example:

"My mother raised me; now I must take care of her."

"She was a good wife, and she would have done the same for me."

"I married him late in life. What responsibility is mine and what responsibility is his children's?"

"He was always hard on me, deserted my mother when I was 10, and he's willed all his money to some organization. How much do I owe him?"

Sometimes expectations are not logical and may not be based on the most practical or fair way to arrange things. Sometimes there have been long-festering disagreements, resentments, or conflicts in the family that are aggravated by the crisis of an illness.

Sometimes family members fail to help as much as they might because it is difficult for them to accept the reality of the person's illness. Sometimes a person just can't bear to face this illness. It is painful, as you know, to watch a loved one decline. Sometimes family members who do not have the burden of daily care stay away because seeing the decline makes them feel sad. However, others in the family may view this as deserting the person who has dementia.

Often one family member assumes most of the care. This person may not tell other members of the family how bad things are. They may not want to burden them, or they may not really want help from others.

Mr. Newman says, "I hesitate to call on my sons. They are willing to help, but they have their own careers and families."

Mrs. King says, "I don't like to call on my daughter. She always tells me what she thinks I am doing wrong."

Often you and other members of the family have strong and differing ideas of how things should be done. Sometimes this happens because not all family members understand what is wrong with the person who has dementia, or why they act as they do, or what can be expected in the future.

Family members who do not share the day-to-day experience of living with a person who has dementia may not know what it is really like and may be critical or unsympathetic. It is hard for people on the outside to realize how draining the daily burden of constant care can be. Often, too, people don't realize how you are feeling unless you tell them.

> **Ultimately, the family must accept that the person who provides most of the care should make the final decisions to use day care, in-home care, or a nursing home**

Occasionally a family member will oppose your efforts to get outside help. If this happens, insist that the family member help take care of the person who has dementia so that you can get some rest. If the family member lives out of town, ask them to attend a support group in their community or to volunteer some time in a program for people who have dementia so that they will better understand what you are facing. Ultimately, the family must accept that the person who provides most of the care should make the final decisions to use day care, in-home care, or a nursing home. Fewer misunderstandings develop when everyone is kept informed about what resources are available and what they will cost.

Your Marriage

When the person who has dementia is your parent or parent-in-law, it is important to consider the effects of their illness on your marriage. Maintaining a good marriage is often challenging, and caring for a person who has dementia can make this much more difficult. It may mean more financial burdens and less time to talk, to go out, and to make love. It may mean being involved with your in-laws, having more things to disagree over, being tired, or shortchanging your children. It can mean having to include a difficult, disagreeable, seemingly demanding person who has dementia in your lives.

> It is important for a caregiving spouse and the person with dementia to find time and energy for each other—to talk, to get away, to enjoy their relationship in the ways they always have

A progressive dementia can be painful to watch. It is understandable that a person may look at their in-law and wonder if their spouse will become like that. Will they have to go through this again?

A son or daughter can easily find themselves torn between the needs of a parent who has dementia, the expectations of brothers and sisters (or the other parent), and the needs and demands of a spouse and children. It's easy to take out frustrations or fatigue on those we love and trust most—our spouse and our children.

The spouse of the person who has dementia may also add to the problems. They may be upset, critical, or ill or may even desert their partner.

Such problems can add to the tension in your marriage and, if at all possible, should be discussed with everyone involved. It is sometimes easier to initiate a solution with your own family members and for your spouse to do so with their own relatives.

A good relationship can survive for a while in the face of stress and trouble, but we believe it is important for spouses to find time and energy for each other—to talk, to get away, and to enjoy their relationship in the ways that they always have.

Coping with Role Changes and Family Conflict

When the family does not agree, or when most of the burden is on one person, it adds to the problems you face. The burden of caring for a chronically ill person is often too much for one individual. It is important to have others to help—to give you "time out" from constant care, to give you encouragement and support, to help with the workload, and to share the financial responsibility.

If you are getting criticism or not enough help from your family, it is usually not a good idea to let your resentment smolder. It may be up to you to take the initiative to change things in your family. When families are in disagreement or when long-established conflicts get in the way, this may be difficult to do.

How do you handle the often complex, painful role changes that are set in motion by a chronic illness that causes dementia? First, recognize these as aspects of family relationships. Just knowing that roles in families are complex and often unrecognized or unacknowledged and that changes in roles can be painful will help you feel less panicked and overwhelmed. Recognize that certain tasks may be symbolic of important roles in the family and that it is the shift in role, rather than the specific issue, that is painful.

Find out all you can about the disease. What family members believe to be true about dementia affects how much help they provide for a person and whether there will be disagreements about caring for them. Family members who live out of town can attend Alzheimer's Association meetings in their community.

Think about the differences between the responsibilities or tasks that a person who has dementia may have to give up and the roles that they may be able to retain. For example, although Mary's illness means she can no longer enjoy candlelit dinners or make many decisions, her *role* as John's loved and respected spouse can remain. They can still celebrate their anniversary but should forego the candles.

Know what the person with dementia is still able to do and what is too difficult for them. Of course, one wants a person to remain as self-reliant and independent as possible, but expectations that exceed the abilities of people who have dementia can make them upset and miserable. (Sometimes such expectations of how well a person can function come from others; sometimes they come from the individual themselves.) If people cannot do tasks independently, try to simplify the job so that they can still do part of it.

Recognize that role changes are not one-time events but ongoing processes. As the illness progresses, you may have to continue to take on new responsibilities. Each time, you will probably reexperience some of the feelings of sadness and of being overwhelmed. This is a part of the grief process that occurs with a chronic disease.

Talk over your situation with other

families. This is one of the advantages of family support groups. You may find it comforting to learn that other families have struggled with similar changes. Laugh at yourself a little. When you have just burned supper or hacked up a turkey, try to see the humor in the situation. Often when families of people who have dementia get together, they share both tears and laughter over such experiences.

Look for ways to help each other. When an adult child has most of the responsibility of daily care for their parent, they may badly need their spouse's help with unfamiliar jobs, whether it is housework, laundry, or minor carpentry. They may need their spouse to sit with the parent while they are out. Spouses will certainly need the love and encouragement of each other. They may also need help from their spouse in dealing with the rest of the family.

You may reach a point where the extent and demands of your job as caregiver are exhausting you. You need to be able to recognize this and to make other arrangements when that time comes. Your responsibilities as decision maker may eventually include making the decision to give up your role as primary caregiver.

A Family Conference

We strongly believe that a family conference is one of the most effective ways to help families cope and plan. Have a family meeting, with help from a counselor or the physician if needed, to talk over problems and to make plans. Together you can make definite decisions about how much help or money each person will contribute.

There are ground rules for a family conference that you might suggest at the beginning: (1) everyone (including children who will be affected by the decision) comes to the meeting, (2) each person has their say, uninterrupted, and (3) everyone listens to what the others have to say (even if they don't agree).

If family members disagree about what is wrong with the person or about how to manage their care, it may be helpful to give them this book and other printed or downloaded materials about the specific disease, or to ask the doctor to talk with them. It is surprising how often accurate information reduces the tensions between family members.

Accurate information can reduce the tensions between family members

---

Here are some questions to ask each other when you get together. What are the problems? Who is doing what now? What needs to be done, and who can do it? How can you help each other? What will these changes mean for each of you? Some of the practical questions that may need to be discussed are the following: Who will be responsible for daily care? Does this mean giving up privacy? not having friends over? not being able to afford a vacation? Does this mean that parents will expect their children to act more grown up because the parents will be busy with the person who has dementia? Who will make the decision to put a parent in a residential or nursing home? Who will be responsible for the person's money?

If the person who has dementia and their well spouse are to move into a son's or a daughter's home, what will the well spouse's roles in the family be? Will they have responsibility for the grandchildren? Will there be two people using the kitchen? An expanded family can be enriching, but it also can create tensions. Anticipating and discussing areas of potential disagreement in advance can make things easier.

It is also important to talk about several other practical areas in which family relationships can get into trouble. It may seem insensitive even to think about matters of money or inheritance when a loved one is sick, but financial concerns are important, and questions about who will get the inheritance are real—if often silent—factors in determining responsibility for a family member. They can be the underlying cause of much bitterness. Money matters need to be brought out in the open. Ask yourself the following questions:

- *Does everyone know what money and inheritance there is*? It is surprising how often one son is thinking, "Dad has that stock he bought twenty years ago, he owns his house, and he has his Social Security. He ought to be quite comfortable." The other son, who is taking care of his father, knows "The house needs a new roof and a new furnace, that old oil company stock is worthless, and he gets barely enough to live on from Social Security. I have to dip into my own pocket to pay for his medicine."

- *Is there a will*? Does someone know or suspect that they have been short-changed in the will? Do some members of the family feel that others are greedy for inherited money, property, or personal possessions? This scenario is not unusual, and it can best be handled when it is openly faced. Hidden resentments often smolder and can emerge as conflicts over the daily care of the person who has dementia.

- *How much does it cost to care for the person who has dementia, and who is paying these bills*? When a family cares for a person at home, there are many "hidden" costs to consider: special foods, medication, security door latches, a sitter, transportation, another bed and dresser on the ground floor, grab bars for the bathroom, perhaps the cost of not working in order to care for the person.

- *Does everyone know what it costs to care for a person who has dementia in a nursing home or an assisted living facility, and does everyone know who is legally responsible for those costs*? (We discuss nursing home costs in Chapter 15.) Sometimes when a daughter says, "Mother must put Dad in a residential or nursing home," she does not realize that doing so may have serious financial consequences.

- *Do some members of the family feel that money has been unequally distributed in the past*? For example:

  •

  "Dad put my brother through college and gave him the down payment on his house. Yet now my brother won't take him, so I get the work—and the cost—of taking care of him."

  •

Families sometimes say, "There is no way you'll get my family together to talk about things like that. My brother won't even discuss it on the phone. And if we did get together, it would just be a big fight." If you feel that your family is like this, you may be discouraged. Although you need your family's help, you may feel trapped because you feel that your family will not help. It is not unusual for families to need the help of an outside professional—a counselor, a religious leader, or a social worker—to help them resolve their problems and help them arrive at equitable arrangements (see page 237).

One of the advantages of seeking the assistance of counselors is that they can listen objectively and help the family keep the discussion focused on the problems it is facing now rather than drifting into old arguments. A nurse, doctor, social worker, or counselor may be able to intervene on your behalf and convince everyone involved of the need for a family conference to discuss issues of concern to them all. Sometimes an attorney specializing in family law can help. If you seek the help of an attorney, select one who is genuinely interested in helping resolve conflict rather than helping you get into litigation against your own family. If your family is having difficulty and you ask a third party to help, the first topic of conversation may be to agree that the third party will not take sides with any one person.

The simple ground rules for a family conference: (1) everyone comes, (2) each person has their say, uninterrupted, and (3) everyone listens to what the others have to say. A counselor can listen objectively and help families keep the discussion focused on the problems they are currently facing rather than on old arguments.

You need your family. Now is an excellent time to put aside old conflicts for the sake of the person who has dementia. Perhaps if your family cannot resolve all its disagreements, you may be able to, through discussion, find one or two things on which you do agree. This will encourage everyone, and the next discussion may be easier.

When You Live Out of Town

"My father takes care of my mother. They live about a thousand miles from us, and it's hard for me to get back home often. I don't think Dad tells me how bad things really are. It's just terribly hard to be so far away: you feel so guilty and helpless."

"I'm just the daughter-in-law, so I can't say much. They haven't gotten a good diagnosis. They keep going to their old family doctor. I worry that there is something else wrong with her. But every time I make a suggestion, they pretend they didn't hear it."

Living far away from both the person who has dementia and the one who provides daily care for them creates special problems. Long-distance family members care just as much as those close to home, and they often feel frustrated and helpless. They worry that they do not know what is really happening, that the caregiver has not obtained the best diagnosis, or that the caregiver should do things differently. They may feel guilty that they cannot be nearby at a time when their family needs them.

In the beginning, it can be more difficult to observe and to accept the severity of a person's limitations if you see them infrequently. People who live out of town often have difficulty recognizing that a problem exists because the subtle problems that occur early in dementia can be masked by the excitement and stimulation of a visit from an out-of-town family member. Later, the shock of seeing how much the person has declined can be heartbreaking.

Your support of the person who provides the daily care is probably the single most important contribution you can make to the family member with dementia. The illnesses that cause dementia usually last for several or many years. You need to build family cooperation for the long haul. If the person who provides daily care rejects your suggestions at first, they may accept them later.

Give the usual caregiver a break. Consider having the person who has dementia spend several weeks with you, or go stay with them while the usual caregiver takes a vacation. Moving a person who has dementia to another home can be upsetting, but, especially early in the illness, it might serve as "vacations" for both the person who has dementia and the caregiver.

If you live a long distance from the person who has dementia, send videos of yourself to keep in touch with them, hire a sitter so their caregiver can go out, send them a weekly card, or call them every day at the same time. Talk for only a minute, just to say "Hello." Don't expect them to be able to carry on a long conversation.

When You Are Not the Primary Caregiver, What Can You Do to Help?

American families do not abandon their elderly members, nor do they abandon each other. Despite differences, families usually resolve their disagreements enough to pull together for the long haul.

There are many things family members can do. One caregiver may need a phone call every day; another may need a sitter so they can go out one night a week; one may need someone who can run over on short notice when things get difficult; another may just need a shoulder to cry on.

Stay in close touch. Maintain open lines of communication with the primary caregiver. This will help you sense when the caregiver needs more help. Caregivers manage better and experience less stress when they feel well supported by their loved ones. It is not solely how much help they receive, but also how well supported they feel that helps them cope better.

Avoid criticizing. Negative criticism usually does not lead to constructive change. None of us like to be criticized. Many of us tend to ignore criticism. If you must say something, be sure your criticism is valid. If you do not live close, are you sure you completely understand the problem?

Caregivers cope better if they have family help and feel well supported

---

Recognize that the primary caregiver must make the final decisions. Although you can offer help and advice, the person who provides care day in and day out should be the one to decide things like whether they can use outside help and whether they can continue to provide care.

Take on the job of finding help. Caregivers are often so overwhelmed that they cannot search for a sitter or a day care program, better medical care, supportive equipment, or help for themselves. Just finding respite can require many phone calls or online searches. Take on this job and be gentle and supportive as you persuade your relative to use respite.

Be informed. You can help most if you understand both the disease and what the caregiver in your family is going through. There are excellent books describing the illnesses that cause dementia, and there are many websites and blogs that focus on caregiving for someone who has dementia. Attend family support group meetings in your community. You may meet other long-distance family members, and you can learn from primary caregivers what *their* long-distance relatives did that helped most. Avoid the temptation to ignore the problem. These diseases are so devastating that the whole family must pull together.

Call the ill person's physician and other health care professionals who have evaluated them. If these professionals are willing, ask direct questions (see Chapter 2). If you have concerns about the diagnosis, the adequacy of the assessment, or the likely course of the disease, ask the professionals who know the person.

Take on tasks the person who has dementia used to do. Cut the grass, take the car to the mechanic, or bring over a home-cooked meal.

Give the caregiver time off. Care for your relative with dementia for a weekend, a week, or a few days so that the primary caregiver can get away. Many local dementia support chapters will teach you the basics of caregiving before you undertake this. Not only will it be valuable for the caregiver to get away, but this will bring you and the person who has dementia closer together. Do things that are therapeutic and fun for the person who has dementia: take walks, go out to dinner, play with the dog together, or go window-shopping.

Arrange for help if you cannot provide it yourself. Arrange for a sitter or adult day care. You can also pay someone to do the grocery shopping, do yard work, or track down resources.

Caregiving and Your Job

Many caregivers are juggling the care of a person who has dementia and a full- or part-time job. The double demands of caregiving and holding down a job can be overwhelming. Some caregivers must take time off from work each time there is a problem. Sometimes, when there is no other choice, caregivers must leave the person who has dementia alone even if this is not absolutely safe. Even caregivers who use an adult day care program or a reliable sitter face extra demands and problems. For example, when the person who has dementia is awake and active at night, the caregiver loses sleep.

If you are thinking about leaving your job to provide full-time care, consider the options carefully. Many caregivers have found that they became more stressed and more depressed after giving up their job. Full-time caregiving may mean that you must put up with the forgetful person's annoying behavior all the time, and it may mean that you will be more isolated and trapped than when you regularly got out of the house and went to work. Leaving your job usually means a significant loss of income. It may mean putting your career on hold and not staying current in your profession. Returning to work after several years of caregiving can be difficult. Will there be a vacancy? Will you have lost seniority or benefits?

If you are thinking about leaving your job to provide full-time care, consider your options carefully

Before you make a decision to leave, discuss your options with your employer. Can you arrange more flexible hours? Work from home? Share the job? Is family leave a possibility? The Family Medical Leave Act mandates leave for people who meet certain criteria. Is a paid or unpaid leave of absence possible? Some loving daughters and sons find that a residential or nursing home is a wiser choice for both themselves and the person who has dementia.

Your Children

Having children at home can raise special problems. They, too, have a relationship with the person who has dementia, and they have complex feelings—which they may not express—about the illness and changing roles in the family. Parents often worry about the effect that being around a person who has dementia will have on children. It is hard to know what to tell a child about a parent's or grandparent's "odd" behavior. Sometimes parents worry that children will learn undesirable behavior from people who have dementia.

Children benefit from an explanation of what is happening to the person who has dementia

---

Children are usually aware of what is going on. They are excellent observers and, even when things are carefully concealed from them, often sense that something is wrong. Fortunately, children are marvelously resilient. Even small children can benefit from an honest explanation of what is happening to the person who has an illness that causes dementia—in language they can understand. This helps them not to be frightened. Reassure children that they cannot "catch" this illness like they can the flu, and that neither they nor their parents are likely to get it. Tell the child directly that nothing they did caused the illness. Sometimes children secretly feel they are to blame for the things that happen in their family.

•

One father put a small pile of dried beans on the table. He took a few beans away from the pile as he gave his young son the following explanation of his grandfather's illness: "Grandpop has a sickness that makes him act like he does. It isn't catching. None of us is going to get like Grandpop. It's like having a broken leg, only little pieces of Grandpop's brain are broken. He won't get any better. This little piece of Grandpop's brain is broken, so he can't remember what you just told him. This little piece is broken, so he forgets how to use his silverware at the table. This little piece is broken, so he gets mad real easy. But this part, which is for loving, Grandpop still has left."

•

It is usually best to actively involve children in what is happening in the family and even to find ways they can help. Small children frequently relate well to people who have dementia and can establish special and loving relationships with them. Try to create an atmosphere in which children can ask you questions and express their feelings openly. Remember that children also feel sadness and grief, but they may be able to enjoy the childlike ways of a person who has dementia without feeling at all sad. The more comfortable you feel in your understanding of this illness, the more easily you will be able to explain it to your child.

Children may need help knowing what to tell playmates who tease them about a "funny" parent or grandparent. It is unlikely that children will mimic the undesirable behaviors of a person who has dementia for long if you don't make a big deal out of it, should it happen, and if the child is getting enough love and attention. Clearly explain (probably several times) to the child that their parent or grandparent has a sickness and cannot help what they do, but that the child can control their own behavior and is expected to do so. Tell the child what to say to their friends.

Small children frequently relate well to people who have dementia and can establish special and loving relationships with them

---

Young people may be frightened by unexplained, strange behavior. Sometimes they worry that something they did or might do will make the person worse. It is important to talk about these concerns and to reassure the young person.

One family with children ranging from ages 10 to 16 shared with us the following thoughts based on their own experience:

- Don't assume that you know what a youngster is thinking.

- Children, even small children, also feel pity, sadness, and sympathy.

- Talk frequently with the children about what is going on.

- The effects of this illness linger long after the person has gone to a nursing home. Get together with the children afterward and continue to discuss things.

- Make an effort to equally involve all the children in the person's care. Children can find it hard to be depended on, or they can feel left out. Sharing in care gives them a sense of responsibility.

- The parent closest to the person who has dementia needs to be aware of the children's feelings and of how their grief and distress may be affecting them. Sometimes, parents can be so overwhelmed by their own troubles that they forget the needs of their children.

Perhaps the biggest problem when there are children at home is that the parent's time and energies are divided between the person who has dementia and the children—with never enough for either. To cope with this double load, you will need every bit of help available—the help of the rest of the family, the resources of the community—and time for you to replenish your own emotional and physical energies. You may find yourself torn between neglecting the children and neglecting a "childish" or demanding person who has dementia.

As the person's condition worsens, so may your dilemma. The declining person may need more and more care, and they may be so disruptive that children cannot feel comfortable at home. You may not have the physical or emotional energy to meet the needs of children or adolescents and the person who has dementia. Children growing up in such a situation may suffer as a result of the person's illness.

You may make the painful decision to place the person who has dementia in long-term care in order to create a better home environment for the children. If you face such a decision, you and your children need to discuss what is to be done. Talk over what the alternatives will mean to each member of the family. "We would have less money for movies, but we wouldn't have Dad shouting all night." "We would move and you have to change schools, but you could bring friends home." Avoid making the children feel that the placement is based only on their needs. Let them know that the decision was made because it was the best thing to do for everyone in the family.

> **You will need every bit of help available—the help of the rest of the family, the resources of the community, and time away for you to replenish your own emotional and physical energies**

The support of your doctor, clergy, or counselor can be helpful at such times. Families often find it easier to make decisions when they know they are not alone.

Teenagers

Adolescents may be embarrassed by "odd" behavior, reluctant to bring friends home, resentful of the demands made on you by the person who has dementia, or hurt by the person's failure to remember them. Adolescents can also be extraordinarily compassionate, supportive, responsible, and altruistic. They often have an unspoiled sense of humanitarianism and kindness that is refreshing and helpful. Certainly they will have mixed feelings. Like you, they may experience the grief that comes from seeing someone they love change drastically at the same time that they may feel resentful or embarrassed. Mixed feelings lead to mixed actions that are often puzzling to other family members. Teenage years can be hard, whether there are problems at home or not. However, many adults, looking back, recognize that sharing in family problems helped them to become mature adults.

Be sure your adolescent understands the nature of the disease and what is happening. Be honest with them about what is going on. Explanations, given gently, help a lot. Children seldom benefit from attempts to shelter them. Involve the adolescent in family discussions, support groups, and conferences with health care professionals so that they, too, understand what is happening.

Arrange for you and your teenager to spend time away from the person who has dementia, when you are not exhausted or cross, to maintain a good relationship with them and to listen to their interests. Remember that they have a life apart from this illness and this situation. Try to find space for them and their friends apart from the person with dementia.

Remember that you may be less patient or more emotional because of all you are dealing with. Again, breaks from caregiving may help you be more patient with your children.

When a grandparent moves into

your home, both the grandparent and the children must be clear about who sets the rules and who disciplines the children. When the grandparent is forgetful, avoid conflicts by letting your children know what is expected of them. The adolescent may say, "Granny says I can't date," or "Granddad says I have to turn off the television." Knowing in advance how you will respond will make it easier for you and your child.

> **When a memory-impaired grandparent moves into your home, make sure your children know who sets the rules and who disciplines them**

When the person who has dementia has adolescent children, these young people are losing a parent at a critical time in their own lives. At the same time, they must cope with the illness and its never-ending problems. They can also feel that they are losing the remaining parent if that person is distracted by grief and fully occupied by caregiving.

In this situation, you face almost insurmountable burdens. You must arrange for enough help to maintain your own mental and physical health and to continue to care for your children. Because adolescents often are more comfortable discussing their problems with an outsider than with a parent, ask a relative, teacher, or coach to assume the role of "special friend." Some Alzheimer's Association chapters offer support groups for young people.

There are books and websites about dementia for children and adolescents. Be sure to read them before you give them to your children.

CHAPTER 12

How Caring for a Person Who Has Dementia Affects You

Family members tell us that they experience many feelings as they care for a person who has dementia. They feel sad, discouraged, and alone. They feel angry, guilty, and hopeless. They feel tired and depressed. They also report feeling hopeful, satisfied, and closer to their loved ones. In the face of the reality of a chronic illness, emotional distress is appropriate and understandable. Sometimes families of people who have dementia find themselves overwhelmed by their feelings.

Human feelings are complex, and they vary from person to person. In this chapter we try to avoid oversimplifying feelings or offering simplistic solutions. Our goal is to remind you that it is not unusual to experience many feelings.

Emotional Reactions

People have different ways of handling their emotions. Some experience each feeling intensely; others do not. Sometimes people think that certain feelings are unacceptable—that they should not have certain feelings or that, if they do, no one could possibly understand them. Sometimes they feel alone with their feelings.

Sometimes people have mixed feelings. One might both love and dislike the same person, or one may want to keep a family member at home and want to put them in a residential or nursing home, all at the same time. Having mixed feelings might not seem logical, but it is common. Often people do not realize that they have mixed feelings.

Sometimes people are afraid of strong emotions, perhaps because such feelings are uncomfortable, perhaps because they are afraid they might do something in haste, or perhaps because they are concerned about how others will view them. These and other responses to our feelings are not unusual. In fact, most of us will have similar responses at one time or another.

We do not believe that there is a "right" way to handle emotions. We think that recognizing how you feel and having some understanding of why you feel the way you do are important, because your feelings affect your judgment. Unrecognized or unacknowledged feelings can influence the decisions a person makes in ways that they do not understand or are aware of. You can acknowledge and recognize your feelings—to yourself and to others—but you have a choice of when, where, and whether to express your feelings and to act on them.

> **Many people don't realize that they have mixed feelings, even though this is very common**

People sometimes worry that not expressing feelings causes "stress-related" diseases. Suppose you know that you are often angry with the behavior of a person who has dementia, but you decide not to yell at them because it only makes their behavior worse. Will you develop migraines, hypertension, or rashes? The idea that it is harmful to keep feelings bottled up is widespread, but there is little evidence to support it. However, the causes of conditions such as headache, high blood pressure, and anxiety are complex. Talk with your own physician about steps you can take—like exercise, relaxation, meditation, and yoga—that will help you. We do believe that as families recognize and acknowledge that the irritating

behaviors of people who have dementia are symptoms of their disease, they feel less frustrated and angry and can care better for them.

> **Recognizing and acknowledging your feelings helps you make better choices about when, where, and whether to express your feelings and whether to act on them**

As you read this section, remember that each person and each family is different. You may not have these feelings. We discuss them to help those family members who do feel angry or discouraged, tired or sad, and so on. Rather than read all this material, you may want to refer to a particular section when you feel it will help you.

Anger

It is understandable that you feel frustrated and angry: angry that this has happened to you, angry that you have to be the caregiver, angry with others who don't seem to be helping out, angry with the person who has dementia for their irritating behavior, angry that you are trapped in this situation.

Some people who have dementia develop behaviors that are extremely irritating and that can seem impossible to live with. You will understandably get angry and may sometimes react by yelling or arguing.

•

Mrs. Palombo felt that it was wrong to become angry with her husband. They had had a good marriage, and she knew that he could not help himself now that he was ill. She says, "We went to dinner at my daughter-in-law's house. I have never felt comfortable with my daughter-in-law, anyway, and I don't think she understands about Joe. As soon as we got in the door, Joe looked around and said, 'Let's go home.' I tried to explain to him that we were staying for dinner, but all he would say is, 'I've never liked it here. Let's go home.'

"We sat down to dinner and everyone was tense. Joe wouldn't talk to anyone and he wouldn't take his hat off. As soon as dinner was over, he wanted to go home. My daughter-in-law went into the kitchen and shut the door and started banging the dishes. My son made me go into the den with him, and all the time Joe was hollering, 'Let's get out of here before she poisons us.'

"My son says I'm letting [his] Dad ruin my life, that there is no reason for Dad to act that way, that it isn't sickness, it's that he's gotten spiteful in his old age. He says I have to do something.

"So we got in the car to go home, and all the way home Joe hollered at me about my driving, which he always does. As soon as we got home, he started asking me what time it was. I said, 'Joe, please be quiet. Go watch television.' And he said, 'Why don't you ever talk to me?' Then I started yelling at him, and I yelled and yelled."

•

Episodes like this can wear out even the most patient person. It seems as if they always start when we are most tired. The things that are most irritating sometimes seem like little things—but little things build up, day after day.

•

Mrs. Jackson says, "I had never gotten along with my mother that well, and since she's come to live with us, it's been terrible.

In the middle of the night she gets up and starts packing.

"I get up and tell her, 'It's the middle of the night, Mother,' and I try to explain to her that she lives here now, but I'm thinking, if I don't get my sleep, I won't be any good at work tomorrow.

"She says she has to go home, and I say she lives here, and every night a fight starts at two o'clock in the morning."

•

Sometimes a person who has dementia can do some things very well and appear unwilling to do other, seemingly identical tasks. Or they will do something when another person asks but not when you do. When you feel that they can do more or are just acting up to "get your goat," it can be infuriating. For example:

•

Mrs. Graham says, "She can load the dishwasher and set the table just fine at my sister's house, but at my house she either refuses to do it or she makes a terrible mess. Now I think it's because I work and she knows I come home tired."

•

Often the person who has most of the responsibility for the care of a person who has dementia feels that other members of the family don't help out enough, are critical, or don't come to visit enough. A lot of anger can build up around these feelings.

You may be irritated with doctors and other professionals at times. Sometimes your anger toward them is justified. At other times you may know that they are doing the best they can, yet you are still angry with them.

People with a religious faith may question how God could allow this to happen to them. They may feel that it is a terrible sin to be angry with God, or they may fear that they have lost their faith. Such feelings may deprive them of the strength and reassurance faith offers at just the time when they need it most. To struggle with such questions is part of the experience of faith.

•

Said a minister, "I wonder how God could do this to me. I haven't been perfect, but I've done the best I could. And I love my wife. But then I think I have no right to question God. For me that is the hardest part. I think I must be a very weak person to question God."

•

Never let a person make you feel guilty for your anger with God. There are many thoughtful and meaningful writings discussing such things as feeling angry with God or questioning how God could allow such a thing as this. Many others have struggled with these questions. Talking honestly with your minister, priest, imam, or rabbi can be comforting.

Remember, it is only human to be angry when faced with the burdens and losses that accompany an illness that causes dementia.

It is only human to feel angry at times when facing the challenges and losses caused by dementia

---

Expressing your anger to the person who has dementia often makes their behavior worse. Their illness may make it impossible for them to respond to your anger in a rational way. You may find that it improves their behavior

when you find other ways to manage both your frustrations and the problems themselves.

The first step in dealing with anger is to know what you can reasonably expect from a person who has dementia and what is happening to the brain to cause the irritating behavior. If you are not sure whether the person can stop acting the way they do, find out from your doctor or other health professional. For example:

•

An occupational therapist discovered that Mrs. Graham's sister had an old dishwasher that her mother had operated before she got sick. Mrs. Graham had a new dishwasher, which her mother could not learn to use because her brain impairment made it impossible for her to learn even simple new skills.

•

It may be possible to change the person's irritating behavior by changing the environment or the daily routine. However, just knowing that unpleasant behavior is the result of the disease and that the person cannot control what they are doing can be reassuring.

It is often helpful to think about the difference between being angry with the person's *behavior* and being angry at the *person themselves*. They are ill and often cannot stop their behavior. Certainly, the behavior can be infuriating, but it is not aimed at you personally. An illness that causes dementia might make it impossible for the person to be deliberately offensive because they have lost the ability to understand the impact of their actions. Mrs. Palombo's husband was not deliberately insulting his family. His behavior was the result of his illness.

It often helps to know that other families and professional caregivers have the same problems.

•

Says Mrs. Kurtz, "I didn't want to put my husband in day care, but I did it. It helped me so much to find out that his constant questions made trained professionals angry too. It wasn't just me."

•

Many families find that discussing their experiences with other families helps them to feel less frustrated and upset. This is one of the major benefits of attending a support group.

It is often helpful to think about the difference between being angry with the person's *behavior* and being angry at the *person*

Sometimes it is helpful to find other outlets for your frustrations: talking to someone, cleaning closets, or chopping wood—whatever ways you have used in the past to cope with your frustrations. Exercising vigorously, taking a long walk, calling a friend, taking a mindfulness break, or taking a few minutes to totally relax may be helpful for you.

Embarrassment

Sometimes the behavioral symptoms of a person who has dementia are embarrassing, and strangers often do not understand what is happening.

•

Said one husband, "Going through the grocery store, she keeps taking things down off the shelves like a toddler, and people stare."

•

Said a daughter, "Every time we try to give Mother a bath, she opens the window and shouts for help. What are we to tell the neighbors?"

•

Such experiences *are* embarrassing, although much of your embarrassment may fade as you share your experiences with other families. In support groups, families often find they can laugh about things like this.

Explaining to your neighbors what is happening usually helps gain their understanding. Your neighbors may well know someone else with one of these diseases. Despite the growing awareness of Alzheimer disease, many misconceptions remain. By telling your neighbors about the illness and the behaviors that it causes, you are helping educate them about the disease.

Much of your embarrassment will fade if you share your experiences with other families

---

Occasionally, some insensitive person will ask a rude question, such as "Why does he act like that?" or "What is wrong with her?" Sometimes a simple response, such as "Why would you ask?" is best.

•

One courageous husband says, "I still take my wife out to dinner. I don't like to cook, and she likes to go out. I ignore other people's glances. This is something we always enjoyed doing together, and we still do."

•

Some families prefer to keep their problems "in the family." This may work best for some people, but friends and neighbors usually know that a problem exists and can be more helpful and supportive if you've told them what the problem is. The illnesses that cause dementia are so overwhelming that it is almost impossible to manage alone. There should be no stigma associated with having dementia.

Being open about what is happening is one way to combat the stigma associated with dementia

---

Helplessness

It is not uncommon for family members to feel helpless, weak, or demoralized in the face of a chronic illness that causes dementia. These feelings are often made worse when you cannot find doctors or other health care professionals who seem to understand such illnesses. We have found that families and people who have dementia have many resources within themselves to help them overcome feelings of helplessness. Although you cannot cure the disease, you are far from helpless. There are many ways to improve life for both the person with dementia and your family. Here are some places to start:

- Things often seem worse when you look at everything at once. Instead, focus on small things that you can change.

- Take one day at a time.

- Be informed about the disease. Read and talk about ways that others manage problems.

- Talk with families who face similar problems. There are online chat rooms and forums where you can read about other families' problems and share your own. Many care facilities, social service agencies, and local Alzheimer's Association chapters have support groups that meet regularly.

- Get involved in exchanging information, supporting research, and reaching out to others.

- Take a break, even for a few hours, from your caregiving responsibilities.

- Discuss your feelings with the doctor, a social worker, a psychologist, or a member of the clergy.

Guilt

It is common for family members to feel guilty—for the way they behaved toward the person with dementia in the past, for being embarrassed by the person's odd behavior, for losing their temper with the person, for wishing they did not have the responsibility of care, for considering placing them in a nursing home, or for many other reasons, some trivial, others important. For example:

"My mother's illness ruined my marriage, and I can't forgive her for it."

"I lost my temper with Dick and slapped him. Yet I know he has dementia and can't help himself."

You may feel guilty about spending time with your friends away from the person with dementia, especially when the person is your spouse and you always did most things together.

You may feel vaguely guilty without knowing why. Sometimes people feel that the person who has dementia *makes* them feel guilty. "Promise me you will never put me in a nursing home" or "You wouldn't treat me that way if you loved me" is something the person who has dementia may say that can make you feel guilty.

You may feel guilty about things you must do that take independence away from the person. Keeping a person from driving or from living alone is a difficult action for a family member to take. Caring for a person who has dementia often makes people feel guilty because it forces them to make decisions for someone who was previously fully able to make decisions for themselves.

You may feel guilty when you know that it is time to put the person in a residential care home or nursing home. Spending your inheritance this way may make you feel even more resentful. Many families experience this same dilemma, but that does not make it any easier.

Guilt is common in family caregivers and has many sources

Sometimes we feel guilty when a person close to us, whom we have always disliked, develops a disease that causes dementia.

•

"I've never liked my mother, and now she has this terrible disease. If only I had been closer to her when I could have been."

•

Families sometimes ask whether something they did or failed to do caused the illness. Sometimes the caregiver feels responsible when the person

with dementia gets worse. You may feel that if only you had taken more time with them or kept them more active, they would not have gotten worse. You may feel that surgery or a hospitalization "caused" this condition.

The trouble with feelings of guilt is that, when they are not recognized for what they are, they can keep you from making clearheaded decisions about the future and doing what is right for the person who has dementia and the rest of the family. When such feelings are recognized, they are not surprising or hard to manage.

The first step is to admit that feelings of guilt *are* a problem. They become a problem when they affect your decisions. If you are being influenced by guilt feelings, you must make a decision. Are you going to go around in a circle with one foot caught in the trap of guilt, or are you going to say, "What's done is done" and go on from there? There is no way to remedy the fact that you never liked your mother or that you yelled at a person who has dementia, for example. However, guilt feelings tend to keep us looking for ways to remedy the past instead of letting us accept it. Make decisions and plans based on what is best now. For example:

•

Mrs. Dempsey had never liked her mother. As soon as she could, she had moved away from home and called her mother only on special occasions. When her mother developed dementia, she brought her mother to live with her. The confused woman disrupted the family, kept everyone up at night, upset the children, and left Mrs. Dempsey exhausted. When the doctor recommended that her mother enter a nursing home, Mrs. Dempsey only became more upset. She could not bring herself to put her mother in a nursing home, even though this clearly would be better for everyone.

•

When the feelings of guilt in a relationship are not acknowledged, they can destructively affect how you act. Perhaps being faced with caring for a person who has a chronic illness is a good time to be honest with yourself about aspects of them that you dislike. You can then choose whether to give the person care and respect without being influenced by not liking them. We have little control over whom we like or love, and some people are not very likable. But we do have control over how we act toward them. When Mrs. Dempsey was able to face the fact that she did not like her mother and that she felt guilty about that, she was able to recognize that she had tried to do what she felt was "right" in spite of her feelings. This realization allowed her to accept that her well-intentioned efforts had failed and that it was best for all concerned to go ahead and arrange for her mother to get good nursing home care.

When the person who has dementia says things like "Promise you won't put me in a nursing home," it is helpful to remember that sometimes the person who has dementia *is unable to* make responsible decisions. When this is the case, you should make the best decisions you can and act on the basis of your responsibility, not on the basis of guilt.

Not all feelings of guilt are over major issues. Sometimes you may feel guilty about little things—being cross with the person who has dementia or snapping at them when you are

tired. Saying "I'm sorry" often clears the air and makes you both feel better. Often the confused person, because of memory impairment, will have forgotten the incident long before you have.

If you worry that you have caused this illness or made it worse, it is helpful to learn all you can about the disease and to talk over the person's illness with their doctor.

In general, Alzheimer disease is a progressive illness. Neither you nor your physician can prevent the progression. It may not be possible to stop or reverse most other causes of dementia, either. Keeping a person active will not stop the progress of such a disease, but it can help the person use their remaining abilities.

A person's condition may first become apparent after an illness or hospitalization, but often, on close examination, the beginning stages of the illness occurred months or years earlier.

If you don't feel right about doing things for yourself and by yourself, remember that it is important for the well-being of the person who has dementia that your life is meaningful and fulfilling outside of caring for them. Rest and the companionship of friends will do much to keep you going.

When feelings of guilt are keeping you from making clearheaded decisions, you may find it helpful to talk the whole thing out with an understanding counselor, clergyperson, close friend, family member, or other families so that you can carry on more easily. Learning that most people do similar things helps to put little nagging feelings of guilt into perspective. If, after doing the best you can, you still feel weighed down by guilt, this may be a symptom of depression. We discuss depression in caregivers and what to do about it later in this chapter.

> When feelings of guilt keep you from making clearheaded decisions, try talking the situation out with an understanding counselor, religious leader, close friend, family member, or other families

Laughter, Love, and Joy

An illness that causes dementia does not suddenly end a person's capacity to experience love or joy or to laugh. And although your life may often seem filled with fatigue, frustration, or grief, your capacity for happier emotions is not gone either. Happiness may seem out of place in the face of trouble, but in fact it crops up unexpectedly. The words of a song written by Sister Miriam Therese Winter of the Medical Mission Sisters reflect this:

> I saw raindrops on my window,
> Joy is like the rain.
> Laughter runs across my pain,
> Slips away and comes again.
> Joy is like the rain.

Laughter might be called a gift to help us keep our sanity in the face of trouble. There is no reason to feel bad about laughing at the mistakes a person who has dementia makes. They may share the laughter, even if they are not sure what is funny.

Fortunately, love is not dependent on intellectual abilities. Focus on the ways you and others still share expressions of affection with the person who has dementia.

Fulfilling one's sense of responsibility can be a source of joy. Studies show that many people report feeling good that they have been able to express their love and commitment by caring for an ill loved one in the face of difficult symptoms.

Feelings of anger, frustration, and fatigue are often intermingled with positive feelings of love and contentment. This should not be surprising since diseases like dementia present many instances of love and pleasure mingled with periods of difficulty and despair.

Grief

As the person's illness progresses and the person changes, you may experience the loss of a companion and a relationship that was important to you. You may grieve for the "way they used to be." You may find yourself feeling sad or discouraged. Sometimes little things make you feel sad or start you crying. You may feel that tearfulness or sadness welling up inside you. Often such feelings come and go, so you alternate between feeling sad and feeling hopeful. Feelings of sadness are often mixed with feelings of depression or fatigue. Such feelings are a normal part of grieving.

We usually think of grief as an emotional experience that follows a death. However, grief is a natural emotional response to loss and so is a normal experience for people who love a person who has a chronic illness.

Grief associated with a death may be overwhelming in the beginning and then gradually lessen. Grief associated with a chronic illness seems to go on and on. Your feelings may shift back and forth between hope that the person will get better and anger and sadness over an irreversible condition. Just when you think you have adjusted, the person may change, and you will go through the grieving experience over again. Whether it is the grief that follows a death or that comes with caring about a person who has dementia, grief is a whole set of feelings associated with losing the qualities of a person who was important to you.

> **Grief is a set of feelings associated with the loss of a person who was important to you. It is a normal emotional response. Caregivers can experience these feelings even when the person who has dementia is still alive.**

Families often say that their own sadness at losing a loved one is made worse because they must watch the suffering of the person as their illness progresses.

Says Mrs. Garcia, "Sometimes I wish he would die so it would be over. It seems as if he is dying a bit at a time, day after day. When something new happens, I think I can't stand it. Then I get used to it, and something else happens. And I keep hoping—for a new doctor, a new treatment, maybe a miracle. It seems like I'm on an emotional treadmill going around and around, and it's slowly wearing me down."

Certain changes that come with a slowly progressive dementia seem especially hard to bear. Particular characteristics of the people we love symbolize for us who that person is: "She was always the one who made decisions" or "He was always such a friendly person." When these things change, it may precipitate feelings of sadness, which are sometimes not understood by people less close to the situation. For example, when a person who has dementia is unable to talk or understand what is being said to them, the family may acutely feel the loss of their companionship.

The husband or wife has lost the spouse they used to have but the relationship persists. This creates a special set of problems, which we discuss below in the section "You as a Spouse Alone."

Another challenge is that the grief that follows a death is understood and accepted by society, while the grief that accompanies a chronically ill spouse is often misunderstood by friends and neighbors, especially when the person who has dementia looks well. Your loss is not as visible as it is with a death. "Be grateful you still have your husband," or "Keep a stiff upper lip," people may say.

> **Grief is eased when it is shared with other people who are close to you or who are also living with a person who has dementia**

There are no easy antidotes for grief. Perhaps you will find, as others have, that it is eased somewhat when it is shared with other people who are also living with the unique tragedy of dementia. You may feel that you should keep feelings of sadness and grief to yourself and not burden others with your troubles. However, sharing these feelings with friends, members of your religious community, support group participants, and other family members can be comforting and can give you the strength you need to continue to care for a declining person.

Depression

Depression is a feeling of sadness and discouragement. It is sometimes difficult to distinguish between depression and grief, or between depression and anger, or between depression and worry. Families of the chronically ill often feel sad, depressed, discouraged, or low, day after day, week after week. Occasionally they feel apathetic or listless. Depressed people may also feel anxious, nervous, or irritable. Sometimes they don't have much appetite and have trouble falling asleep at bedtime. The experience of being depressed is painful—we feel miserable and wish for relief from our sad feelings.

A slowly progressive illness that causes dementia takes its toll on our emotions and provides reasons for feeling low. Sometimes counseling helps reduce the depression you experience, but counseling cannot change the situation that has made you depressed—it can only help you deal with it. Many families find that it helps to share experiences and emotions with other families in support groups. Others find that it helps to get away from the person who has dementia and spend time on hobbies or with people they enjoy. When you are unable to get enough rest, fatigue may make your feelings of discouragement worse. Getting help

so that you can rest may cheer you up. Still, the feelings of discouragement and depression may stick with you, understandably.

For a few people, depression goes beyond—or is different from—the understandable feelings of discouragement or demoralization caused by long-term caregiving. If any of the things listed on pages 235–37 are happening to you or someone else in the family, it is important to find a physician who can help you or refer you to a counselor. Such professionals can help significantly.

Caregivers sometimes use alcohol, tranquilizers, or sleeping pills to keep themselves going. Alcohol or medication may increase your fatigue and depression and can sap what little energy you have left. If you find this happening to you, you are not alone: many other caregivers have done the same, but it is important that you *seek help now* (see Chapter 13).

Isolation and Feeling Alone

Sometimes family members feel they are facing the stresses of caregiving alone. "Despair," one wife said to us. "Write about that feeling of being alone with this." You may feel very much by yourself when the one person with whom you could share things is no longer able to participate in a meaningful conversation.

This is a miserable feeling. We are all individuals, and no one else can truly understand what we are going through. The feeling of being alone is not uncommon when people are facing dementia. Staying involved with others—your family, your friends, other people with relatives who have dementia—can help you feel less alone. Sharing experiences with them will help you to realize that others have similar feelings of aloneness. While you may feel that you can never replace the relationship you had with the person who has dementia, you may gradually find that friends and family are offering love and support.

Worry

Who doesn't worry? We could fill many pages with things we all worry about, but you already know them. These can be serious concerns. Worry is a fact of life for families dealing with dementia. It can combine with depression and fatigue to make each of these worse. Each person has their own way of coping with worries: some people seem to shrug off serious problems while others seem to fret endlessly over trivial things. Most of us fall somewhere in between. Most of us have also discovered that the kind of worrying we do when we lie awake at night does not solve problems, but it does make us tired. Some of this kind of worrying is inevitable, but if you are doing a lot of it, you need to look for other ways to manage your problems.

•

A woman who faces some real and terrible possibilities in her life has tried this approach to worry: "I ask myself what is the worst thing that could happen. We could run out of money and lose our home. But I know people wouldn't let us starve or go homeless. It seems like I don't worry as much once I've faced what the worst could be."

•

Being Hopeful and Being Realistic

As you struggle with the person's illness, you may find yourself chasing down every possible hope for a cure and at other times feeling discouraged and defeated. You may find yourself unable to accept the bad news that doctors have given you. Instead, you may seek second, third, and even more medical opinions at great expense to yourself and the person who has dementia. You may find yourself refusing to believe that anything is wrong. You may even find yourself giggling or acting silly when you really don't have anything to laugh about. Such feelings are normal and are usually a part of our mind's efforts to come to terms with something we don't want to have happen.

Sometimes, of course, ignoring the problem can endanger the person who has dementia (for example, if they are driving or living alone when they cannot do so safely). Seeking many medical opinions can be futile, exhausting, and expensive, but sometimes seeking a second opinion is wise.

This experience of a mixture of hope and discouragement is common to many families. The problem is complicated when professionals give conflicting information about dementia.

Most families find reasonable peace in a compromise between hope and realism. How do you know what to do?

Know that we may be a long way from a major research breakthrough or we may be close. Miracles do happen, and yet not often.

Ask yourself if you are going from doctor to doctor hoping to hear better news. If your reaction is making things more difficult or even risky for the person who has dementia, you need to rethink what you are doing. Are you ignoring their impairments? Are they endangering themselves by driving, cooking, or continuing to live alone?

Put the person who has dementia in the care of a physician or a memory clinic that you trust. Make sure they are knowledgeable about dementia and keep abreast of current research.

Avoid quack "cures." Know that what is in the news may be overstated or lack detail.

Keep yourself informed about the progress of legitimate research. The website of the National Institute on Aging (www.alzheimers.gov) is a good source of information, as is the website of the Alzheimer's Association (www.alz.org).

Mistreating the Person Who Has Dementia

"Sometimes I couldn't stand it. My wife would get to me so, always on me about something, and the same thing over and over. Then I would tie her into her chair and go out for a walk. I felt terrible about it, but I couldn't stand it."

"My mother would scratch at herself in one spot until it bled. The doctor said we had to stop it. I tried everything until one day I guess I snapped: I grabbed her and shook her and I screamed at her. She just looked at me and began to cry."

"I never hit my wife, but I would get so mad at her, it was like I would get spiteful: I would tell her I was going to put her in a nursing home if she didn't behave. It would make her cry. I know she couldn't help what she did and I don't know why I did that."

Caregiving is difficult, and frustration is understandable: caregivers endure overwhelming burdens. Perhaps you have found yourself hitting or slapping or screaming at the person

you care for. Perhaps you have promised yourself it will never happen again, but somehow it does.

> Losing your temper is a warning sign: hitting, shoving, shaking, or tying down a person is evidence that you have lost control. Each of these indicate that you need help with your burden.

In itself, losing your temper is not terrible. But it is a warning that you need help with your burden. Anger is common in caregivers. Yelling at the person who has dementia is also common, but it is a warning sign that your frustration is building. However, hitting, shoving, shaking, or tying down a person is a sign that you have lost control and need help. Even if this has happened only once, it is a danger signal. You may need regular time away from the person. You may need someone you can talk to, someone who can help you talk about your frustrations.

You may need to turn the tasks of full-time care over to someone else, perhaps an assisted living facility or nursing home. If you lose your temper and do things you wish you had not, then you *must* ask for the help you need. To continue in silent isolation *is* mistreating the person.

Call the nearest chapter of a dementia support agency like the Alzheimer's Association. Most of the people who answer telephones or lead support groups have heard many such problems—or have been through them personally. Most will understand and help you find sitters or other outside help (see Chapter 10).

Not everyone has the capability to be a full-time caregiver. If the person who needs care is someone you did not like or who mistreated you, you may have mixed feelings about caregiving. Sometimes the most responsible thing you can do is to recognize that someone else should provide the day-to-day physical care.

Physical Reactions

Fatigue

People who care for a person who has dementia are often tired simply because they are working hard all day and not getting enough rest at night. However, being tired can add to feelings of depression. At the same time, being depressed may make you feel more tired. Always feeling tired is a problem for many people who care for a person who has dementia.

Do what you can in little ways to help yourself be less exhausted. For example:

•

Mrs. Levin says, "He gets up in the night and puts his hat on and sits on the sofa. I used to wear myself out trying to get him back to bed. Now I just let him sit there. If he wants to wear his hat with his pajamas, it's okay. I don't worry about it. I also used to think I had to do my windows twice a year and my kitchen floor every week. Now I don't. I have to spend my energy on other things."

•

It is important to your health that the person who has dementia sleep at night or at least be safe at night if they are awake. (We discuss this problem in more detail in Chapter 7.) If you are regularly up in the night and still caring for the person all day, your body is paying a price in exhaustion, and you will not be able to keep up such a routine indefinitely. We know that you cannot always get enough rest. However, you should recognize your own limits. We make suggestions throughout this book that will help you find ways to avoid complete exhaustion.

> If you are regularly up during the night and still caring for the person all day, your body is paying a price in exhaustion. You will not be able to keep up such a routine indefinitely.

Illness

Illness often follows depression and fatigue. It often seems that people who are discouraged and tired are sick more frequently than others. And people who aren't feeling well are more tired and discouraged. When someone else is dependent on you for care, your illness can become a serious problem. Who takes care of the person when you have the flu? You, probably. You may feel that you have no choice but to keep on dragging yourself around and hope you don't wear yourself out.

Our bodies and minds are not separate entities, and each has a great influence on the other. They both make up a whole person, and that whole person can be made less vulnerable—but not invulnerable—to disease by taking care of both the mind and the body.

Do what you can to reduce fatigue and to get enough rest. Eat a well-balanced diet. Get enough exercise.

Arrange to take a vacation or to have some time away from your duties as caregiver.

Avoid abusing yourself with alcohol, drugs, or overeating. Ask an expert—a good physician—to check you routinely for hidden problems, such as high blood pressure, anemia, and cancer.

Few of us do all that we can to maintain good health even when we have no other serious problems. When you are caring for a chronically ill person, there is often not enough time, energy, or money to go around, and it is yourself that you most often cut short. However, for your sake and, very importantly, for the sake of the person who has dementia, you must do what you can to maintain your health.

Sexuality

It can seem insensitive to think about your own sexuality when there are so many pressing worries—a chronic illness, financial concerns, and so forth. However, people have a lifelong need to be loved and touched, and sexuality is a part of our nature. It deserves to be considered. Sometimes sex becomes a problem in dementia, but sometimes it remains one of the good things a couple still enjoys. This section is for those couples for whom it has become a problem. Do not read this *expecting* a problem to develop.

If Your Spouse Has Dementia

Even today, most people, including many physicians, are uncomfortable talking about sex, especially when it involves older people or people with a disability. This embarrassment, combined with misconceptions about human sexuality, can leave the spouse or partner of a person who has dementia alone in silence. Many articles on sex are no help. The subject often cannot be discussed with one's friends, and if one works up the courage to ask a doctor or nurse, they may quickly change the subject.

At the same time, sexual problems, like many other problems, are often easier to face when they can be acknowledged and talked over with an understanding person.

The spouse of a person with an impairment may find it impossible to enjoy a sexual relationship when so many other aspects of the relationship have drastically changed. For many people their sexual relationship can only be good when the whole relationship is good. You may be unable to make love with a person with whom you can no longer enjoy sharing conversation, for example. It may not seem "right" to enjoy sex with a person who has changed so much.

When you are feeling overwhelmed by the tasks of caring for a person who has dementia, when you are tired and depressed, you may be totally uninterested in sex. Sometimes the person who has dementia is depressed or moody and loses interest in sex. If this happens early, before the correct diagnosis has been made, it can be misinterpreted as trouble in the relationship.

You may not be comfortable making love to a person for whom you must also provide physical care.

Sometimes the sexual behavior of people with brain disorders changes in ways that are hard for their partner to accept or manage. When impaired people cannot remember things for more than a few minutes, they may still be able to make love, and may want to make love, but will almost immediately forget when it is over, leaving their spouse or partner heartbroken and alone. A few such experiences can make you want to end this aspect of life forever.

Sometimes the person you have cared for all day may say, "Who are you? What are you doing in my bed?" Such experiences can be heartbreaking.

Memory loss can sometimes cause a formerly gentle and considerate person to forget the happy preliminaries to sex. This, too, can be discouraging for the partner.

> **Sexual problems are easier to face when they can be acknowledged and talked over with an understanding person**

Occasionally a brain injury or brain disease will cause a person to become preoccupied with sexual thoughts or to become sexually demanding. This is most common in people who have frontotemporal dementia (see Chapter 17). It can be devastating to a spouse when a person who needs so much care in other ways makes frequent demands for sex. While rare, this problem is difficult to treat when it occurs. Medication is very rarely helpful because most that are used only sedate the person. If the problem persists, you should think about placement outside the home. When the sexual behavior of a person who has dementia changes, this likely relates to the brain injury or brain damage and is something the person cannot help. It is not a purposeful affront to your relationship.

Often what people miss most is not the act of sexual intercourse but the touching, holding, and affection. Sometimes, for practical reasons, the well spouse chooses to sleep in a separate room. Sometimes a formerly affectionate person will no longer accept affection when they develop dementia.

•

Mr. Bishop says, "We always used to touch each other in our sleep. Now, if I put an arm across her, she jerks away."

•

What can you do about problems of sexuality? Like many of the other problems we discuss, there are no easy answers.

It is important that you understand from your spouse's physician the nature of the brain damage and how it affects this and all other aspects of behavior. If you seek help with this problem, be sure the counselor is qualified. Because sexuality is such a sensitive issue, some counselors are not comfortable discussing it, or they give inappropriate advice. The counselor should have experience addressing the sexual concerns of disabled people and should clearly understand the nature of dementia. They should be aware of their own feelings about sexual activity in elderly or disabled people. There are excellent counselors who have talked about sexuality with many families and who will not be shocked or surprised at what you say. There are also some insensitive people posing as sex counselors whom you will want to avoid.

If a Parent Who Has Dementia Lives with You

So far, we have discussed the problems of the spouse of a person who has an illness that causes dementia. However, if your ill parent has come to live with you, and you have your own spouse, the sexual aspect of your marriage can be badly disrupted, and this can affect other areas of your relationship. You may be too tired to make love, or you may have stopped going out together in the evening and thus lost the romance that precedes lovemaking. Your parent may wander around the house at night, banging things, knocking on your door, or shouting. The least little noise may rouse the parent you tried so hard to get to sleep. Lovemaking can turn into hurried sex when you are too tired to care, or it can cease altogether.

Relationships are enriched by all their facets: talking together, working together, facing trouble together, making love together. A strong relationship can survive having things put aside for a while, but not for a long time. It is important that you find the time and energy to sustain a good relationship. Make yourself find ways to create the romance and privacy you need at times when neither of you is exhausted.

The Future

It is important that you plan for the future. The future will bring changes for the person who has dementia, and many of these changes will be less painful if you are prepared for them.

Some husbands and wives discuss the future while both of them are well. If you can do this, you will feel more comfortable later, when you have to make decisions for your spouse. Helping the forgetful person talk about the future and how they would like to bestow their possessions can help them feel that this is still their life and that they have some control over their final years. Other people will not want to think about these things and should not be pressured to do so.

Members of the family may also want to discuss what the future will bring, perhaps talking it over a little at a time. Sometimes, thinking about the future is too painful for some members of the family. If this happens, you may have to plan alone.

Here are some of the things you will want to consider:

- What will the person be like as their illness progresses and they become increasingly physically disabled?

- What kind of care will they need?

- How much will you honestly be able to continue to give to this person?

- At what point will your own emotional resources be exhausted?

- What other responsibilities do you have that must be considered?

- Do you have a spouse, children, or a job that also demands your time and energies?

- What effect will this added burden have on your marriage, on growing children, or on your career?

- Where can you turn for help?

- How much help will the rest of the family give you?

- What financial resources are available for this person's care?

- What will be left for you to live on after you have met the expenses of care? It is important to make financial plans for the future, especially if you and the person who has dementia have a limited income. The care of a severely ill person can be expensive (see Chapter 15).

- What legal provisions have been made for the person's care?

- Will the physical environment make it difficult for you to care for a disabled person? (Do you live in a house with stairs that the person will eventually be unable to manage? Do you live in an apartment building that is not accessible? Do you live a long way from stores? Do you live in an area where crime is a problem?)

As time passes, you, the caretaker, may change. In some ways you may not be the same person you were before this illness. You may have given up friends and hobbies because of the illness, or you may have changed your philosophy or your ideas in the process of learning to accept this chronic illness. What will your future be like? What should you do to prepare for it?

You as a Spouse Alone

We know that spouses think about their futures and how they will deal with changes in their relationship. There is no one "right" answer. Each person is unique. What is right for one person is not right for another, and only you can make those decisions. However, as you think through these things, there are several factors you will want to consider.

Your status changes. Sometimes a spouse feels that they are neither part of a couple (because they can no longer do many things together, talk together, or rely on each other in the same ways) nor single.

When the time comes that you are alone, you will need friends and interests of your own

---

Couples sometimes find that friends drift away from them. This is a particularly difficult problem for the well partner. "Couple" friends often drift away simply because the friendship was based on the relationship among four people, which has now changed. Establishing new friendships can be difficult when you can no longer include your spouse and when you have the responsibility for their care. You may not want to make new friends alone.

You may face a future without the person who has dementia. Statistics indicate that these illnesses shorten the life of those who develop them. There is a good chance that your spouse with dementia will die before you do or that they will become so ill that they need nursing home care. It is important that, when the time comes that you are alone, you have friends and interests of your own.

•

A husband told of trying to write an account of what it is like to live with someone who has dementia. He said, "I realized that I was telling the story of my own deterioration. I gave up my job to take care of her, then I had no time for

my hobbies, and gradually we stopped seeing our friends."

•

As the illness progresses and the person needs more and more care, you may find yourself giving up more and more of your own life in order to care for them. Friendships are lost, there is no time for hobbies, and you can find yourself alone with a person who is severely impaired.

What then happens to you after the person has become so ill that they must be placed in a nursing home or after they die? Will you have "deteriorated"— become isolated, without interests, lonely, used up? You need your friends and your hobbies through the long illness to give you support and a change of pace from the job of caregiver. You are going to need them even more after you are left alone.

Even though placing a person in a residential or nursing home means that others will provide the day-to-day care and that you will have more free time, you may find that you feel as burdened and distressed after the person's placement as you did before. Place reasonable limits on the amount of time you spend at the nursing home. Be prepared for an adjustment period and make plans to resume your interests and contacts with friends (see Chapter 15).

The problems of being alone but not single are real. Usually the relationship between spouses changes as the dementia progresses. For many caregivers, the relationship continues to have meaning. For some this means a continuing commitment to a changed relationship. For others it means establishing a new relationship with another person.

•

One husband said, "I will always take care of her, but I've started dating again. She is no longer the person I married."

•

A wife says, "It was a terribly difficult decision. For me, the guilt was the hardest part."

•

Another husband said, "For me, caring for her, keeping my promise, is most important. It is true that she is not the same, but this too is a part of our marriage. I try to see it as a challenge."

•

Sometimes it happens that a person falls in love with someone else while still caring for their ill spouse. If this happens to you, you face difficult decisions about your own beliefs and values. Perhaps the "right" decision is the decision that is "right" for you. Perhaps you will want to talk this over with people close to you. Family members often find that their children and in-laws are very supportive.

Not all marriages have been happy. When a marriage was so unhappy that a spouse was already considering divorce when the person developed dementia, the illness can make the decision more difficult. A good counselor can help you sort out your mixed feelings.

In any event, should you be faced with questions about new relationships, divorce, or remarriage, you are not alone. Many others have also faced—and resolved—these dilemmas.

When the Person You Have Cared for Dies

Caregivers often have mixed feelings when the person they've been taking care of dies. You may feel glad in some ways that the person's suffering and your responsibilities are over, but sad at the same time. There is no "right" way to feel after the death of someone who had dementia. Some people have shed their tears long before and feel mostly relief. Others are overwhelmed by grief.

Talking about your feelings with someone you trust can be helpful. Sometimes, saying things out loud helps clarify your feelings and thoughts. If you find your feelings changing over time, remember that this too is normal.

When much of your time and emotional energy were focused on the person's care, often for many years, you may find yourself at loose ends after their death. You may have lost touch with friends and given up your job or your hobbies. No longer carrying the responsibility you had for so long may bring feelings of both relief and sadness.

One wife said tearfully, "I don't have to tell anyone how they can reach me when I'm away."

CHAPTER 13

Caring for Yourself

The well-being of the person who has dementia depends directly on *your* well-being. It is essential that you find ways to care for yourself so that you will not exhaust your own emotional and physical resources.

When you care for a person who has an illness that causes dementia, you may feel sad, discouraged, frustrated, or trapped. You may be tired or overburdened. While there are many reasons for feeling fatigued, the most common is not getting enough rest. You may put aside your own need for rest, friends, and time alone in order to care for the person who has dementia. If you have multiple responsibilities—family, job, children—your own needs have probably been greatly shortchanged.

Even if you are not caring for the person full-time, you may have little time for yourself. You may be going to an assisted living facility or nursing home after work several days a week or spending the weekend providing care so the full-time caregiver can get some rest. Whatever your direct care responsibilities may be, you probably feel anxious, saddened, and frustrated at times. Throughout this book we offer suggestions for ways to address challenging and annoying behaviors. While addressing the person's behavioral symptoms will help considerably, it is often

not possible to eliminate all behavioral symptoms, and these may get on your nerves. To be able to cope, you will need to get enough rest and will sometimes need to get away from the person who has dementia.

Your mood can affect the person's behavior. When you are rushed, tense, or irritable, they may sense your feelings.

We have emphasized that behavioral symptoms are caused by interactions between the brain damage and the environment. Among the environmental issues is *your* mood. When you are rushed, tense, or irritable, a person with dementia may sense your feelings. They may become more anxious or more irritable, move more slowly, or begin a behavior that annoys you. When you are rested and feel better, the person with dementia may manage better and feel better too.

To be a caregiver, you need to take care of yourself. You need enough rest and time away from the person who has dementia. You need friends to socialize with, to share your problems with, and to laugh with. You may find that you need additional help to cope with your feelings of discouragement or to sort out the disagreements in the family. You may decide that it will help you to join other families to exchange concerns, to make new friends, and to advocate better resources for people who have dementia.

Take Time Out

"If only I could get away from Alzheimer disease," Mrs. Murray said. "If only I could go someplace where I didn't have to think about Alzheimer disease for a little while."

It is absolutely essential—both for you and for the person with an illness that causes dementia—that you have regular times to get away from the twenty-four-hour care of the chronically ill person. You must have some time to rest and to be able to do some things *just for yourself.* This might be sitting down uninterrupted to watch television, or it might be sleeping through the night. It might mean going out once a week or taking a vacation. We cannot overemphasize the importance of this. The continued care of a person who has dementia can be an exhausting and emotionally draining job. It is quite possible to collapse under the load.

> **We cannot overemphasize the importance of taking time to rest and do things just for yourself**

It is important that you have other people to help you, to talk with, and to share your problems. We know that it can be difficult to find ways to care for yourself. You may not have understanding friends, your family may not be willing to help, and it may seem impossible to take time away from the person who has dementia. They may refuse to stay with anyone else, or you may not be able to afford help. Finding ways to meet your own needs often takes effort and ingenuity. However, it is so important that it must be done.

If the resources you need to give yourself time off are difficult to find, perhaps you can piece together a respite plan. For example:

Mr. Cooke could only afford to have his wife go to the day care center twice a week, even with a discounted rate. His son, who lived out of state, agreed to pay for a third day. His neighbor, a longtime friend of his wife's, agreed to come over and help get her dressed on those mornings.

You may also have to compromise and accept a plan that is not as good as you would like. The care others give may not be the same as the care you try to give. The person who has dementia may be upset by the changes. Family members may complain about being asked to help. Paying for care may mean financial sacrifices. But be persistent in your search for help, and be willing to piece things together and to make compromises.

Taking time out, away from the care of the person who has dementia, is one of the single most important things that you can do to make it possible for you to continue to care for them.

•

Mrs. Murray said, "We had planned for a long time to go to France when he retired. When I knew he would never be able to go, I went alone. I left him with my son. I was scared to go alone, so I went with a tour group. He would have wanted me to, and when I came back I was rested—ready to face whatever came next."

•

Give Yourself a Present

Could you use a "lift" once in a while? An occasional self-indulgence is another way to help you cope. Some people may buy themselves "presents"—a magazine or a new dress. Listen to a symphony or the ball game (use headphones), stand outside and watch the sunset, or order your favorite restaurant meal as takeout.

Friends

Friends are often marvelously comforting, supportive, and helpful. The support of good friends will do much to keep you going through the hardest times. Remember that it is important for you to continue to keep up with your friends and social contacts. Try not to feel guilty about maintaining or establishing friendships on your own.

Even the person who can talk quite reasonably and hide any sign of mental deterioration may not be remembering names or really following conversations. Many people who have dementia retain the social aspects of speech long after they have lost the ability to express themselves or accurately understand what others are saying. You will need to explain to friends that forgetfulness is not bad manners but something the person cannot avoid.

It can be painful to tell old friends what is happening, especially those who do not live nearby and have not seen the gradual changes dementia causes. Some families have solved this problem by composing a holiday or end-of-year letter, lovingly and honestly sharing this illness with distant friends.

Avoid Isolation

What can you do if you find yourself becoming isolated? It takes energy and effort to make new friends at a time when you may be feeling tired and discouraged. But this is so important that you must make the necessary effort. Start by finding one small resource for yourself. Little things will give you the guidance and energy to find others. Call your nearest dementia support organization chapter, join a support group for families, or start one yourself. Maintain or renew ties with your place of worship. Your religious leader can offer you comfort and support, and members of your religious community can offer friendship. Many houses of worship have some resources to provide practical help for you.

As you find time for yourself away from the person you are caring for, use that time to do things with other people: pursue a hobby or attend discussion groups. New friends are most easily made when you are involved in activities that you have in common with other people.

> We make new friends most easily when we are involved in interests that we share with other people

You may become friends with other people who are or have been caregivers for someone who has dementia. You may find that widows and widowers understand what you have been going through and that you share a special bond with them.

We know that it is difficult to find the time or energy to do anything beyond the necessary care of the person who has dementia. Some activities can be put on the "back burner" while you are burdened with care, but they must not be completely stopped. This is important. When the time comes that you are no longer responsible for the day-to-day care of this person, you will need friends and activities.

•

"I like to go to the Masonic lodge. I still go once a month. When Alice has to go to a nursing home, I'll probably get more involved—volunteer to run the Christmas drive or something. I still have my friends there."

•

"I play the violin. I can't play with the quartet anymore, but I keep in touch with them and I still practice a little. When I have more time, there will be a place for me in the community symphony."

•

You may also choose to become involved in new activities, such as joining a local Alzheimer disease organization or volunteering for an agency whose work you value. Putting the effort into finding new interests is often difficult but worth it.

•

"My wife got Alzheimer disease just about the time I retired. All I was doing was taking care of her. I thought I should get some exercise, so I joined a senior citizens' exercise group. The days I take my wife to the day care center are the days I work out."

•

Find Additional Help If You Need It

Fatigue, discouragement, anger, grief, despair, guilt, and ambivalence are all normal feelings that may come with caring for a chronically ill person. Such feelings may seem overwhelming and almost constant. The burden you carry can be staggering. Sometimes one's coping skills are overwhelmed and things can drift out of control. You may want to seek professional help if this happens.

Recognize the Warning Signs

Mrs. Scott says, "I worry that I am drinking too much. John and I used to have a cocktail when he got home in the evening. Now, of course, he doesn't drink, but I find I have to have that cocktail and another one or two more later on or at bedtime."

•

Each individual is different, and we all have our own ways of responding to problems. A healthy response for one person may be unhealthy for another. Ask yourself the following questions: Do I feel so sad or depressed that I am not functioning as I should? Am I often lying awake at night worrying? Am I losing weight due to the stress? Do I feel overwhelmed most of the time? Do I feel isolated and alone with my problem? While depression and discouragement are common feelings for families of people who have chronic diseases, if your answer to any of these questions is "yes," you need some help to keep your feelings manageable.

Am I drinking too much? While the amount of alcohol that is too much for one person may not be too much for another, you should ask yourself how your drinking is affecting your life. Is my drinking interfering with how I function with my family or friends, my job, or other aspects of my life? Is my drinking adversely affecting my health? Am I ever drinking too much to care properly for the person? Are others—my coworkers, for example—having to "cover" for me? If the answer to any of these questions is "yes," you are drinking too much. Ask your doctor or nurse if they can recommend someone who can evaluate you. Alcoholics Anonymous (available on the internet) is a good self-help organization. Often the group will help you solve the practical problems like transportation and finding a "sitter" so that you can get to the meetings. Call them, explain your special circumstances, and ask for their assistance.

Am I using pills to get me through each day? Tranquilizers, pain pills, and sleeping pills should be used only under the careful supervision of a physician and only for a short time. Stimulant pills should never be used to give you an energy boost. If you are already using tranquilizers, sleeping pills, pain pills, or stimulants on a regular basis, ask a doctor to help you give them up or refer you to a treatment program. Some of these drugs create a drug dependency. Abrupt withdrawal can be life-threatening, so discontinuing them must be supervised by a doctor.

Suppose you are surviving the stressors of your life by using alcohol, marijuana, pain medications, or other drugs. You have joined the ranks of thousands of other ordinary people. You may have a problem with one or several of these substances for the first time under the stress of caring for someone who has dementia. There is no reason to be ashamed. There *is* a reason to get help *now*.

Am I drinking too much coffee, tea, or caffeinated soda each day? While nowhere nearly as serious as amphetamine or stimulant abuse, excessive caffeine can be hard on your body and can reduce your ability to manage stress.

Am I screaming or crying too much?

Am I often losing my temper with the person who has dementia? Am I hitting them? Do I find myself more angry and frustrated after I talk with my friends or family about these problems? Do I find that I am becoming irritated with more than just one or two people—friends, family, the doctors, my coworkers—in my life?

How much screaming or crying is too much? One person may feel that any crying is too much, while another feels that crying is a good way to "get things out of my system." You probably know already if your emotions are exceeding what is normal for you.

Anger and frustration are normal responses to caring for a person whose behavior is difficult. However, if your anger begins to spill over into many relationships, or if you take your anger out on the person who has dementia, find ways to manage your frustrations so that they do not drive people away from you or make the person's behavior worse.

Am I thinking about suicide?

•

Mr. Cameron said, "There was a time when I considered getting a gun, killing my wife, and then killing myself."

•

The thought of suicide can come when a person is feeling overwhelmed, helpless, and alone. When people feel that they cannot escape an impossible situation or that they have irrevocably lost the things that make life worth living, they may consider suicide. Suicide may seem like the only alternative when people feel that the situation they face is hopeless, when they feel that there is nothing either they or anyone else can do. The present can seem intolerable and hopeless, and the future may appear bleak, dark, empty, and meaningless.

•

One family member who attempted suicide said, "Looking back, I don't know why I felt that way. Things have been hard, but I'm glad I didn't die. My perceptions must have been all mixed up."

•

It is not uncommon for us to *perceive* things to be bleaker than they really are.

If you are feeling hopeless, try to find a friend or professional (a counselor, psychologist, or psychiatrist) whose perception of the situation may be different and with whom you can talk.

Do I feel that I am out of control of my situation or at the end of my rope? Is my body telling me that I am under too much stress? Do I often feel panicky, nervous, or frightened? Would it help just to talk the whole thing over with someone who understands? If the answer to any of these questions is "yes," it may be that you are carrying too heavy a burden without enough help. You should seek professional help as soon as possible. If you are thinking about suicide, call the national suicide hotline at 1-800-273-8255, or go to the nearest emergency room. Beginning in 2022, dialing 988 will connect to a suicide hotline.

Counseling

It may be that all you need is more time away from a seemingly demanding, difficult person or more help in caring for them. But perhaps you see no way to find more help or more time for yourself. Perhaps you see yourself trapped by your situation. We feel that talking these problems over with a trained person is one good way to help you feel less pressured. You and the counselor can sort out the problems you face a bit at a time. Because therapists are not as caught up in the problems as you are, they are able to see workable alternatives you had not thought of. At the same time, you will know that you have a lifeline in this person that you can turn to if you begin to feel desperate. Family or friends can be of help as well, but if they are too close to the situation, they may not be able to see things objectively.

Should you seek counseling? Do you need "help"? People who use counseling are not "sick," "crazy," or "neurotic." Most are healthy individuals who sometimes have trouble coping with real problems. They may feel overwhelmed or discouraged or find that they are thinking in circles. Such a person may find that talking over feelings and problems helps to clarify their options.

> **A good counselor can help people who are trapped by feelings of demoralization or who are thinking in circles**

We believe that most people most of the time do not need counseling. However, we know that counseling is sometimes a great help to families struggling with dementia. Such help may come from discussion groups, an objective friend, a social worker, a nurse, a clergyperson, a psychologist, or a physician.

The first step in seeking outside help is often the hardest. One's reasoning sometimes goes around and around in circles.

"I can't get out of the house because I can't get a sitter. He's terrible to anyone in the house but me. I can't afford counseling because I can't get a job because I can't leave the house, and a counselor couldn't help me with that anyway."

This kind of circular thinking is partly the product of your situation and partly the way you, in your discourage-ment, see the problem. A good counselor can help you objectively separate the problem into more manageable parts. With the help and support of a counselor, most people can begin to make needed changes a little at a time.

Sometimes people feel that it is a sign of weakness or inadequacy to go to a counselor. Given the degree of burden you carry in coping with an illness that causes dementia, you can use all the help you can get. Taking this step is not a reflection of your strength of character.

People sometimes avoid counseling because they think that the therapist will delve into their childhood and "analyze" them. Many therapists begin directly by helping you in a matter-of-fact way to cope with "here and now" concerns. Others help you take control of your emotions and frustrations. Still others can help you learn the skills you need to solve your problems. Find out in advance the approach preferred by the therapist you select. If you decide to seek counseling, the kind of counselor you choose may be influenced by availability, what you can afford, and who is knowledgeable about dementia.

Psychiatrists are physicians, and they are able to prescribe medications. They have a good understanding of physical problems that accompany psychological problems. Advance practice nurses with special training in mental health can prescribe medications and provide counseling. Psychologists, social workers, psychiatric nurses, and some other professionals can have excellent therapeutic or counseling skills. If they do, they may be a good choice for counseling. You will want to select a person who is knowledgeable about dementia, whose services you can afford, and with whom you feel comfortable.

You have a responsibility to discuss with all professionals, including counselors, any concerns you have about your relationship with them. If you are worried about your bill, if you don't like their approach, or if you wonder whether they are telling your family what you have said, you should openly and directly raise your concerns.

There are several ways to find a counselor. Ask the staff or participants in your local dementia support chapter. If you have an established relationship with a religious leader or a physician with whom you feel comfortable, ask if they can counsel you or refer you to someone who they feel is a good counselor. If you have friends who have had counseling, ask them if they liked the person they consulted. If you are a member of a family support group and need more help, ask other group members whether they have consulted someone.

If you cannot find someone through such recommendations, counseling services or referrals are available from the community mental health clinic or from religious-affiliated service agencies like Jewish Family Services, Catholic Charities, or Pastoral Counseling (these agencies usually serve people of all religions). County and state medical and psychological societies can give you the names of local practitioners.

Not all counselors are equally good, nor are they all knowledgeable about dementia. Select a counselor as carefully as you would any other service you seek. Ask about the person's credentials as a therapist. If, after a period of time, you do not think that the counselor is helping you, discuss this and then consider trying a different therapist.

Joining with Other Families: The Alzheimer's Association and Similar Organizations

The Alzheimer's Association was founded by family members. Local chapters are present throughout the United States. Some parts of the country have similar organizations that are not affiliated with the Alzheimer's Association. These organizations promote research and education about dementia and provide support, information, care consultation, and referrals for families. Many local chapters have a telephone helpline, and the Alzheimer's Association has a 24/7 contact center at 1-800-272-3900. They are good places for you to start, whether you are looking for specific information or just an understanding person.

These organizations have excellent websites, and many provide printed and online educational materials. Many local chapters offer support groups that meet during the day and in the evening.

Local chapters often sponsor speakers on a wide range of topics related to dementia. They often can suggest physicians, memory evaluation programs, respite services, attorneys, social workers, and residential and nursing homes that other families have found to be knowledgeable about dementia. There is no charge for calling helplines or attending a support group. Some chapters offer special programs such as assistance to persons with Alzheimer disease who live alone, rural or multicultural outreach, care coordination services, and training programs for families and professionals. The national Alzheimer's Association provides extensive information on its website (www.alz.org) as does the National Institute on Aging's website (www.alzheimers.gov).

> There is no charge for calling the Alzheimer's Association helpline or attending support groups

Telephone helplines put you in contact with people who will listen supportively to your concerns. Many of them have been caregivers themselves and have been trained to work with caregivers. You usually do not need an appointment for a phone conversation, and there is no charge. You can usually reach someone quickly during regular business hours. People manning helplines offer understanding and suggestions on how to find help. They are usually not trained professionals; they cannot offer therapy or prescribe medications.

Some support groups are independent charities. They may be sponsored by nursing homes, hospitals, state offices on aging, or family service agencies.

Support Groups

"I did not really want to go to a group, but my mother was driving me crazy and so finally I went. The speaker talked about power of attorney—until then I didn't realize I had to get one if I want to take care of my mother's property. Then over coffee I was talking to three other women. One of them told how her mother was driving her crazy hiding the silverware in the dresser. She said one day she suddenly realized it didn't matter where they kept the silverware. Up until then I thought I was the only one dealing with things like that. I told them about my mother and these other women understood."

•

"There are usually more women than men in groups, you know. I didn't want to go to a hen party, but there was this other fellow there whose mother-in-law lives with them, and he really understood what I'm going through. Going to that support group saved my marriage."

•

Thousands of family members have had the same experience: people in support groups *understand* each other. Many support groups meet once a month, but schedules vary. They may have a speaker or show a video, followed by coffee and a social period. Meetings may be led by a professional or by family members.

People from all walks of life attend support groups: men and women, adult children, spouses, long-distance caregivers, office workers, manual laborers, retired people. Some support groups provide help for young children of people who have dementia. Some support groups have been established for people with dementia, particularly those in the early stages.

> **People in support groups understand each other because they have been through similar experiences**

The diseases that cause dementia strike people of all groups and all races. No matter what their background, people who attend support groups share similar struggles with grief, exhaustion, behavioral symptoms, and limited available services. Families of all ethnic backgrounds are doing all they can to care for their loved ones—the problems they struggle with are universal.

The Alzheimer's Association or the local Agency on Aging will have the resources to help you start a group. However, you must guide them in setting up a support group that meets the special needs of your community—when and where the group meets, how it is structured, the role of the group leader, and so on.

Excuses

When we are overwhelmed and tired, we find excuses for not joining a support group. We don't have the energy, or we don't feel up to facing a room full of strangers. Here are some answers to those reasons cited by family members for not going to support groups.

I'm not a group type of person. The families we know say, "Go anyway," even if this is the only group you ever attend. These diseases are so terrible and last so long that our usual methods of coping are not sufficient. We all can use suggestions on how to cope. Just hearing that someone else deals with similar problems can renew your energy. No one is "forced" to talk.

I can't leave the person who has dementia. Fatigue can lead to inertia. It is easier just to stay home than to find a sitter or to put up with the objections of the person who has dementia. Ask the organization running the group if it can help you find a sitter, set up a program that the person who has dementia can attend at the same time, or ask a friend or a relative to stay with them for a few hours. If the person who has dementia objects, ask the sitter to visit a few times while you are there. Reread pages 151–52, 176, and 180–83. You may have to just ignore the person's objections.

I can't talk to strangers. The people in support groups have faced similar problems and won't remain strangers long. If you are shy, just listen the first few times.

I can't drive at night. Ask if there are daytime groups. If not, ask the group leader if someone can pick you up. Although problems like these are real concerns, letting them keep you from getting the support you need indicates your depression and fatigue. There are ways around these problems if you are determined. Ask about the availability of an online group or chat room.

Sometimes a particular support group is not right for you. For example, if all the members have their family member at home and yours is in a nursing home, you may feel as if you don't fit in. Many communities have several support groups. Visit another group, or attend an Alzheimer's Association chapter meeting and ask around for a group that has concerns similar to yours.

Support groups aren't for everyone. Some people do not need the extra support these groups give. Others find it more comfortable to talk individually with a knowledgeable person. Before you decide that you don't need to attend a support group, we suggest that you try one a few times.

Advocacy

Alzheimer disease and the related dementias are widely recognized, and research into treatments and prevention is ongoing. However, much remains to be done. Although public funding for research and for care is increasing, it is still limited. There is only enough money to fund about 20 percent of the good research projects that seek funding. Diagnosis and follow-up care are not available everywhere. The federal- and state-funded respite programs are few and far between—most families are still unable to obtain financial assistance for day care or help at home—and in many places the dementia support organization, helpline, and support groups are understaffed, with most of the work being provided by a few hardworking volunteers. Many long-term care facilities and programs fall short of what people who have dementia need. Although federal and state laws mandate that the staff of these organizations have some training, the training is often inadequate and not specifically geared to the daily care needs of people who have dementia. Chapter 15 discusses these issues in more detail.

Families often tell us that participating in advocacy efforts is a way to fight back against this terrible disease. Perhaps you will want to become involved too. Here are some ways you might contribute:

- Participate in research projects (see Chapter 18).

- Answer telephones or assist with office work at a local dementia support program.

- Volunteer your skills. Can you balance the books for a small, volunteer-run day care program? Can you fix the plumbing for a struggling caregiver?

- Lead a support group. Often the best group leaders are those who have been caregivers.

- Locate and reach out to other caregivers who need support. If you have ties to minority groups, you might contact them and let them know that they are not alone.

- Participate in fundraising. Even small amounts of money make big differences. There are many skills needed in fundraising and good books on how to do it.

- Teach your local elected officials or agency leaders about dementia. Write your congressional representative or your newspaper.

- Spearhead a movement to establish a day care or home care program in your area. Many of the respite care programs for people who have dementia have been created by the families who needed them.

- Work for a local political candidate who supports long-term care services.

- Advocate for a particular need in your community, such as help for people who have dementia who are living alone or help for rural families.

Families tell us that participating in advocacy efforts is a way to fight back against this terrible disease. Perhaps you will want to become involved too.

There is much to be done, and you can find a volunteer position or task that fits your talents and available time. Many exciting things are going on in dementia support communities—coordinate your efforts with others, and learn what other communities are trying so that you do not have to reinvent the wheel. Well-informed caregivers are the grass roots that make a difference to those affected by dementia.

CHAPTER 14

Financial and Legal Issues

A detailed discussion of the financial and legal issues that may arise around the care of a person who has dementia is beyond the purpose and scope of this book. However, we have outlined some of the key factors for you to consider. You may need to seek professional financial and legal advice. Some attorneys with elder-law expertise specialize in conserving estates and in managing the affairs of people who have dementia.

Your Financial Assessment

Providing care for the person with a chronic illness can be costly. In addition, an older person may be living on a fixed income, and inflation can be expected to continue to eat into that income. It is important that you assess both available financial resources and potentially increasing costs of care and make plans for the person's financial future. Some people in the early stages of dementia can be involved in planning. If you are a spouse, your own financial future may well be affected by decisions and plans you make now. Many factors must be considered in assessing your financial future, including the nature of the illness and your individual expectations.

If you are in a domestic partnership, consult an attorney as soon as possible. Laws vary on the rights of partners, and there may be local laws and policies that can deny you visiting privileges, decision-making rights, and many other things. Act while the person is still legally competent, if possible.

> Consider getting professional financial and legal advice. Some attorneys with elder-law expertise specialize in conserving estates and in managing the affairs of people who have dementia.

The costs of residential or nursing home care are discussed in Chapter 15. If there is any chance that your family member will need nursing home care, you must read that section and plan ahead. Planning can save you money and anguish. Whether you have little income or are affluent, *it is most important that you plan ahead for the person's financial future.*

Potential Expenses

Lost income

- Will the person who has dementia have to give up their job?

- Will someone who would otherwise be employed have to stay at home to care for them?

- Will the person who has dementia lose retirement or disability benefits?

- Will the purchasing power of a fixed income decline as inflation rises?

Housing costs

- Will you or you and the person who has dementia have to move to a home that is without stairs, closer to services, or easier to maintain? Will you move a parent into your home? This may involve the expenses of renovating a room for them.

- Will the person who has dementia enter a life care facility, foster care home, assisted living facility, or skilled nursing facility?

- Will you have to make modifications to your home (new locks, grab rails, safety devices, a wheelchair ramp)?

Medical costs

- Will you need
  - visiting nurses?
  - doctors?
  - medical insurance?

- evaluations?
- occupational therapists?
- physical therapists?
- medications?
- medical equipment and appliances (a hospital bed, a special chair, a wheelchair)?
- disposable care supplies (adult diapers, moisture-proof pads, egg-crate pads, petroleum jelly, tissues, cotton swabs, and so on)?

Costs of help or respite care

- Will you need
  - someone to clean?
  - someone to stay with the person?
  - someone to help with care?
  - day care?

Food costs

- Will there be costs of having meals prepared or eating out or ordering in?

Transportation costs

- Will you need someone to drive if you cannot?

- Will there be costs for taxis, rideshares, or a driver?

Taxes

Legal fees

Miscellaneous costs

- Will there be costs for easy-to-use clothing, ID bracelets, home modifications that manage wandering, or various devices for safety or convenience?

Nursing home costs

- In addition to basic costs, you may be charged for adult diapers, laundry, medications, disposable supplies, therapies, and hair care.

Residential care home costs

- Unless the person receives Medicaid, there is no state or federal program to pay the costs of residential care or board and care in most cases. The person may have to sell their home or use up other assets to pay for such care, or the burden may fall on their children, although no laws require children to pay for a parent's care.

Potential Resources

Resources of the Person Who Has Dementia

Determine the assets and financial resources of the person who has dementia. Identify pensions, 401(k) accounts, Social Security income, savings, mutual funds, stocks, real estate, automobiles, long-term care insurance, and other potential sources of income or capital.

Some people become secretive about their finances. At the end of this chapter, we list some of the potential available resources a person may have and where to look for the relevant documents.

Resources of the Person's Spouse, Children, and Other Relatives

Laws regarding the financial rights and responsibilities of family members, particularly when they apply to nursing home care, are complex. Not all social workers, tax accountants, or lawyers understand them. The local chapter of a dementia support program will be able to refer you to professionals with expertise in this area. In addition, family members have feelings of obligation to each other. With obligation comes dilemmas:

> "Dad put me through college. Now it's my turn."

> "I want to help my mother, but I also have a son to put through college. What do I do?"

> "I know Mom would be better off if I could get dentures for her, but my husband's job depends on his truck, and right now the engine has to be rebuilt. I don't know what to do."

These are difficult questions, and families often disagree over how money should be spent. With few public programs to help families, diseases that cause dementia can be financially devastating, particularly for the well spouse.

Life Insurance

Find out what life insurance policies the person has and whether these can be a resource if funds are needed now. Some insurance policies waive the premiums if the insured becomes disabled. This can be a significant savings.

Long-Term Care Insurance

If the person who has dementia has long-term care insurance, it may help pay for home care, adult day care, hospice, and residential care. Policies vary, and each state regulates them differently. These policies can be a helpful resource for many people but not for everyone. People pay into the policy for a number of years (defined by the policy) until they need care. If the person needs home care, you locate and pay an agency that supplies caregivers, and the insurance plan reimburses you for the caregiving expenses. This gives you the freedom to select and train a person with the skills and temperament to work with a person who has dementia.

> **Get legal advice from someone who is knowledgeable before taking any steps to protect your financial assets**

The insurance company makes its profit by taking in more in payments than it pays out in reimbursements. Thus, they have motivation to limit payment for services. You should monitor whether they are appropriately reimbursing you each month for the amount of service you need.

With few exceptions, relatives other than a spouse are not legally responsible for the support of a person who has dementia, but adult children and other relatives often contribute to the cost of care. The legal responsibility of the spouse is defined in two separate bodies of law: the laws governing Medicaid (see Chapter 15, especially pages 271–72) and the family responsibility laws of each state. Both federal and state laws shape Medicaid. Family responsibility law is completely under state control; thus, the law is different in different states. You will need legal advice before taking any steps to protect your financial assets.

Medicare

Medicare is a federal program that provides health insurance for people age 65 and over and for some disabled people. Medicare is explained in the booklet *Medicare & You*, which is mailed to all Medicare recipients every year and can be found on the program's website (www.medicare.gov). In this book we will cover only some of the issues with Medicare that families have told us have caused them problems.

Medicare does not pay for nursing home care except for short periods following an acute illness, usually after a hospitalization.

Medicare Part A covers inpatient hospital care, acute rehabilitative care, some inpatient care in a skilled nursing home, hospice care, and some home health care. Staying overnight or even several nights in a hospital—even if a person is in a bed, in a room, getting tests, or being administered treatments—doesn't always mean they are inpatients. You should always ask if a person is an inpatient or outpatient during their stay since that affects what is owed for the hospital stay and whether a person will qualify for Part A coverage in a skilled nursing facility.

> **Medicare does not pay for nursing home care except for short periods, usually following an acute illness or a hospitalization**

Discharge from a hospital can seem abrupt. People may still be receiving IVs and getting treatments when you are told that they are being discharged. You may have only a few hours to plan. Start planning as soon as the person gets admitted. Will you need help getting them home? What help awaits you there? Will someone be able to go to the pharmacy to fill new prescriptions for you? Medicare may pay for up to two weeks of home help if the person needs dressing changes (bandages) and medication management. You may have to press for this. If the person has a broken hip or pelvis, insist that the hospital determine whether they are eligible for transfer to a rehabilitation center.

> **Start planning for discharge as soon as a person gets admitted to the hospital**

Medicare Part B covers doctor visits, outpatient services, home health services, durable medical equipment, and other medical services such as tests used to diagnose a problem.

Part C is the Medicare Advantage plans such as HMOs (health maintenance organizations) and PPOs (preferred provider organizations).

Medicare may deny a claim for home health care because they argue that the person is not confined to the home. They may deny physical therapy, occupational therapy, speech therapy, or mental health treatment because they argue that a person who has dementia cannot benefit from it, even though you, the therapist, and the doctor can see that it is beneficial. These decisions can be appealed.

Medicare Part D provides prescription drug coverage. If you are choosing a Plan D for a person who has dementia, ask yourself the following:

- Does the plan cover the Alzheimer drugs the person takes? in the doses that are prescribed?

- Check the formulary (the list of prescription drugs your plan covers). Does it limit coverage of the person's Alzheimer drugs or their more costly drugs by requiring prior authorization or that a person try a similar but less expensive drug?

- What will the plan cost? premiums? deductibles? cost sharing?

- Is the plan available at the pharmacy you prefer?

- Is mail order an option?

If people are on medications and are stable but the insurance plan now denies coverage of those medications, their representative or physician can request an "exemption" to cover a nonformulary prescription (see www.alz.org).

Nationwide, Medicare has a number of low-cost programs. For example, Extra Help is a Medicare program to help people with limited income and resources pay for Medicare prescription drug costs. PACE is a Medicare and Medicaid program offered in many states that allows people who otherwise need nursing home level care to remain in the community.

The Medicare/hospital/nursing home system does not well serve people who have a combination of dementia and another serious illness such as diabetes, congestive heart failure, cancer, pneumonia, and so forth that got them into the hospital. Hospitals are under pressure from Medicare to discharge people as soon as they no longer need the intensive care provided by a hospital. You may be given no time to select—or even check out—a nursing home if the person is to be discharged to a facility from the hospital. The hospital social worker will assign the person to the next available nursing home bed. You may be given a chance to visit it. Medicare law requires that nursing homes be equipped to meet the level of care the person needs. The law requires that the facility have a registered nurse on duty, but the nurse may be caring for too many patients or be responsible for multiple floors of the facility.

> **Medicare law requires nursing homes to be equipped to meet the level of care their clients need**

You should keep records of your expenses for tax purposes. If you ever need to place the person in a nursing home and they eventually need Medicaid, this documentation of money paid for care from their assets and income counts toward their eligibility for Medicaid.

Expenses for which you should keep documentation include modifications to the home, adaptive gadgets, medications, and insurance fees. If you use your home computer or tablet to keep these records, you will already be halfway there, but you still need hard copies of bills and receipts. If you don't use a computer program for this kind of record keeping, buy a notebook with "pockets" and keep it handy. Records of thousands of dollars worth of small expenditures can disappear easily if you are not diligent. Allowable deductions

for medical expenses change over time, but you don't want to regret that you didn't keep records of your expenses.

•

Mrs. Worth said that keeping records of minor expenses was impossible. "I just pick up a few things—a couple of boxes of diapers and wipes—when I get his prescriptions and then, when I get home, Joe is yelling and I have to put the food in the freezer. I can't just run to the computer."

•

She solved the problem by putting a shoebox on the counter and, as she emptied her bags, tossing the receipts into it. A friend came over once a week, and they sorted through the box for tax-deductible items.

Medicaid

Medicaid is a federal- and state-funded health care program for people with low income and few assets. Depending on the state, it covers visits to doctors, hospital care, outpatient care, home health care, medications, and nursing home care. In some states, it may also cover other services, such as medical day care. Look into the person's eligibility for Medicaid if they have little or no income, receive Supplemental Security Income (SSI), or have no savings or assets other than their home and car (see Chapter 15). Some people qualify for both Medicare and Medicaid and are referred to as "dual-eligible." Medicaid eligibility is determined by individual states and continues to change. Check with the Medicaid office in your state or see their website for current eligibility rules. If the person has some assets, they will be required to spend them before becoming eligible for Medicaid.

Tax Breaks for Elderly Persons or for the Care of Persons Who Have Dementia

Elderly and disabled persons are eligible for various tax breaks. General information about these can be found in the IRS publications for older Americans, such as the *Tax Guide for Seniors*.

Tax deductions for the care of a person who has dementia can make a significant difference to families. You are entitled to medical deductions for someone who is your dependent. Whom you may claim as your dependent for medical deductions and tax credits may differ from whom you can claim as a dependent in other circumstances.

> **If you work and must hire someone to care for your disabled dependent, you may be entitled to a tax credit for part of the cost of their care**

Some nursing home costs that are not covered by Medicare or Medicaid may be deductible. The definitions of what part of nursing home care can be deducted and when it can be deducted are complex, and you may want to review carefully the IRS and tax court definitions of whom you can claim as your dependent and what deductions you can take.

Tax laws are being examined by family organizations and some legislators who are urging tax relief for families who care for a disabled elderly person. You may want to look into the most recent federal and state legislation concerning your individual situation. If you are uncertain about your rights, a tax consultant may be helpful to you. You do not have to accept as final the information given to you by the IRS staff.

State, Federal, and Private Resources

State, federal, and private funds support a range of resources, such as day care centers, Meals on Wheels, food stamps, sheltered housing, mental health clinics, social work services, recreation centers, and outpatient memory centers. The funding source usually defines the population to be served in specific terms (such as only people 65 and over or only people with income under a certain amount).

Pilot programs are programs funded for a brief period to determine their effectiveness. The person in your care may qualify to take part in such a program. Find out about pilot programs in your area. The local Agency on Aging should know whether there are programs in your area.

Research programs are programs in which participants are studied in specific ways. Such programs sometimes offer excellent free or low-cost services. They usually have specific criteria for eligibility. Most research programs must meet exacting standards to assure that the research does not harm the subjects. You will be asked to sign a consent form that explains exactly what research is being done; what risks, if any, are involved; and what benefits are possible. You must be given the option of withdrawing from the study at any time.

Where to Look for the Forgetful Person's Resources

Sometimes, people who have dementia forget what financial resources they have or what debts they owe. They may have shared financial information with a confidant before the illness but then made changes or hid assets in the early stages of the disease. People may be private about their finances or disorganized in recording them. Sometimes suspiciousness is a part of the illness, and the individual has hidden money and other financial assets. Family members may not know what resources the person has that could be used to provide for their care.

Finding out what resources a person has can be difficult, especially when documents are in disarray or are hidden.

Debts usually turn up on their own, often in the mail. Some businesses will be understanding if a debt or a bill is not paid on time. When you do find a bill, call the company, explain the circumstances, and arrange how and when the bill will be paid. Request that future bills be sent to you.

Assets may be harder to find. Review recent mail. Look in the obvious places, such as on a desktop and in desk drawers, an office, and other places where papers are kept. Look under the bed, in shoeboxes, in pockets of clothes, in old purses, in teakettles or other kitchen items, under rugs, and in jewelry boxes. One wife asked the grandchildren to join her in a "treasure hunt." The children thought of obscure places to look. Look for bank statements, canceled checks, bankbooks, savings books, passbooks, or checkbooks; keys; address books; insurance policies; receipts; business or legal correspondence; and income tax records for the past four to five years. If the person has a computer, ask them where they keep passwords and look for financial programs, emails from financial organizations, and online purchases. (A spouse filing a joint return or a person possessing a power of attorney for finances or guardianship of property can obtain copies from the IRS. The power of attorney must meet IRS standards or be completed on the IRS form.) These various clues can be used to piece together a person's resources.

There are many kinds of assets.

Bank accounts. Look for bankbooks, bank statements, checkbooks, savings books, passbooks, statements of interest paid, and joint accounts held with others. If you have access to a person's online accounts, you can obtain needed information directly. Most banks will not release information about accounts, loans, or investments to anyone whose name is not on the account. However, they may give limited information (such as whether there is an account in an individual's name) if you send a letter to the bank from your doctor or lawyer explaining the nature of the person's disability and the reason you need the information. Banks will release information about the amount in an account or about current transactions only to a court-appointed guardian or other properly authorized person. However, often you can piece together what you need to know from papers and notes you can find.

Stock certificates, bonds, certificates of deposit, savings bonds, and mutual funds. Look for the actual bonds, monthly statements from stockbrokers or mutual fund companies, the kind of bonds that one clips coupons from, notices of payments due, notices of dividends paid, earnings claimed on income tax, regular amounts paid out from a bank account, and receipts. Mutual funds are accounts held in the name of the person; look for canceled checks, correspondence, or receipts from a broker. Look for records of purchase or sale.

Insurance policies (life insurance, disability insurance, and health insurance). These are among the most frequently overlooked assets. Life insurance policies and health insurance policies may pay a lump sum or other benefits. Look for premium notices, policies, or canceled checks that give you the name of the insurer. Contact the company for full information about the policy. Some insurers will release this information upon receipt of a letter from a physician or attorney; others will need proof of your legal right to information. Look for receipts or bills for long-term care and also for deductions listed on the person's income tax returns.

Safe deposit boxes. Look for a key, a bill, or a receipt. You will need a court order to be permitted to open a safe deposit box.

Military benefits. Look for discharge papers, dog tags, and old uniforms. Contact the military branch to determine what benefits are available to the person. Parkinson disease and amyotrophic lateral sclerosis (ALS) are now considered service-connected disabilities for veterans who served in the Vietnam Era. Dependents of veterans may be eligible for benefits.

Real estate property (houses, land, businesses, and rental property, including joint ownership or partial ownership of such property). Look for regular payments into or from a checking account, gains or losses declared on income tax returns, keys, and fire insurance premiums (on houses, barns, businesses, or trailers). The insurance agent may be able to help you. Look for property tax assessments. Ownership of real estate property is a matter of public record; the tax assessor's office may be able to help you locate properties if you have some clues.

The tax assessor's office or the county clerk's office can tell you whether there are liens against property or whether a foreclosure is pending on a house.

Retirement or disability benefits. These are also often overlooked. An application is required for Social Security Disability Income (SSDI), Supplemental Security Income (SSI), veterans' benefits, or railroad retirement if the person is eligible. Spouses and divorced spouses may also be eligible for benefits. Federal and state government employees, union members, the clergy, and military personnel may have special benefits. Check into possible retirement or disability benefits from *all* past employers. Look for an old résumé, which will list previous jobs. Look for benefit letters.

Collections, gold, jewelry, cash, loose gems, cars, antiques, art, boats, camera equipment, furniture, and other negotiable property. In addition to looking for such items, look for valuable items listed on property insurance policies. Some of these items are small enough to be easily hidden. Others may be in plain sight and so familiar as to be overlooked.

The tax assessor's office or the county clerk's office may list a luxury tax on boats or luxury cars. This is useful if you are trying to find out whether the person owns such items.

Wills. If the individual has made a will or established a trust, it should list their assets. Wills, if not hidden, are often kept in a safe deposit box, recorded by the court, or kept by a person's attorney.

Trust accounts. Look for statements of interest paid.

Personal loans. Look for withdrawals, payments, correspondence, and alimony payments (occasionally divorce settlements provide for payment of alimony if the spouse should become disabled).

Foreign bank accounts. Look for statements of interest paid and bank statements.

Inheritance. Find out whether the person who has dementia is someone's heir.

Cemetery plot. Look for evidence of purchase.

If the person belonged to a benevolent organization like the Masons, the organization may help you find resources. The person may also have insurance through such an organization.

Legal Matters

The time may come when a person who has dementia cannot continue to take legal or financial responsibility for themselves. This may mean that they can no longer manage their finances or that they have forgotten what financial assets or debts they have. It may mean that they are unable to decide responsibly what to do with property or to give permission for needed medical care.

Usually these abilities are lost gradually, rather than all at once. A person who is unable to manage their money may still be able to make a will or accept medical care. However, as their impairment increases, they will likely reach the point where they cannot make any significant decisions for themselves. At that point, someone else will have to assume legal responsibility for them.

People must make legal arrangements early, *before they become unable to make their own decisions*. All adults are *competent*, that is, have the ability to make decisions for themselves, unless a judge finds that they are not. Competency to write a will, called *testamentary capacity*, means that the person knows, at that time and without prompting, the purpose of a will, how people usually distribute their assets, the nature and extent of their property (sometimes referred to, legally, as "bounty"), and that they have the ability to state how they want their assets distributed. An attorney may be able to assess a person's competency, but if there is any doubt the attorney should ask that a professional with expertise in capacity assessment be involved.

> We should all make legal arrangements when we're healthy, before we become unable to make our own decisions

The most efficient way to prepare for an eventual disability (which could happen to any of us) is for all of us to make plans *before* we reach the time when we cannot do so. Such plans usually include making a will and executing a durable power of attorney (see below).

Families sometimes find it difficult to face these issues when the person still seems quite able. Sometimes a person who has dementia resists these steps. Unfortunately, waiting until the person cannot participate in decision-making may cost thousands of dollars later or may result in decisions that no one would have wanted.

We believe that people who have dementia should discuss the plans they want to make with a lawyer. A lawyer with estate planning expertise can advise people about how best to protect their wishes if they lose the capacity to make decisions. However, the relevant laws (particularly those governing the financial responsibility of families) are very complex. Lawyers who have not specialized in this area may not have the best information. Ask your local dementia support program or an elder-law center for a referral.

Lawyers specialize in different areas of law (criminal law, corporate law, divorce law, civil law). You have a right to know what you can expect from a lawyer and what their fees are. Misunderstandings can be avoided by discussing what they charge and what services you will get for that fee. Find out if they practice this sort of law and are knowledgeable about it.

In addition to making a will, a person who is still able to manage their own affairs (by the above definition) may sign a *power of attorney*, which gives a spouse, a child, or some other person who has reached legal age authority to manage their property. A power of attorney can give broad authority to the specified person, or it can be limited. A limited power of attorney gives the designated person authority to do only specific things (sell a house or review income tax records, for example).

However, a power of attorney becomes void if the person who granted it becomes mentally incapacitated. This means that if you have a power of attorney to do your mother's banking, you will no longer have that authority when she develops dementia. Thus, a power of attorney is of little use to the family of a person who has dementia. Because of this, all states and the District of Columbia have passed laws creating *durable powers of attorney*. These authorize someone to act on behalf of a person *after* they become unable to make their own decisions. You can tell which kind you have: a durable power of attorney must state that it can be exercised even if the person becomes disabled.

All states and the District of Columbia have passed laws creating *durable powers of attorney*

Most states now accept *MOLST (Medical Orders for Life-Sustaining Treatment)* or *POLST (Physician Orders for Life-Sustaining Treatment) forms.* These are documents that people complete when they have a chronic, progressive illness from which recovery is not likely, when death is expected within one or two years, or when they have a terminal illness. MOLST forms list the types of care a person does and does not want for specific issues such as feeding difficulties, inability to breath independently, and resuscitation. The form is filled out by a health care professional after consulting with the person or the person's representative (if they have a legally recognized surrogate).

Some financial organizations now require that a person fill out a form that the organization has devised, while the person is competent, that gives a substitute the ability to access the person's accounts if the person becomes incompetent. These organizations will not accept the durable power of attorney document. While the person is competent you should ask all institutions in which the person has money whether they will accept a durable power of attorney for finances or will require that

different form, which must have been filled out before the person became incompetent.

Some states recognize more than one type of durable power of attorney. For example, many separate the power of attorney to make medical decisions from the power of attorney for financial matters. Find out what the laws are in your state. Ask your attorney or the state's attorney's office. Many state's attorney's offices have websites, and some have the forms available online.

A general power of attorney becomes void if the person who granted it becomes mentally incapacitated. A *durable power of attorney* authorizes someone to act on behalf of a person *after* they become incapacitated and unable to make their own decisions.

Because a power of attorney authorizes someone to act on another person's behalf, the person granting such power must be sure that the person selected will, in fact, act in their best interests. Someone who holds a power of attorney is legally responsible to act in the other person's best interests. Once in a while someone abuses this responsibility. The risk of abuse is small in a limited power of attorney, but a durable power of attorney transfers greater responsibility and requires greater trust. A person who wants to plan ahead for their eventual disability must consider this decision carefully.

By making a will and granting a durable power of attorney while they are still able to do so, people who feel that their memory may be beginning to fail can be sure that if it gets worse, their life will continue the way they intended and that their property will be distributed as they would have wanted rather than in a way imposed by a court or by state law. People who prepare durable powers of attorney continue to manage their own affairs or part of them until such time as the designated person must take over. Then the appointed person will usually not need to take further steps before being legally empowered to take over the management of the affairs of the person who has dementia. State laws vary, but when you prepare and sign a durable power of attorney for health care, you designate the person (referred to as the "attorney") to make major health care decisions for you. You can designate specific wishes and circumstances in the document, or you can appoint a person and not describe your wishes in specific circumstances. Either way, choosing a person you trust is crucial. This person will be involved in all medical decisions, including whether heroic measures to postpone death will be used at the end of life.

Choosing a trustworthy person to be your durable power of attorney is crucial

Some people are unwilling to sign a power of attorney document, have no one that they trust to represent their wishes, or are already too impaired to do so. Others have chosen not to appoint someone even though they were aware of the ability to do so. If this is the case, you may need to take steps that require the help of an attorney. If the person is currently unable to effectively manage their property and affairs because of their disability, a *guardianship of property* procedure (also called a conservatorship) may be necessary. In this procedure, the lawyer must file a petition in court. After a hearing, a judge determines whether the person is no longer legally competent to manage their property or financial affairs. When a judge finds that the person lacks financial decision-making capacity, they appoint a legal guardian to act for the person in financial matters only. This guardian must file financial reports periodically with the court.

Reassure a person who is beginning to have memory problems that writing a will and preparing durable power of attorney documents ensure that their life will continue the way they intended and that their property will be distributed as they wish

In some states, laws provide a mechanism by which family members or friends can automatically be granted health power of attorney if a person becomes incompetent. Check with an attorney or your state's attorney's office to find out the law in your state.

If a home is owned jointly by a husband and wife and one of them becomes impaired, the well spouse will need a power of attorney or guardianship of the property in order to sell the home.

> **If a person is unable to manage their property and affairs because of their impairments, a *guardianship of property* (also called a conservatorship) may be necessary**

Sometimes people who have dementia become unable to care for their daily needs and must have someone else make decisions about needed medical or nursing home care. Most states specify by law that certain close relatives may make medical decisions without going to court and having a legal determination of incompetency. This usually requires two practitioners with medical or psychological expertise to attest that the person has become incompetent to give consent for medical procedures. If there is no one available or if there is disagreement among interested parties, a petition must be filed in court to request a *guardianship of the person*. The judge may then appoint a guardian of the person, order the needed care, or send the person to a hospital.

CHAPTER 15

Long-Term Care Arrangements

Sometimes a family is unable to care for a person who has dementia at home, even if relief services are available. A number of other living arrangements may be considered. These include sheltered settings where the person can manage with minimal support for a time, settings where a couple may be able to manage more easily together, and settings where the person receives complete care.

There is no right time to place a family member in a nursing home or other residential care facility, and there is no single reason that leads most people to take this step. For some, the time has come when the caregiver is just worn out. Other demands, children, a spouse, or a job may make it impossible for anyone in the family to be a full-time caregiver. A common reason for placement is that the person needs more care than the family can provide. There may be no way to pay for enough care in the home. Older adult children and spouses are likely to have health problems of their own and may no longer be able to provide the amount of care a person who has dementia needs. In both single- or dual-income households, it may be financially impossible for a family member to stay at home and care for the person who has dementia.

Caregivers often wait too long to place a family member. Both you and the person who has dementia may find it easier if you discuss and plan for placement before you are exhausted and while the person still has the ability to adjust to a new setting.

If the person does well in a residential setting, you will have more time and energy to be with them as a loved one rather than as a care provider

---

Placing your family member in a nursing home or other residential facility can be a difficult decision to make, and it often takes time. Families usually try everything else first. However, the time may come in the process of caring for a person who has dementia when placement is the most responsible decision the family can make.

Family members may feel great sadness and grief at having to accept the inevitable decline of their spouse, parent, or sibling. They frequently have mixed feelings about placing a person in an assisted living facility or nursing home. They may experience a sense of relief that a decision has finally been made and that part of the care will be assumed by others, yet feel guilty for wanting someone else to take over these burdens. Family members may feel angry that no other choices are available to them. The caregiver and others may feel considerable guilt over the decision to place the person, especially when one of the reasons for placement is that the caregiver can no longer manage a behavior problem.

> **The time may come in the process of caring for a person who has dementia when placement is the most responsible decision the family can make**

Many people believe that loved ones should be cared for at home, and many have heard that American families "dump" unwanted old people in institutions. Not all families care lovingly for their elderly members, but statistics clearly demonstrate that families are *not* dumping their elderly in nursing homes, that most families do all they can to postpone or prevent placement, and that they *do not* abandon their elderly members after placement. Instead, most families regularly visit the person in the new residence.

We tend to think of the "good old days" as a time when families took care of their elderly at home. In fact, in the past not many people lived long enough for their families to be faced with the burden of caring for a person who had dementia. The people who did become old and sick were in their 50s or 60s, and the sons and daughters who cared for them were considerably younger than you may be when your parent or spouse needs care in their 70s or 80s. Today many children of an ailing parent are themselves in their 60s or 70s.

It is not unusual for family members to disagree about placement plans. Some members of the family may want the person to remain at home, while others feel that the time has come for the person to enter a nursing home or other residential setting. It is helpful if all the involved family members discuss the problem together. Misunderstandings and disagreements are often worse when not everyone has all the facts. All the family members who are involved should discuss at least these four topics: (1) why it is best for the person to move, (2) the cost of care in the long-term care setting and where that money is to come from (see page 270), (3) the characteristics of the facility you select (see pages 272–73), and (4) the changes that placement will make in each person's life.

Types of Living Arrangements

In many parts of the country, people who have dementia arrange for full-time support in their home or move to a residential care facility or assisted living facility instead of or before moving into a nursing home. There are advantages and disadvantages to this arrangement. Continuing to care for people at home requires the resources to sustain in-home support long term but has the advantage of allowing people to remain in a familiar place. Residential care may feel more homelike to people who have dementia, and they may be freer to move about and participate in appropriate activities. Some assisted living facilities have special dementia units or specialize in what they refer to as "memory care." There is usually no state or federal funding for the care of people who have dementia in any long-term care setting unless there are specific waiver programs or the person meets criteria for Medicaid support. Nursing home care allows people to receive the medical services that are needed if they are so disabled as to be unable to care for themselves.

We urge you to plan for long-term care, whether it is at home, in a residential building, in an assisted living facility, or in a nursing home, even if you hope it will not be necessary. Investigate financial issues and select one or more homes that you like. You may never need nursing home care, but the difficulties associated with trying to locate a good home are enormous, so planning ahead will make a big difference. Many families end up losing money or using homes they do not like because they did not anticipate the need.

There is a serious shortage of facilities suitable for people who have dementia. If you find a facility that you believe offers exceptional care, get on the waiting list well in advance. If you delay until you must place your family member quickly (for example, following a hospitalization), you may have to take whatever is available, at least for the short term, even if it does not offer the quality of care you want. You can always withdraw from the application process if you wish.

In 2019, the cost of nursing home care in the Unites States averaged more than $100,000 per year. The cost of assisted living was less, averaging $60,000 per year. There is no public source of funding designed to assist with this cost. Payment comes from the resident's own income (such as a pension) and assets (such as a home, savings, and investments), the family's financial help, long-term care insurance (limited), Medicare, and Medicaid. Medicare pays only for short periods of care for the treatment of serious and acute illnesses. Medicaid pays only for the care of people who are impoverished. With such high costs, middle-class people in nursing homes deplete their resources within a short time and will need Medicaid. Federal and state policies are very restrictive, but some allow spouses to retain some funds if they continue to live in the community. *It is essential that you plan as far in advance as possible for ways to pay for long-term care, whether the person has some financial resources or no financial resources* (see page 270).

We briefly discuss each of several residential options, including retirement communities and senior citizen apartments or condominiums, adult foster care, board and care (also called domiciliary care), assisted living, memory care, continuing care retirement communities, nursing homes, skilled nursing facilities, and hospice. The labels used to identify the different types of care are confusing because they vary from state to state.

We urge you to plan for long-term care, even if you hope it will never be necessary

---

Continuing Care at Home (CCAH) programs are relatively new. They use the model developed by continuing care retirement communities, that is, guaranteed care for the rest of a person's life that is supported both by fees paid at admission and by monthly fees. The services are provided in the person's home rather than in a separate facility and range from meals only to twenty-four-hour supervision.

Retirement communities and *senior citizen apartments or condominiums* are planned for retired people who can live independently. If a person who has dementia moves into such a facility alone, there will not be adequate care for them when they need supervision and personal care. Such a living arrangement may be appropriate for people with mild cognitive impairment.

In senior citizen apartments, the resident pays rent. Ask whether a portion of the cost is subsidized under one of several state or federal programs, such as Section 8 of the Department of Housing and Urban Development (HUD). There is often a waiting list for subsidized housing, so plan ahead if you think you might need it.

In an *adult foster home*, the person who has dementia lives, for a fee, with an individual who provides a room and sometimes also personal care. Ideally, foster homes care for their guests as members of the family and provide meals, a room, transportation to the doctor, access to social work assistance, and supervision. Many adult foster homes will not accept people who have dementia. Those that do may provide nothing more than food and a bed. A few adult foster homes specialize in the care of people who have dementia and provide excellent care, but these are rare. The regulation of foster care varies widely from state to state. If you use such a program, you should plan on assuming full responsibility for monitoring the quality of care given. The quality of care may decline rapidly if the management or staff changes or if the condition of the person receiving care changes.

Boarding or domiciliary homes (also called homes for the aged or personal care homes) provide less care than nursing homes. They are not covered by Medicare or Medicaid. They usually offer a room, meals, supervision, and some other assistance. A few specialize in dementia and offer excellent care. Some of the best special care programs are homes for the aged. Other programs may take advantage of the vulnerable person who has dementia and of lax regulations. They may call themselves "Alzheimer facilities" but provide inadequate or dangerous care. These facilities may serve only a few people. They usually serve specific populations, such as the developmentally disabled, mentally ill, or people who have dementia. As you search for a facility, identify what population it serves. An internet search will help you with this task.

People who have dementia manage best when there are others nearby who can provide assistance and reassurance. You need to monitor both the long-term care provider and the person who has dementia.

There are no federal quality assurance standards for these facilities, and state oversight ranges from good to nonexistent. If you use such a program, you must assume full responsibility for ensuring that good care is provided. Fees vary widely. States may supplement the federal Supplemental Security Income (SSI) pension to help pay for boarding or domiciliary care. Some homes accept Social Security Disability Income (SSDI) as full or partial payment; however, neither source of assistance may be adequate to purchase good care.

If your family member takes medication or has an unstable medical condition, be sure that the facility can provide the care that is needed. Can its staff manage wandering? Food quality and quantity, sanitation, fire safety, control of communicable diseases, and cleanliness may or may not be adequately supervised by the state.

You must check these things yourself. People who have dementia usually cannot recognize a fire alarm or leave the building independently. Is there enough staff, particularly at night, to assist everyone in leaving the building in case of a fire? Ideally a facility will have smoke detectors, fire alarms, fire barrier walls and doors, and a sprinkler system. However, these things are expensive and are not required in many domiciliary and foster care settings. Programs that use such systems usually must charge more.

If you consider having the person who has dementia live in any new setting, carefully evaluate their ability to do so and watch for any decline that limits their ability to continue to live there. Keep on monitoring the facility, especially when staff or management changes. Our experience has been that people who have dementia do not manage well unless there are others nearby who can provide extensive assistance and reassurance.

Assisted living facilities (also called *residential care communities*) provide a room, meals, supervision, activities, and assistance with tasks such as dressing, eating, and bathing. Some provide nursing or medical care, but many do not. Many supervise medication, and some have daytime medical care available in the building. Many require that residents be able to walk and participate in their own care. These facilities may be more homelike and less like a hospital than a nursing home. They may also be less expensive. Some of them are an excellent option for people who have dementia, but others are not. Some specialize in care of people who have dementia and advertise that they provide "memory care."

Many states have regulations that govern the quality of assisted living facilities, but state standards (and inspections) vary. Facilities may be certified by the state or by an industry group. However, you have the primary responsibility to ensure that the person you place in an assisted living facility continues to receive good care. The facility may discharge a resident who becomes unable to walk, who needs frequent or regular nursing care, or whose behaviors are considered dangerous.

Life care facilities, also called *continuing care retirement communities (CCRCs)* or *life plan communities*, provide an array of care that ranges from independent living to long-term care. Many provide a set number of meals per month as part of the basic care package. Most people entering the facility live independently, but if they decline, they will be moved to a part of the facility that provides the level of care that is required. This may include assisted living or skilled nursing care. For a facility such as this, you should expect to pay a monthly fee in addition to an initial down payment and/or an entrance fee.

The retirement communities may be set up as rental units or as condominiums. In a condominium, the resident pays an entry fee that covers their apartment cost and also pays a monthly fee for services such as the maintenance of buildings and grounds, recreation facilities, security systems, and transportation to shopping areas. Some communities require an entrance fee that is refundable upon discharge, others charge a fee that is not refundable, and still others return part of the fee depending on how long the person has lived there. Find out whether the CCRC is accredited by CARF, the Commission on Accreditation of Rehabilitation Facilities (www.carf.org), which acquired the Continuing Care Accreditation Commission. However, even this accreditation is not a guarantee that the facility will be able to meet the needs of the person who has dementia.

A spouse may choose to move with the person who has dementia into a continuing care community. This option makes assistance available in a place where they can continue to live together. However, some life care communities screen applicants and do not accept people who have developed even mild dementia. Others charge higher entrance fees if dementia is already present. Some such facilities are not-for-profit, while others are owned by for-profit corporations that invest the initial payment and expect to earn more than the resident's care costs.

Before moving to a CCRC or life plan community in which you live with the person who has dementia, investigate it carefully. Once you have put your financial resources into such a program, you have little flexibility to change your mind or get a refund. Among the questions you need to ask beforehand are these:

- What kind of state or industry certification does the facility have? Is it inspected, and if so, how often?

- Will the entrance fee or part of it be returned to the resident's estate if they die before a given time period? Does the initial investment build equity for the resident?

- What will become of the resident's investment if the facility goes bankrupt?

- Is an additional entrance fee or monthly fee charged if a resident develops dementia?

- What services and activities are included in the monthly fee? Is participation in community meals or activities required? What if a resident doesn't like the food or activities?

- Does the facility have assisted living rooms, and are enough available so that a person who needs one is able to move there when they need to?

- Does the facility have a nursing unit? Do you like the nursing unit? Does the nursing unit accept people who have dementia? Is the staff trained to care for people who have dementia? Is there an extra charge on the nursing unit for people who have dementia? Are you satisfied with the quality of care offered? Review the guidelines for choosing a long-term care facility on pages 272–73.

- Can people who have dementia be asked to leave? If a resident is later found to have had a preexisting dementia, which you did not know about at the time of admission, can they be asked to leave? Under what other circumstances can a person or a couple be asked to leave?

- How are other medical, dental, and vision needs met? Does the facility have its own physician? If so, is it required that all residents use this physician? If this is not required, what will happen in the case of an emergency? Is transportation to medical providers available? How are medical needs met in the nursing unit? Do the physicians who work in the facility have expertise in geriatrics, and do they understand the medical needs of people who have dementia?

Your state may have regulations governing life care fees, but you must carefully examine the policies and the quality of services before making an investment. Check with the state consumer protection office or the office of the attorney general.

Moving with the Person Who Has Dementia

If you choose to move to a residence where you can continue to live with the person who has dementia and receive some help, there are some things you will want to consider. We discuss ways to help a person who has dementia accept a move in "Moving to a New Residence" in Chapter 4. In addition, ask yourself the following questions:

- What are the financial costs of moving, such as the cost of a new residence, moving costs, closing costs, and the capital gains tax on property you sell?

- Will moving mean less property for you to clean or maintain? Will help, such as meal preparation or house-cleaning, be provided for you?

- Will moving bring you close to doctors, hospitals, shopping centers, or recreation areas?

- What kind of transportation will you need? If you will use a facility's transportation service, can you manage the person who has dementia in the car, van, or bus?

- Will moving put you closer to or farther from friends and family who can help you?

- Will moving affect your eligibility for special programs or financial assis-

tance? (You may not be eligible for some programs until you have lived in a state for a given period of time.) If you have sold your house, you may be required to spend most of your capital from the house on nursing home care before you are eligible for Medicaid.

- Will moving provide a safe environment for the person who has dementia (call bells, a ground-floor bathroom, supervision, no stairs, a lower crime rate)?

- What will you do if your financial or physical health circumstances change?

Nursing Homes

The term *nursing home* brings negative images to many people's minds, but often nursing homes give good care and are the best alternative for a person who has dementia. *Skilled nursing facilities* (sometimes called SNFs) accept people who are medically ill and who need specific medical services such as feeding tubes or total assistance with feeding. They may also accept less-disabled people. They may—or may not—be certified to accept Medicare and/or Medicaid reimbursement for care. Medicare patients must have an acute condition for which they need skilled nursing for a short period of time. Often these are people who are being discharged from a hospital.

Be sure to find out what levels of care and reimbursement the facility accepts. If the person is to be admitted at one level of care or payment type, can they remain in the facility if the funding source or level of care changes?

If the facility accepts either Medicare or Medicaid, it will be licensed and inspected by the state. However, this does not guarantee quality. Some nursing homes do not meet the standards set by the state. When you visit the facility, ask to see the most recent inspection report.

The Medicare website (www.medi care.gov) provides (or will mail you) information about Medicare and how to select a facility. You will find a checklist you can print out and take with you to help you evaluate the facility. This checklist is useful even if the person who has dementia will not be covered by Medicare in the nursing home.

Use the interactive Medicare website (www.medicare.gov/care-compare) to compare the nursing homes you are considering with one another and with the average scores of nursing homes in your area and in the nation. It uses a five-star rating system to help you compare nursing homes and identify topics you'd like to ask questions about. Nursing homes with five stars are considered to have quality much above average, and nursing homes with a one-star rating are considered to have quality much below average. The health inspection rating contains information from the last three years in which the state inspectors have visited the facility. If a nursing home has a low rating, ask what is being done to correct it.

Pay special attention to the staffing ratios. This ratio considers the differences in the level of care needed by residents. For example, a nursing home with residents who have more severe needs would be expected to have more nursing staff compared to the number of residents than a nursing home where residents' needs are not as high. About 90 percent of care in a nursing home is provided by certified nursing aides (CNAs). A high staff-to-resident ratio means more individual time can be given to each resident.

> **The best way to ensure that your family member continues to receive good care is to visit often and to stay in close touch with the staff**

The quality rating measures many aspects of resident safety, such as the presence of pressure sores or changes in a resident's mobility. These measures do not assess kindness, knowledge about good dementia care, or types of appropriate activities. You should ask whether staff are available to meet the resident's individual plan of care? Is there enough staff to prevent incontinence through an individualized toileting schedule? How are anxiety and depression managed? How is pain monitored and managed?

There is often rapid turnover of ownership, administration, and staff in long-term care. Therefore, the quality of care can change quickly. The best way to ensure that your family member continues to receive good care is to visit often and to stay in close touch with the staff.

Memory Care Units

Across the nation, facilities offering varied types of care have opened *memory care units* or *special dementia care units* for people who have dementia. They are also sometimes called *Alzheimer units*. These units are most often features of assisted living facilities and nursing homes. Dementia care units range from those that are advertised as Alzheimer units but offer no specialized care to those that provide excellent care that meets the unique needs of a person who has dementia. Here are some of the issues you will want to consider:

- What is really special (as opposed to just good) about the care the facility offers?

- Does the program offer care that will be helpful to your family member? Do not assume that it will be better for your family member just because it is called *special*. Some people do not need special care, and some "special care" facilities are not offering care that meets the needs of people who have dementia.

- Are there a range of regularly scheduled activities that people who have dementia of varying levels of severity would enjoy participating in?

- Does this care cost more? If so, is the difference worth the price? Increased fees do not necessarily mean better care. Does the facility require that you pay privately? Can you afford it? If your family member will need to change to Medicaid after a few years, will the facility keep them?

- Is the facility close enough that you and others can visit easily? Seeing you frequently may be better for the person than whatever special care is offered.

- Are people moved off the unit if their condition declines? If so, is this satisfactory to you? Do you like the unit to which the person would be transferred? Would they be transferred within the same home?

Find out exactly what services are provided. Many of the recently developed special dementia programs have a more social approach to care and are excellent settings for people who have dementia.

Ask what positive changes the staff observe in the residents. The amount and type of positive change that excellent dementia care can produce are controversial. No large studies have documented particular benefits, but many programs in the United States and abroad report positive changes in the social function and behavior of people who have dementia who receive good care, even though the relentless progress of the disease continues. Some things that occur in most but not all residents and indicate good care are minimal use of behavior-controlling medication, increased enjoyment of activities, decreased agitation and wandering, evidence of pleasure in daily life, better control of continence (through staff assistance), evidence that the person feels that they belong, increased tendency to sleep through the night without sleeping medications, and little or no screaming. Good programs care for people who have challenging symptoms of dementia without using physical restraints. Residents in these programs smile and laugh more easily, appear more alert and responsive, and establish eye contact more often and for a longer part of their illness.

If you are able to place your family member in a good care facility, you may observe that they do better than they did at home. Families sometimes have mixed feelings about this—while they are pleased to see their family member doing well, they are sad that they could not bring about this change at home. However, it is easier for the staff to create a therapeutic program since they can leave the resident at the end of an eight-hour shift and are not doing the caregiving alone. When the person is doing well in a residential setting and you are free of the other demands of care, you have more time and energy to give them the love and sense of family that no one else can give.

Good care improves the quality of life for a person who has dementia at every stage of the disease

---

Some people who have dementia are depressed or anxious and require *mental health care* (see Chapter 8). Often they do not get good care for depression, anxiety, or other mental health needs in a nursing home or other residential setting. Ask the Alzheimer's Association or the local ombudsperson to help you advocate for psychiatric care. You may have to pay privately for mental health care in the setting or transport the person to a psychiatrist, social worker, or psychologist. Mental health needs should not make a person who has dementia ineligible for nursing home care. However, when a person has both dementia and a mental illness, such as depression, you may need expert help to get the person admitted to a nursing home.

Hospice can significantly improve the quality of life of people who have late-stage dementia

---

The Department of Veterans Affairs (VA) is obligated to serve people with service-related illnesses first, then other veterans as space and availability of services permit. Occasionally a veteran who has dementia will be admitted to a VA long-term care hospital or a VA contract nursing home but may be discharged later. A few VA facilities offer respite or family support services. Policies vary among VA hospitals. What is available in one area may not be available in another. Your congressional representative may be able to help you obtain services through the VA.

Medicare covers *hospice care* for people whose condition is expected to be terminal within six months. Hospice care is usually provided at home or in a nursing home, but it can be provided in a hospice facility in certain circumstances when the person is close to death. Hospice care is designed to keep people comfortable and maximize their quality of life. It does not aggressively treat the underlying disease unless it is leading to discomfort. Palliative care also focuses on patient comfort but is not a specific Medicare benefit.

Finding a Long-Term Care Setting outside the Home

The process of finding a facility will depend on whether you are planning in advance and whether the person who has dementia enters the nursing home from home or from the hospital. If the person enters a nursing home from the hospital, the hospital social worker will help you find a placement quickly. Hospital social workers are caught between their professional commitment to help you and the pressure on hospitals to discharge people as soon as possible. The social worker will know which homes have a bed available on the day the person is to be discharged. You may not be able to delay more than a day while you evaluate a home, and you can lose the bed of your choice in the course of that day. We recommend that you not rely solely on hospital social workers' word about the quality and reliability of a facility since they may never have visited the facility. If possible, visit any facility you are referred to. You may have little choice of facilities. By planning ahead, you can accept admission to whatever facility is immediately available but remain on the waiting list of the home you prefer. You can then decide whether to move the person when there is an opening in the preferred home.

If you have some time to plan, ask the local chapter of the Alzheimer's Association if they have a list of homes that families have liked or if they can refer you to members who have used the homes you are considering. The Association is the source most likely to have good, current information about how a facility manages people who have dementia. However, Alzheimer's Association chapters are lay organizations and usually cannot give you more than personal observations.

Many states have nursing home ombudspersons who have information about nursing homes that have failed to meet state or federal standards. Federal law requires that this information be publicly available. However, this information may not be the best reflection of a home's current status. Your own eyes, ears, and nose over several visits will be your best guide. See pages 272–73 for guidelines on choosing a facility.

Some local dementia support organizations such as Alzheimer's Association chapters or local offices on aging have staff who can advise you on the application process and provide you with a list of facilities in your area. Family service agencies have social workers, and in larger cities you can find the names of geriatric care managers or private social workers online. Agency social workers may be prohibited from recommending some facilities over others, or they may not have visited all facilities. So, their recommendations usually do *not* imply a judgment about the quality of a facility. In contrast, a geriatric care manager who works for you can visit homes and help you evaluate them.

Good facilities may be known to other families in your community or your doctor. Always get more than one opinion. If you have friends or acquaintances who have placed a loved one in a long-term facility, ask them about their experience. Favorable recommendations from others who have direct experience with a facility are often the best way to identify providers of good care.

> One of the best ways to identify providers of good care is to get recommendations from other families who have direct experience with a facility

When you have a list of possible facilities, call to make an appointment to see the administrator and/or the director of nursing of each home. Visit as many as you can. There are some fundamental questions you might want to ask over the phone even before you visit. First, you will need to find out whether the home has openings (if you need it immediately) or a waiting list. Second, you will need to find out if the home accepts the funding sources you are planning to use. When you visit the home, observe and ask questions. Take a friend or family member with you. This person will be less emotionally involved and can help you observe the facility and think through your decision. We recommend visiting more than once if there is time. On the second visit, you will notice things you missed on the first. Many families have told us that the things you notice when you first enter a home may not be the ones that matter as time goes on. Allow plenty of time to visit, talk to alert residents and the staff, and try to picture how your relative would fit in.

When Art first visited Sunhaven Assisted Living Facility, he was favorably impressed. He was struck by the spacious lobby and the long, clean corridors with the residents' names on their doors. He observed several staff members all in fresh uniforms, and he liked the sunny rooms and well-equipped bathrooms. Later, after visiting his father several times at Sunhaven, Art noticed that no residents used the lobby. He decided that what mattered most was whether the aides were friendly to his father and whether they came and helped him in the bathroom when he needed it. His father had always enjoyed meals, and the bland, lukewarm food depressed him. Art wished the home had spent more money on a cook and less on the lobby. His father had always liked to stay up late at night and to sleep late in the morning, but the facility required that everyone be in bed by 8:30 p.m. and up by 7:00 a.m.

Paying for Care

Care in long-term care facilities is extremely expensive (see the box on page 260). Care in other settings, while sometimes less expensive, may still be beyond the means of the person who needs it. Sources of payment include the following:

- the person's own income (for example, Social Security or a pension)

- the person's assets (for example, savings, real estate, or investments)

- financial help from family members

- the person's long-term care insurance

- Medicare (Medicare does not pay for long-term care in nursing homes or other settings)

- Medicaid (medical assistance)

- the Department of Veterans Affairs (see page 268)

The person's own *income* will almost certainly have to be spent on their care. For most people, it will not be enough to cover the entire cost of care. In addition to income, the person will need to begin spending their *assets* to pay for care. If the person has any assets, consult a tax accountant or the person's broker for advice on which assets to spend first and to help you make a plan for converting assets to liquid funds.

Some *family members* may be able to help with the cost of the person's care and be willing to do so. We recommend that family members discuss this openly.

Some people have purchased *long-term care insurance* in advance of the time that they become ill. Find out if a long-term care policy exists, and read it carefully. Some policies will pay part of the cost of care in the person's home, which might enable you to keep the person who has dementia at home if you wish to do so. Some pay for care only in specific kinds of long-term care facilities and may have certain exclusions. Most will pay only a portion of the daily cost of long-term care. While such insurance helps, you will probably need other sources of funding as well.

Medicare pays for care in a skilled nursing facility for brief periods of time (usually less than ninety days) for people who have an acute illness and who need inpatient skilled nursing care or rehabilitative therapy. Dementia is usually not considered to warrant this kind of care, but if the person has a co-existing condition, you should inquire whether Medicare will cover rehabilitation or intensive nursing care. Only care in a Medicare-certified facility will be covered.

Medicare does not pay for long-term care

Medicare therefore is not a major resource for paying for long-term care. It is important that you not overestimate Medicare benefits. (Medicare Parts A, B, and D will help pay for hospital care, outpatient care, and drug costs if the person transfers from a nursing home to the hospital or if the person lives in a foster home, a board and care facility, or an assisted living facility.)

Long-term care is so expensive that many middle-class people exhaust their resources and must turn to Medicaid to pay for it

---

Medicaid (Medi-Cal in California) pays for nursing home care for people who have no other means of support. Medicaid is based on legislative policy that tax money should be spent only for people who cannot otherwise obtain care. This is a federal program that is administered at the state level. Because long-term care is so expensive, many middle-class people quickly exhaust their financial resources and must turn to Medicaid. Thus, the person must spend all other resources (such as savings and investments) before becoming eligible for Medicaid. Medicaid makes up the difference between a set base amount and any income and long-term care insurance. The nursing home or hospital social worker will help you apply for Medicaid. Finding a placement for a person who will need Medicaid has become increasingly difficult, and Medicaid policy has become increasingly restrictive.

You may have strong feelings of discomfort about taking what some people call "welfare." In fact, Medicaid pays for at least part of the care for about two-thirds of nursing home residents.

If Medicaid requires that people use up their income and assets before they become eligible, what becomes of the well spouse who continues to live in the community? Federal law has become increasingly restrictive, and state policies vary widely. However, there are some provisions for dividing assets between spouses so that the well spouse is not immediately impoverished. For example, a spouse may be able to remain in the home and not be required to sell it, but when that spouse dies the state may require that the money be applied to the person with dementia's long-term care costs.

If you apply for Medicaid, it is important that you receive fair and equitable consideration. You may have a lot of difficulty getting accurate information about your eligibility. Not all lawyers are knowledgeable about this complex law, and social workers and nursing homes may have incorrect or out-of-date information. Information

can be obtained from the Alzheimer's Association, its local chapters, the National Citizens' Coalition for Nursing Home Reform, and other advocacy groups. There is an appeals system, but it may be burdensome.

Guidelines for Selecting a Long-Term Care Facility

We have provided a list of questions you may want to ask as you visit potential places to move to. These questions will help you evaluate the quality of care they provide. When you meet with the facility's administrators, you should feel free to ask questions about accreditation and fees and whether the facility meets state standards for the quality of care. Do not take anything for granted. If there are things you do not understand, don't hesitate to ask. All financial agreements should be in writing, and you should have a copy of the final agreement. If the staff is reluctant to answer your questions, this may be an indication of how you will be treated after placement. Take this checklist with you when you visit the facility.

> Do not take anything for granted when selecting a long-term care facility. If there are things you do not understand, don't hesitate to ask.

There are three vital questions to ask first:

1. Does the home have a current license from the state?

2. Does the administrator have a current license from the state?

3. Does the home meet or exceed state fire regulations? Because it is difficult to evacuate frail elderly people in case of fire, sprinkler systems and fire doors are important.

If any of these questions cannot be answered yes, do not use the home. If you will use Medicare or Medicaid, is the home certified to accept it? (If you will pay from another source initially and then switch to Medicaid, you need to know whether the home is certified for it and whether it will keep the resident.)

Are the agreed date of admission and the care to be provided set forth in the written contract?

Under what conditions could the resident be asked to leave (decline in health, behavioral symptoms, problems walking, incontinence)? How much notice must the facility give you? If their condition changes (either improves or declines), will the facility move them? And if so, will it be to another part of the same home?

Carefully review the fine print of the contract. Ask a lawyer if you don't understand it.

Convenience of Visiting

Is the home close enough that you can visit frequently? Is there adequate parking or public transportation? Does the home have long and convenient visiting hours? (When a facility restricts visiting hours, one wonders what goes on when no family members are around.) May children visit? Can you spend extra time in the beginning to help the person adjust? (See pages 278–80.) Will you feel comfortable visiting here?

Some facilities strongly recommend or require that family not visit the person for days or weeks after a person moves in. We do not believe there is a single policy that is best for all people who have dementia. Some people become so upset by visitors that it is best to minimize contact for a week or two, but the majority do well with frequent visits from the beginning.

Meeting Regulations

What is the home's most recent rating in the five-star rating system, and when was it received? The most recent inspection must be posted in the facility. Ask to see it. If you are considering a home that has been cited for failure to meet federal or state standards (and many have), ask what the failures were and what has been done to correct them. Some violations are quickly remedied. Some relate to minor issues that have no real relevance to quality of care, but other violations indicate serious problems. If the staff evades your question, you may not wish to use the facility.

Costs

Do you clearly understand what costs are included in the basic charge? Obtain a list of extra charges, such as laundry, television, radio, medications, haircuts, incontinence pads, special nursing procedures, and behavior management procedures. Ask how residents' personal funds are handled. Will the resident receive a refund of the advance payments if they leave the facility? How does the home protect cash and assets that have been entrusted to it? Is a receipt given to you or the resident? Are withdrawals noted by signed receipt so that you can keep track of the account? If the resident enters the hospital or goes home for a few days, what charges are involved? Will the resident be able to return to the same facility?

Cleanliness and Safety

Is the home clean? Look at bathrooms and the food preparation area.

A facility can be clean and still have a warm, comfortable atmosphere. Highly waxed floors and shiny surfaces create glare, which can confuse people who have dementia and may not be the best indicators of cleanliness.

Are bathrooms and other areas equipped with grab bars, handrails, nonskid floors, and other devices for residents' safety? Are the height differences between rooms limited to minimize fall risk?

What provisions are made for the safety of people who wander or become agitated? Can staff members spend individual time with someone who becomes upset? Are doors secure (either disguised, locked, or equipped with a system to alert the staff that someone has gone out)? Are physically frail residents protected from stronger, more mobile people who have dementia? Is the facility well lit, the furniture sturdy, and the temperature comfortable?

It is difficult to balance independence and maximal function for people who have dementia with the things needed to ensure their safety. Ask how the home addresses this. Do the policies seem reasonable to you? For example, how does the staff manage unsteady people who still try to walk?

Staff

Ask whether there is enough staff to assist your family member individually or to wait while they slowly do some things for themselves. The larger the staff, the higher the cost of care is likely to be, but some individual assistance should be available. How many people does each aide take care of? Does this seem reasonable, given the severity of the residents' impairments? How is the facility staffed on evenings and weekends? How well trained are supervisory nurses? Observe how residents are handled. Are they asking for help and not getting it? Do the aides seem rushed?

Does the staff seem happy and friendly? Happy personnel indicate a well-run institution. Also, contented staff are less likely to take out their personal frustrations on people who are receiving care. Ask staff members how staff turnover rates compare with those at other local homes. The staffs of good nursing homes recommend this as an excellent clue to the level of staff satisfaction.

Ask what training the nursing staff, including nursing assistants, has received. Have nurses, aides, social workers, and activity directors had training in the care of people who have dementia? Staff members need to know how to manage catastrophic reactions, suspiciousness, wandering, and irritability. How willing are they to accept information from you on how to manage your family member?

Ask about the extent of professional training the social worker and the activity director have had. These two people make a significant contribution to the quality of resident care. Ask to meet them. Ask them how much of their time is spent with people who have dementia. Ask to see some care plans. Do they seem to have been filled out by rote, or do they describe individual needs the home is really addressing?

Does the facility have a consultant with whom they work if severe behavioral problems develop? Do they have the skills needed to maximize the person's quality of life and minimize the use of antipsychotic drugs?

Care and Services

Federal law mandates that nursing homes (but not other types of facilities) have an individual care plan for each resident. Ask to see what things are considered in the care plan. Are you welcome to participate in care planning? Do the activity director and the social worker participate?

What things will the home want to know from you about the resident? In addition to many questions about medical history, financial resources, and the like, does the home want to know about the person's likes and dislikes, habits, how you manage behavioral symptoms, and what abilities the person still has? This information is essential for good care.

How much of the time does the facility involve people who have dementia in activities? Long hours of inactivity indicate poor care. Do the activities offered seem dignified and adult? Will they interest your family member? Do they have a variety of activities available so that people can continue to participate even if they decline significantly? Ask to observe activities. Do the residents appear to be interested and

content, or are they dozing off or wandering away? Are programs available to keep residents alert and involved, within the limits of their abilities?

> Federal law mandates that nursing homes have an individual care plan for each resident. Ask to see the plan and do your best to attend care plan meetings.

Is supervised daily exercise provided? Even people who are confined to a wheelchair or bed need exercise, and those who can walk should be doing so. Exercise may reduce the restlessness of people who have dementia.

Are there creative and effective planned social activities? A television room is not enough. People who have dementia need structured programs, such as music programs, recreation groups, visiting or resident pets, and outings to keep them as involved in interpersonal activities as they are able to be.

Are physical therapy, speech therapy, and occupational or recreational therapy available to residents who need it?

Do clergy visit regularly, and can residents attend religious services?

Do residents wear their own clothes and have a locked, private storage space? Is the privacy of their mail and phone calls respected? Can they have privacy with visitors, and is private space provided for visits from a spouse or multiple family members?

Ask to see the home's written policy on the use of restraints. Look around. Do you see people wearing vests or belts or sitting in furniture they cannot get out of? Restraints should not be used unless all other measures to control the person have failed and they are necessary to protect them from harm. Experienced staff members can almost always manage wandering and agitation without restraints.

People who have dementia need structured programs to stay as involved as they are able

Geri Chairs are occasionally used to make people comfortable or to restrain people, but they should be used only when other options are not safe. If such chairs are present, are people being released, repositioned, walked, and taken to the bathroom frequently?

Ask to see the home's written policy on using psychoactive drugs to manage difficult behavior. Ask how many of their residents are taking such medications. A high proportion (more than 20 percent) of residents on psychoactive medications can indicate staff levels are too low to manage behavioral symptoms in other ways. What does the staff do before resorting to medications for behavioral or psychiatric symptoms? What behaviors do they treat with medication (see "Using Medication to Manage Behavior" in Chapter 7)? If your family member were to need medications to control behavior, mood, or sleep, will you be consulted *before* the medications are started? How frequently will a physician see the person to review their status, attempt to lower the dose, and try to discontinue the medication? Ask what strategies the facility will try in the attempt to

reduce the need for medication and/ or restraints. If your family member is depressed, ask how the facility manages depression and whether a mental health professional will be involved in their care. Does the home have a consulting nurse, psychiatrist, or psychologist who can see the person if they develop serious behavioral symptoms or become depressed? How will the facility handle these problems?

Ask who is responsible for the person's medications. How will medical care be handled? Will their own physician visit them, or does the facility have a physician who sees all the residents? How frequently will this physician see the resident? Will this physician meet with you when you have concerns? Can you meet with them ahead of time? Do they have training in geriatric medicine? People who have dementia need close, skilled medical supervision, and their medical care requires special skills. In the absence of such a physician, does the home employ specially trained nurses or physician's assistants? If the facility is not a nursing home, who will take the person to the doctor? How are medical emergencies handled? Does the facility have arrangements for the transfer of acutely ill people to a hospital? Is this hospital satisfactory to the family?

If the person is bedfast or has serious health problems, has the staff had special training in these areas?

How is incontinence managed? Nursing management, such as individualized scheduled toileting or even the use of absorbent pads, is preferred over the use of catheters for ambulatory people who have dementia. Look around. Do you see more than a very few people who have catheter bags hanging from their wheelchairs or beds?

> **Like all of us, people who have dementia are sensitive to the way they are treated. Observe how the staff treat residents.**

Ask the staff or the ombudsperson about the frequency of pressure sores (also called decubitus ulcers). More than an occasional pressure sore may indicate poor care.

Like all of us, people who have dementia are sensitive to the way they are treated. Observe how the staff treat residents. Do they address them as adults or as if they were children? Do they stop and pay attention to residents who approach them? Do they greet people before providing care? Do they explain what they are about to do? Do they seem sensitive to needs for privacy and dignity?

The Physical Environment

Is the home pleasant to be in and well lit? Is the furniture comfortable? Are residents' personal possessions in sight in their rooms? A nursing home that looks like a hospital is not necessarily a pleasant place in which to live. Pleasant surroundings and a kind, patient staff are important to a person who has dementia. Also, you need to feel comfortable when you come to visit.

Do you think your relative will feel comfortable here? There are "homey" facilities that have worn furniture but seem more like home to some people. Other people will feel more comfortable in a newer-appearing facility. Is it too noisy and confusing for your family member, or too quiet and boring? Does it allow private time for those who seek it and provide social activities for outgoing people?

Glare, noise, and dim light all add to the difficulties a person who has dementia experiences. If these things bother you, chances are they will also create unnecessary stress for a person who has dementia.

Policies on Terminal Care

What is the home's policy regarding life-sustaining measures? Ask to have a statement recording the person's preferences readily accessible in addition to having their living will, advance directives for health care, and MOLST (Medical Orders for Life-Sustaining Treatment) form placed in the chart. Although this is a painful subject to think about at the time of the person's admission, facilities are required to ask about it. This is a step toward assuring that a person's wishes about end-of-life care and resuscitation are respected.

Meals

Visit at mealtime and ask to eat a meal there. Does the food look appetizing? Are meals adequate? Are individual diets available? Are snacks available?

Is the food wholesome, attractive, and suitable for elderly people? Are people who have dementia served in a small, quiet area or in a large, noisy dining room? Do you observe aides helping people who cannot feed themselves? If so, do they seem to be pacing their feeding to a rate that the person who has dementia is comfortable with?

Are people with swallowing problems closely supervised? Feeding tubes should not be used as a long-term substitute for voluntary eating if good nursing management will enable the person to eat.

Rights

Is there a resident council that can take problems and complaints to the administrator? To whom can you take concerns? Is there a family council?

Ideally, all facilities should be able to respond positively to these questions. In reality, high-quality care is hard to find. If the person who has dementia is difficult to manage, or if you must rely on Medicaid funding, you may not be able to find an ideal home. Use these questions as a guide to help you decide which things are most important to you and which ones you are willing to compromise on.

Moving a Person to a Residential Care Facility

Once a facility has been found and financial arrangements have been made, the next step is the move. It involves many of the things that are important whenever a person who has dementia changes residence (see "Moving to a New Residence" in Chapter 4).

Tell the person where they are going if you think there is any chance that they will understand. If they become very upset and cannot discuss the reasons with you, it likely means they lack the ability to comprehend such a complicated issue. It is then better not to discuss it further until close to the time to move.

Take familiar items the person is fond of (pictures, mementos, a blanket, a radio). Label them. If possible, have the person help select these items. Even a person who is upset or severely impaired needs to feel that this is their life and that they are still important.

You may have to close your ears to the person's accusations if they blame

you for this move. If they repeatedly become upset when the home is mentioned, it is not helpful to keep reminding them. You may need to go on matter-of-factly with arrangements. Try to avoid dishonest explanations such as "We are going for a ride" or "You are going for a visit." This can make the person's subsequent adjustment in the home more difficult.

> **Visiting almost always improves after a few weeks**

Most states have procedures by which clinicians can declare a person unable to make their own medical decisions if they have lost the capacity to do so. Most hospitals are experienced at handling this delicate issue. If there are problems, you should consult an attorney.

Many people who have dementia will adjust better to the facility if the family visits frequently in the early weeks. People vary though, and some residents need some time on their own before they begin to join in facility activities. Use the ill person's behavior as a guide. If they become very distressed during your visit or every time you begin to leave, then it is better to limit your visits at the beginning. Almost every person who has dementia does better over time, so regular visiting is always best after a few weeks.

If the person continues to be uncomfortable in the facility, ask yourself whether your own tension and anxiety are making it more difficult for them to relax in the new surroundings. Avoid a facility that always recommends that you stay away until the person gets used to their surroundings. This can increase their feeling of being lost. You may be exhausted at this point, and the person may greet you with accusations or beg you to take them home with you. Remember that these may be the only words they can find to express their understandable anxiety and unhappiness. Offer reassurance and affection, and avoid being drawn into arguments. After the first weeks, you may want to taper your visiting to fewer hours. Find a schedule that both supports the person and allows you to recharge your own resources.

We encourage people to write up information about the person for the staff. Do they prefer to bathe in the morning or at night? Do they go to bed early or late? Who are the people in their life that they may ask for? What do certain words or behaviors mean? How do you respond to things they often do? What will comfort them? What will trigger outbursts?

You may not find a facility you really like, or you may feel that the staff is not giving the person who has dementia the kind of care they should receive. However, you may have no alternative but to leave them in that facility. The director of an excellent home suggests that you carefully consider all your complaints and do all that you can to establish a friendly relationship with the staff. This may mean a compromise on your part, but it may well encourage their cooperation. Offer them information about dementia.

If you are moving the person to the nursing home from a hospital, you may have had little or no time to search for a home and to plan an orderly transition. You may be exhausted by all that had to be done in a few hours or days. If this happens, at least try to go with the person to the home and to have some familiar things waiting there for them.

Adjusting to a New Life

The changes imposed by living in a nursing home or other residential care facility require major adjustments for most people. Making these adjustments takes time and energy for staff and family, as well as for the person who has dementia, and it can be a painful process. Remember that a move does not mean the end of family relationships. In fact, many people find that their relationship with the person improves. Your relative can continue to be a part of the family even though they have moved into a setting that better meets their needs. There are some practical suggestions for things that you can do to make the adjustment to the new home easier. However, we know that the most difficult part of the adjustment may be the feelings you and your relative have about it.

Visiting

It is important to your family member that you visit. Even if they do not recognize you or do not seem to want you there, your regular visits help on some level to sustain their awareness that they are a valued part of the family. Frequent visits from family can also prompt better care from the staff. Sometimes people beg to be taken home or cry when family leaves after a visit. It's tempting to avoid such scenes by visiting less often, but usually the benefits to everyone from the visit far outweigh the upset that comes at the end. Expressing grief and anger at being in a nursing home is understandable.

You may be distressed by the atmosphere of the nursing home or by the other sick people you see there. Family members find it painful to see a loved one so impaired. Because dementia interferes with communication and comprehension, families can have difficulty thinking of things to do when they visit. There are things you can do to make visiting easier.

You can help your relative orient themselves in their new home. While you are visiting, explain again why they are there (for example, say, "You are too sick to stay at home"). Review what the daily routines of the home are, and make a schedule for the person if they are able to read it. Help them find the bathroom, the dining room, the television, and the phone. Help them find their things in their closet. Think of a way to identify the door of their room as theirs. Decorate their room with things that are theirs.

> **Your loved one can continue to be a part of the family even though they have moved into a setting that better meets their needs**

Tell them exactly when you will visit next, and write this down for them so they can use it to remind themselves. Some families write a letter to the resident, mentioning highlights of the most recent visit and the day and time of the next one. The staff can read the letter with the resident between visits to reassure them that you do come frequently. Try to continue to involve them in family outings. If they are not acutely ill, take them for rides, shopping, home for dinner or overnight, or to religious services. Even if they resist going back to the facility, they may eventually come to accept this routine and will benefit from the knowledge that they are still part of the family. Select activities that do not overly stress or tire them. Occasionally, it continues to be difficult to get the person to return. In this instance, it is better to visit them at the facility rather than take them to your house.

Help them remain a part of special family events such as birthdays and holidays. Even if they are depressed or confused, they usually should still be informed of sad events.

Phone calls between visits help a forgetful person keep in touch and remind them that they are not forgotten. Don't expect the person to be able to remember to call you. Landline phones are becoming a thing of the past and are not always available in people's rooms. The facility office should have a telephone and be willing to help the person call or receive calls if they are unable to do so on their own.

Take an old photograph album, an old dress from the attic, or some other item that may trigger memories of the past, and encourage the person to talk about things they remember from long ago. If they always tell you the same story, accept this. It is your listening to them and your presence that communicate that you still care about them.

Include the person in special family events such as birthdays and holidays when possible

Talk about the family, neighbors, gossip, the local sports team. Even if they are not fully aware of the issues, they can enjoy the act of listening and talking. Being together is what is most important to both of you. Exactly what you talk about is not so important. People who have dementia may not be interested in some topics, such as current events. If the person seems rest-

less, do not insist on bringing them up to date on information.

Be sympathetic about the person's complaints. Listening to the things they complain about tells them that you care about them. They may make the same complaint over and over because they forget that they have told you. Listen anyway—it is your empathy that is most important. Investigate any complaints thoughtfully before you complain to the staff, act on them, or decide not to pursue them further. Remember that the person's perception of things may not be accurate, although there might be an element of truth in the complaint.

What you talk about is not as important as being together

Sing old, familiar songs. Don't be surprised if other residents drift by to listen or participate. Music is a wonderful way to share. Nobody will care if your singing isn't very good. Take along recordings of the family or children.

Make a personal history scrapbook telling the story of the person's life—where they grew up, when they married, their children, job, hobbies, and so on. Write in large letters. Decorate it with photographs, clippings, bits of fabric, medals, and so on. Making a scrapbook can occupy both of you for several visits. Reviewing it may help the person recall their past. Even if they do not remember, they may be reassured that they *have* a past.

Make a personal history box. Put in items that are safe and will trigger memories: treasured keepsakes, antique kitchen tools, assorted nuts and bolts for a handyman, or spools of thread for a seamstress. Look for items with interesting colors, weights, textures, and sizes. The person may enjoy sorting and touching the things in this box. You and the staff can use it to trigger memories. Include a card that gives information about the items: "This is an old-fashioned apple corer like the one Mother used when she made apple butter for her five children," or "Dad wore these dancing shoes until he was 70."

If there is no place to store a scrapbook or box, just bring it with you on visits. Use it for something to do with your family member.

Avoid too much excitement. Your arrival, news, and conversation may overexcite the person and could trigger a catastrophic reaction.

Do things that show the person that you are interested in their new home. Walk around it together, read the bulletin board to them, talk to a roommate or other residents and staff. Remind the person to smell the flowers and see the birds when you walk around outside.

Help the person care for themselves. Eat a meal together, do their hair, rub their back, hold hands, help them get some exercise. Bring a treat that you can eat together while you are there. Avoid bringing food the staff must store. If the person has difficulty eating, you may want to come at mealtimes and help feed them. If other confused or upset residents interrupt your visit, you may be able to tell them gently but clearly not to talk with you now. If necessary, ask where there is a more private place for you to visit. Sometimes visits go more smoothly if you include one or two other residents in a simple activity.

If the person enjoys it and if it does not cause a catastrophic reaction, take along children (one at a time) or a pet (ask the staff in advance). Seeing the person in a facility is usually helpful for children. You can prepare the child by talking about the things they might see, such as catheters or IV tubes, and explaining that these things help sick people maintain their bodily functions.

> **Help the person care for themselves. Remind them to smell the flowers and see the birds when you go outside together.**

Sometimes a person is so ill that they can no longer talk or recognize you or respond to you. It may be hard to know what to say to such a person. Try holding hands, rubbing the person's back, stroking their face, or singing. One minister said this about his visits:

"I've grown in these visits. I am so used to doing, doing, doing, that it took me a long time to accept that there is nothing I can do for people who have dementia. I've learned to just sit, to just share being and not to feel I have to do or talk or entertain."

It is not easy to share family life and love a person who is in an institution and who is in the late stages of dementia, but perhaps you will find your own meaning in doing so, as this man has.

Repeating the same conversations or activities may get boring, but keep in mind that many people who have dementia have such severe memory impairment that they do not remember what they did five or ten minutes ago. Repetition of enjoyed activities may give them pleasure, even if it is frustrating for you.

Your Own Adjustment

You also will have changes in your life when a family member has moved to a new care setting. If the person lived with you, and especially if they are your spouse, the adjustment may be difficult. You may be tired from the effort of arranging for the placement, and on top of your fatigue, you may feel sad at the changes that have occurred. The move may intensify your feelings of grief and loss. At the same time, you may wish that you could somehow have kept the person at home, and you may feel guilty that this was not possible. You may have mixed feelings of relief and sorrow, guilt and anger. It *is* a relief not to have to carry the burden of care, to be able to sleep or read uninterrupted. Still, you probably wish things were different and that you could have continued to care for this person yourself.

Families often tell us that in the first few days they feel lost. Without the usual demands of caring for a sick person, they cannot decide what to do with themselves. At first you may not be able to sleep through the night or relax enough to watch television.

The trips to the facility may be tiring, especially if it is some distance from where you live. The visits may be depressing. Sometimes people who have dementia are temporarily worse until they adjust to a new setting, and this can upset you. Sometimes, too, the other people in the home are depressing to see.

Staff members are geared to provide care for many people, and you may not feel that your loved one is receiving the individual care that you would like. Other things about the home or the staff may upset you. It's not unusual for family members to feel angry with the staff from time to time. If you are upset with the home or the staff, you have a right to discuss your concerns with them, to be given answers, and not to jeopardize the person's care or status in the home by doing this. It is against federal law for a nursing home to discharge a resident because their family raised questions about their care. If there is a social worker in the home, they may help you work through your concerns. If there is no social worker, discuss your concerns in a calm, matter-of-fact way with the administrator or director of nursing.

> **Placing a person who has dementia in long-term care may intensify your feelings of grief and loss, guilt and anger**

Often things are better after placement, especially when the person with dementia has been difficult at home. With other people responsible for daily care, you and the person can relax and enjoy each other again. Because you are not always tired, and because you can get away from their irritating behaviors, you may be able to enjoy your relationship for the first time in a long while.

If other family members do not visit, it may be because they find it very hard to face visiting their relative in a nursing home or don't know what to talk about. If people in your family react this way, try to understand that this may be their way of grieving and that you may not be able to change them. Tell them what you have been through emotionally and what you have learned from your visits—that the most important thing you can do is be with the person and that what you say or do matters much less.

Sometimes family members spend many hours at the facility helping with the resident. Only you can decide how much time you should spend visiting. Ask yourself if part of your reason for being there has to do with your loneliness and grief, and if it might be better if you spent less time there so the resident can better adjust to their new home.

> **Tell reluctant family members what you learn from visiting: that being with the person matters more than what you say**

Time does pass, and gradually the acute phase of adjustment also passes. As time goes on, you will settle into a routine of visits. It is natural for you gradually to build a life apart from the person who has changed so much.

When Problems Occur in the Nursing Home or Other Residential Care Facility

Sometimes serious problems about patient care do arise.

•

Mr. Rosen says, "My father has Alzheimer disease, and we had to put him in a nursing home. He got terribly sick and was transferred to a hospital, where they said his condition was made worse because he was dehydrated. Apparently, the home failed to give him enough fluid. I feel like I am guilty of not checking up on this, and I feel like I can't send him back to a home that neglects him."

•

As you know, people who have dementia can require a lot of care, especially in the late stages of the disease. Mr. Rosen may feel that complaining to the nursing home staff will only make them angry. If he decides to move his father to another home, he may find that there are no other homes any better or that no home will accept a person with his father's needs who has Alzheimer disease or someone who is receiving Medicaid.

The dilemma you, Mr. Rosen, and many other families face lies not so much with one home but with national policy, value systems, federal training budgets, and so forth. These things are gradually changing through the efforts of organizations such as the Centers for Medicare & Medicaid Services, the Alzheimer's Association, and the National Consumer Voice for Quality Long-Term Care.

We hope you will not encounter

problems like these. If you do, first take time to consider what kind of care you can reasonably expect. You should expect that the person will be kept as healthy as possible, well fed and hydrated, protected from obvious risks, and clean and comfortable. You should also expect that the person's wishes will be known to the staff and accommodated as much as reasonably possible. They should be engaging in activities that are appropriate for their level of illness and should not be ignored. Concurrent illnesses should be recognized, and residents should be watched for drug reactions and interactions. However, dementia care can present challenges, and sometimes the facility can be "wrong if they do and wrong if they don't." It is often not possible to solve every problem or to treat every condition completely. For example, allowing a person to walk independently may be good for their heart, fitness, and self-confidence but may result in a fall. Asking the staff about the risks and benefits of the care they are providing and how they balance these sometimes conflicting goals can help you decide what risks you are willing to take.

Staff problems are a frequent cause of inadequacy in care. A facility cannot give the kind of individual care to one person that you could give at home. However, if there are not enough staff members to keep residents clean, comfortable, and fed and to monitor their medical needs, then something is wrong. The National Consumer Voice for Quality Long-Term Care publishes information about laws governing nursing home quality. Reading this material

will help you judge what you can expect from a home.

Talk over your concerns honestly but calmly with the facility administrator, director of nursing, or social worker and offer them the information you have about the care of people who have dementia. How do they respond? Do they thank you for talking to them and say they will address the problem, or do they make excuses or brush you off? If a physician or other professional should be aware of the problem, ask for that person's support in correcting the situation.

•

Mr. Rosen said, "The doctor at the hospital was so helpful. She called the nursing home and talked to them, explaining that his fluid intake needed to be monitored even when he kept assuring them that he was drinking because people who have dementia can easily become dehydrated."

•

If talking with people at the facility does not solve the problem, contact the local nursing home ombudsperson (usually in the office on aging). They have resources to investigate the issue and help you. As a final resort, report the problem to the state nursing home inspector's office. However, problems are usually successfully solved by working informally with the administrator and the staff of the home.

The problem may be that the staff needs more information about how to care for people who have dementia. The Alzheimer's Association has information about training resources. Encourage all levels of staff, from the nurses and administrator to the aides, to get training.

It is against the law for a facility to discharge a resident because the family has made a complaint. It is also against the law to mistreat a resident whose family has complained. You must closely monitor the care your family member receives.

Sexual Issues in Nursing Homes or Other Care Facilities

Sometimes people who have dementia undress themselves in public, masturbate, or make advances to staff members or other residents. The sexual needs and behaviors of residents in nursing homes raise controversial issues. Sexual behavior in a nursing home differs in significant ways from such behavior at home—it no longer is a private matter if it has an impact on other residents, the staff, and the families of residents. Sexual behavior also raises the ethical issue of whether people who are impaired can or should retain the right to make sexual decisions for themselves.

While our culture seems to be saturated with talk about sex, it is usually the sexuality of the young and beautiful that is being discussed. Many people are uncomfortable considering the sexuality of the old, the unattractive, the disabled, or those who have dementia. Nursing home staff members also often feel uncomfortable discussing sexual issues.

If the staff reports what is considered inappropriate behavior to you, remember that much of the behavior that at first seems sexual may be behavior of disorientation and confusion. You and the nursing home staff can work together to help the person know where they are, when they can use the toilet, and where they can undress. Often all that is needed is to say, "It isn't time to go to bed yet. We'll put your pajamas on later." Distractions, such as offering a glass of juice, are helpful.

People who have dementia may become close friends with another resident, often without a sexual relationship. Friendship is a universal need that does not stop when one has dementia. Occasionally, one hears stories about people getting in bed with other residents in a nursing home. This is not hard to understand when we consider that most of us have shared a bed with someone for many years and have enjoyed the closeness this sharing brings. The person may not realize where they are or whom they are with. They may not realize that they are not in their own bed. They may think they are with their spouse. Remember that assisted living facilities and nursing homes can be lonely places where there is not much opportunity for being held and loved. How you respond to such an incident depends on your attitudes and values and on the response of the nursing facility.

Some residents masturbate. The staff usually ignores such behavior if it occurs in the privacy of the person's room. If it occurs in public, the resident should be quietly returned to their room.

Flirting is a common and socially acceptable behavior for men and women. In a long-term care setting, a person may flirt to reinforce old social roles. It makes them feel younger and more attractive. Tragically, dementia may cause a person to do this clumsily, making offensive remarks or inappropriate gestures. Inappropriate remarks and behaviors that are sexual in nature are more common in people who have frontotemporal dementia and occur because disinhibited behavior is a common result of damage to the brain's frontal lobes.

When the staff is trained to remind the person matter-of-factly and kindly that this behavior is not acceptable, it sometimes fades away. If it persists, the person may need to be placed in an area where contact with others can be observed by staff. Residents can be provided with other opportunities to re-experience their social roles.

The question of sexually intimate behavior occurring between residents has legal implications because it requires that both parties are competent to consent and agree to participate in sexual activity. When either staff or family raises a concern about potential sexual activity, it is appropriate to involve a professional who can determine whether the parties are competent. While this might seem intrusive, the presence of dementia raises the significant possibility that a person lacks capacity (is incompetent) to give knowing consent. However, even when people are found to be competent, family members might be upset. If this occurs, we recommend that facilities convene a meeting that includes the person who has dementia, the family, competency experts, and appropriate facility staff to discuss the issue.

Sexual intimacy between married couples raises other issues in long-term care. If there is no objection, then there seem to be no grounds to raise a concern. However, if the person who has dementia appears distressed, then the facility should follow the steps discussed in the prior paragraph. This issue is more likely to be contentious when stepchildren are involved. The right of adults to engage in sexual intimacy is considered a privacy right that is protected by the Constitution, but when cognitive impairment is present, there is also an obligation to protect the vulnerable. Ideally, these issues can be discussed with all the appropriate parties and a solution can be reached that is acceptable to all involved. Legal adjudication is very rarely necessary.

CHAPTER 16

Preventing and Delaying Cognitive Decline

Several recent studies have reported that dementia is declining in frequency. The reasons for this encouraging finding are unknown. The most likely explanation is that the steps people have been taking to lower their risk of developing Alzheimer disease are working.

One of the challenges in studying prevention is the need to distinguish between age-associated changes in

> Dementia is declining in frequency, possibly because people have been taking steps to lower their risk of developing Alzheimer disease and vascular dementia

thinking that seem to be normal and the earliest symptoms of dementia.

Usual Age-Associated Changes

To begin, we reemphasize what we state throughout this book: cognitive decline that impairs the ability to carry out everyday activities is not inevitable. Many people live into their late 90s with fully intact mental function. In fact, wisdom and accumulated knowledge *increase* as we age.

•

Jane worries because she finds herself doing things like walking into the kitchen and then not being able to remember why she went there.

This kind of absentmindedness, sometimes called "a senior moment," is not a sign of impending dementia.

Recalling Words and Speed of Mental Performance

Two changes in thinking are a part of usual or "normal" aging. These changes begin as early as people's 40s but are often noticeable only when we reach our 60s or 70s. The first is a slowing of mental processing. As we age, the brain remains as able as ever to process information, evaluate its meaning, and decide on a course of action based on what it has processed. But it does so more slowly. This partly explains why it takes longer to remember words and facts in later life. It is best dealt with by taking one's time and not being rushed when trying to remember something or making a decision.

> **A person with a normally aging brain uses hints to retrieve information from memory. Hints do not help a person who has dementia remember better.**

Difficulty coming up with names and words is the other change asso-ciated with normal aging. The "senior moment" that Jane experienced is an example. With time, the name, thought, or word "pops into" memory, but it may take seconds or even minutes. Studies have repeatedly shown that "hints," "clues," and having choices ("Did you come into the kitchen to get a snack or a cookbook?") improve this difficulty in memory recall. This improvement with hints tells us that the word or name is still in our memory but is harder to access or "retrieve." In contrast, the memory loss seen in Alzheimer disease is permanent. The memory is "gone" and does not significantly improve with hints or cueing.

Risk Factors for Dementia

One approach to preventing or delaying the onset of Alzheimer disease and other dementias is to identify risk factors for developing these conditions. Here we discuss several categories of risk factors that have been identified and the evidence that addressing them lowers the risk of developing dementia.

Cardiovascular Factors
High blood pressure in midlife, blood lipid abnormalities (such as high cholesterol), and obesity are risk factors for developing Alzheimer disease and vascular dementia. Recent studies have demonstrated that lowering blood pressure into the desirable range decreases the risk of dementia. It has yet to be proven that addressing blood lipid abnormalities or obesity lowers the risk of developing Alzheimer disease, but treating them clearly lowers the risk of having a heart attack or stroke.

> **Lowering blood pressure into the desirable range decreases the risk of developing dementia**

Physical Exercise
Many studies show that people who develop dementia had been less physically active in the prior five to ten years than people who did not develop dementia.

This is indirect support for the idea that physical exercise prevents or delays the onset of cognitive decline, but it does not prove it. It is also possible that lower rates of exercise are a result of the brain changes that precede dementia. Studies in animals genetically programmed to develop Alzheimer brain changes show that exercise can lessen the development of the plaques that are characteristic of Alzheimer disease, a finding that supports the importance of exercise in prevention. Studies in humans have shown that exercise can lessen the cognitive declines that accompany usual aging, but none have shown that exercise prevents dementia.

To reduce the risk of heart attack, stroke, and dementia, the CDC recommends thirty minutes of physical exercise five days a week for everyone who can do so

---

The benefits of physical exercise in preventing heart attack and stroke are well established. If exercise also lowers the risk of developing Alzheimer disease, then a regular exercise program would have a triple benefit—lowering the risk of stroke, heart attack, and Alzheimer disease. For this reason, the Centers for Disease Control and Prevention (CDC) recommends thirty minutes of physical exercise five days a week for all people able to participate.

After checking with your doctor to make sure it is safe to exercise, gradually build up to the CDC recommendation. Even a short walk every day is good for you. Exercise is also a part of weight-loss programs. Since being overweight is another risk factor for Alzheimer disease, regular exercise

may prevent Alzheimer disease through multiple mechanisms.

Social and Intellectual Activity

Studies comparing people who do and do not develop dementia have shown that those who are more socially active are less likely to develop dementia. Just as with physical activity, these studies do not allow us to determine whether very early cognitive decline causes people to be less socially active or if less social activity leads to dementia. It is possible that the very beginnings of dementia cause people to be less socially and intellectually active.

Studies of mice and rats genetically programmed to develop the plaque lesions of Alzheimer disease in their brains have found that being raised in a stimulating environment decreases the number of plaque lesions in the brain, leads to less brain shrinkage (as seen on MRI), and results in less memory impairment.

Contrary to what was long thought, we now know that humans continue to make new brain cells throughout life. These new cells form in the hippocampus, the part of the brain essential for the formation of new memories. This exciting finding has spurred the development of many memory stimulation programs, particularly computer-based activities. Long-term studies have shown that mental exercises can improve performance on a specific cognitive test, but there is no evidence that cognitive or social stimulation programs lower the risk of developing dementia.

One of the challenges in studying mental and social stimulation is that the changes in the brain that lead to Alzheimer disease begin fifteen to twenty years before symptoms become noticeable. This means that prevention would be most effective if begun in people's 40s and 50s. Many people who are physically, mentally, and socially active throughout their lives develop dementia, so these actions cannot completely override the other genetic and environmental factors that cause dementia. The Food and Drug Administration (FDA) has fined companies for claiming that computer programs prevent dementia, but if you find mentally and socially stimulating games fun and can afford them, there is no harm in trying them.

There are many other ways to remain mentally active. Even if such activities do not prevent dementia, they may improve quality of life. Reading, traveling, and participating in hobbies you have long enjoyed are all mentally stimulating. Even if you develop health issues that limit participation, you can often modify an activity and remain active. For example, when the painter Henri Matisse's health declined in old age and left him unable to paint, he continued to create artworks by cutting large shapes out of colored paper. These bold designs are among his most beautiful works.

Diet

Several studies have found that following a Mediterranean diet delays the onset of dementia. This diet emphasizes eating fruits, vegetables, and healthy fats such as olive oil or canola oil, consuming very little red meat, and eating fish or shellfish twice a week. It also encourages the use of herbs and spices instead of salt to season food, eating nuts, and drinking red wine in moderation. This diet also lowers the risk of heart attack and stroke.

There are many websites and cookbooks that can help you plan a Mediterranean diet. If you begin a new diet program, ask yourself if you can afford it. Can you maintain it over time? Starting and then stopping within days or weeks will have no long-term effect on your health.

> **Studies support the idea that following a Mediterranean diet delays the onset of dementia**

Vitamin B12, folic acid, calcium, vitamin D, and fish oil have been promoted as reducing the risk of developing dementia, but there is no evidence that they are effective in preventing Alzheimer disease. Vitamin B12 can improve and sometimes totally reverse the dementia caused by pernicious anemia, a disease that results either from an inability to absorb the vitamin or from very low intake of the vitamin, but pernicious anemia is a rare cause of dementia today (although it should always be checked during an evaluation of new onset dementia). Vitamin B1 prevents the development of amnestic (Korsakoff) syndrome, a rare cause of memory impairment.

Antioxidants are also promoted as potential dementia preventers. No studies have shown them to be preventive, but they are known to prevent brain damage in studies of animals and cell cultures. Fruits, such as blueberries, that are high in antioxidants are part of a Mediterranean diet.

Ginkgo biloba, turmeric, and ginseng have long been promoted as cognition enhancers and dementia preventers. Ginkgo has been widely studied and has not been shown to prevent dementia. Ginseng and turmeric are less well studied, but there is no evidence that they are beneficial. In recent years coconut oil and jellyfish fluorescent protein have also been promoted as preventing and treating dementia, but no well-designed studies support these claims.

Education

Many studies show that receiving more education early in life is associated with a lower risk of developing dementia. Sometimes this research is cited as supporting the claim that mental stimulation might be preventive. Whether this finding is explained by the benefits of early-life schooling or is attributable to the fact that it is harder to detect the beginnings of dementia in better-educated people has not been determined.

Diabetes

Diabetes is a well-established risk factor for developing Alzheimer disease and vascular dementia. The mechanisms by which this occurs are under intense study. It is not known whether better control of blood sugar will prevent dementia.

Depression

Depression in early and midlife is a risk factor for developing dementia and Alzheimer disease. The mechanism is unknown. It is not known whether early treatment of depression lowers the risk. Depression occurring for the first time in later life is sometimes the first symptom of a progressive dementia.

Toxins

Lead can cause permanent intellectual impairment in children and can cause dementia in adults. Many other heavy metals, including manganese, mercury, thallium, and arsenic, are also toxic to the brain and can cause permanent damage.

Organic solvents can cause permanent nervous system damage, including dementia. Avoiding exposure to these toxins when possible and following safety precautions when they are used in the workplace will reduce the risk they pose.

Aluminum has been found in larger-than-expected amounts in the brains of some people who have Alzheimer disease. It now seems most likely that this is a *result* of whatever is causing the dementia, rather than a cause of the dementia. People sometimes wonder if they should stop taking antacids, stop cooking in aluminum pans, or stop using deodorant—all sources of aluminum. There is no convincing evidence that the use of these products is a cause of dementia. Treatments that promote the elimination of aluminum and heavy metals from the body do not benefit people who have Alzheimer disease, and some of these treatments have serious adverse side effects.

Head Injury

Repeated concussions are known to increase the risk of dementia. Evidence for this first emerged in the 1920s in studies of boxers who were described as "punch-drunk." They were found to have widespread tangles, one of the two lesions characteristic of Alzheimer disease, throughout their brains.

It is now clear that people with multiple concussions from any cause are at increased risk of developing dementia. The most common autopsy finding in the brains of people who develop dementia after multiple concussions is chronic traumatic encephalopathy (see page 299). This condition has been most widely studied in individuals who suffered concussions in contact sports such as American football, hockey, and soccer. Soldiers exposed to high-energy explosions are also at risk of developing chronic traumatic encephalopathy. It is not clear whether helmets or other protective headgear lower the risk in athletes or soldiers, but their use is still recommended.

Repeated concussions increase the risk of dementia

Age
Older age is the strongest risk factor for developing Alzheimer disease. The reasons for this are unknown. It is not yet known whether control of many of the risk factors discussed in the previous paragraphs will lower this age-associated risk or if there is some other yet undiscovered aspect of aging that predisposes people to cognitive decline.

Genetics
Genetics contributes from 35 to 65 percent of the risk of developing Alzheimer disease and frontotemporal dementia. Genetics contributes less to dementia with Lewy bodies and to dementia due to Parkinson disease. The genetics of Alzheimer disease is discussed in "Heredity and Dementia" in Chapter 18.

In the past, genetic risk was seen as discouraging because it was thought that "nothing could be done." We now know that the negative consequences of some gene abnormalities can be modified if treatment is begun early enough. For example, cognitive impairment due to phenylketonuria (PKU), a disease for which all newborns are screened, can be prevented by placing children who inherit two copies of the abnormal gene on a specific diet that prevents the disease from developing.

Medications

Aduhelm, whose scientific name is aducanumab, is the first drug approved by the FDA to treat mild cognitive impairment (see pages 295–96) and early Alzheimer disease. Aducanumab works by reducing the amount of beta amyloid protein (see pages 298–99 and 312–13) in the brain. Since beta amyloid is one of the abnormal proteins present in the brains of all people with Alzheimer disease, it is thought by many scientists to be involved in causing the disease.

Aducanumab is given intravenously at monthly intervals. This requires a visit to a center that provides the drug. Two controversies surround the FDA's approval of this medication. First, there is little evidence that the drug improves memory, thinking, or the ability to do everyday activities. Second, the drug can cause both small areas of bleeding and swelling in the brain, two potentially dangerous side effects. Even though the FDA has approved aducanumab, it is requiring the company that makes the drug to conduct more studies to determine if the medication can improve memory and daily function over time.

The drugs previously approved to treat Alzheimer disease—cholinesterase inhibitors (such as Exelon, Razadyne, and Aricept) and memantine (Namenda)—do not prevent or slow down the biological progression of the disease.

Summary

Preventing dementia and delaying its onset are major focuses of research. Treating high blood pressure is the only approach currently supported by scientific evidence, but indirect evidence also supports the benefits of physical and mental activity. Since Alzheimer disease likely has multiple causes, it is quite possible that several or many different preventive therapies will be identified in the future.

CHAPTER 17

Brain Disorders and the Causes of Dementia

Sometimes the brain does not work as it should. The problem may be called intellectual disability, dyslexia, dementia, or psychosis, to name a few. It may be caused by an injury to the brain before or after birth, a genetic abnormality, chemicals in the environment that damage the brain, interruption of the supply of oxygen to the brain, and many other things.

Never conclude that a person has dementia without having them evaluated by a physician

---

Doctors and scientists group the different things that can go wrong with the brain by the symptoms they cause and how those symptoms start and change over time. Just as fever, cough, vomiting, and dizziness are symptoms of many different diseases, memory loss, confusion, personality change, and problems with speaking are also symptoms of several diseases. In this chapter we explain how dementia differs from other problems of the brain, describe some of the most common causes of dementia, and describe some of the other conditions that can impair thinking. The most important thing to learn from this chapter is that you should take the person who has dementia to a specialist who can determine the exact cause of the dementia.

Mild Cognitive Impairment

A diagnosis of *mild cognitive impairment*, usually referred to as "MCI," requires a person to report thinking difficulties and to have a mild, measurable thinking impairment but to not have a decline in their ability to work or perform their everyday activities. People with MCI do not meet the criteria for dementia (described below). While impairment in the ability to form new memories is the most common measurable difficulty, thinking problems in other areas such as reasoning, judgment, and language are also common.

MCI increases the likelihood that a person will develop dementia in the future. In each year after the diagnosis of MCI has been made, 5 to 12 percent of people develop dementia, a rate about ten times greater than that of same-aged people in the general population. This means that after five years, 40 to 50 percent of people diagnosed with MCI either remain in the MCI category (that is, their symptoms have stayed the same) or have improved and returned to normal cognition. Presumably, people who had been diagnosed with MCI and then returned to normal after the diagnosis was made had a reversible cause of their thinking difficulties such as a short-term illness, a medication side effect, or depression.

Dementia

Dementia is the medical term for a group of symptoms defined by three characteristics: (1) two or more areas of intellectual ability are impaired to such a degree that daily functioning is interfered with, (2) the symptoms begin in adulthood, and (3) the person is awake and alert, not drowsy, intoxicated, or unable to pay attention.

The declines in intellectual functioning can affect any mental process. These include mathematical ability, vocabulary, abstract thinking, judgment, language, memory, and the ability to perform actions that have multiple steps. "Not feeling quite as sharp as you used to" does not mean that you are developing dementia. The person's ability must decline enough from what was normal for them to interfere with daily functioning. Dementia is different from what used to be called *mental retardation* and is now labelled *intellectual disability*. A person with intellectual disability is impaired from infancy, while a person who has dementia declines from their baseline thinking ability during adulthood.

Between 10 and 12 percent of people over age 65 suffer from dementia. At age 65 the rate is only about 1 percent, at age 75 the rate is about 10 percent, at age 80 the rate is 20 to 30 percent, and by age 90 the rate is 40 to 50 percent. Dementia beginning before age 60 is rare.

The symptoms of dementia can be caused by many diseases, probably more than one hundred. Some of these diseases are treatable, but many are not. In some of these diseases, the dementia can be stopped, in some it can be reversed, and in others its progression cannot be changed. Some of these diseases are rare. Others are more common but only rarely cause dementia. Do not assume that dementia is the inevitable result of having such a disease. However, some diseases, like Alzheimer disease, always cause dementia.

Most research indicates that about 50 to 60 percent of the cases of dementia are caused by Alzheimer disease, 10 percent are caused by vascular (multi-infarct) disease, 10 percent are caused by a combination of Alzheimer disease and vascular disease, 5 to 15 percent are due to Lewy body dementia, and 5 percent are caused by frontotemporal dementias. About 10 percent of the cases of dementia are caused by other conditions.

> Alzheimer disease and frontotemporal lobar degeneration always cause dementia. There are many other diseases that sometimes cause dementia.

This chapter describes the most common diseases, in alphabetical order, that cause dementia. Other brain disorders that impair thinking but do not cause dementia are discussed at the end of the chapter.

If you already have a diagnosis, you may want to read only the section describing the disease that you or the person you are caring for has.

Alcohol Use Disorder–Associated Dementia

People who have a history of drinking problems are at increased risk of developing dementia, though we don't know why. The cause may be a combination of multiple nutritional deficiencies, repeated head trauma from falls and fights, and, perhaps, the alcohol itself. The symptoms of dementia due to alcohol use disorder are usually different from those of Alzheimer disease. The person can express themselves well (language is rarely affected), but memory impairment, personality change, irritability, and explosiveness are common. These symptoms can be difficult and frustrating for families.

Therefore, it is important for caregivers to recognize these differences and try approaches aimed at this form of dementia.

The first step is to ensure that the person has been treated for their substance use disorder and no longer has access to alcohol. When there are questions about how disabled the person is or whether their behaviors are deliberate or manipulative, neuropsychological testing is helpful. If the family has painful memories of the person's misuse of alcohol, family counseling is helpful. The coping strategies that the family learned to use while the person was drinking heavily may no longer be appropriate when dementia enters the picture. Some aspects of dementia due to alcohol use disorder are reversible if the person abstains from alcohol, eats a well-balanced diet, takes thiamin (vitamin B1) supplements, and avoids head injury.

Alzheimer Disease

Alzheimer disease was first described by a German psychiatrist, Alois Alzheimer, in 1906, and the condition was named for him. The disease that Dr. Alzheimer originally described affected a woman in her 50s. It was initially called *presenile dementia* because she was so young. Clinicians now believe that the dementia that occurs in elderly people is the same as or very similar to the presenile condition, but younger onset cases are much more likely to have specific genetic causes. Regardless of the age of the person who has the disease, it is usually called *Alzheimer disease* (AD).

The symptoms of Alzheimer disease usually develop very gradually, even imperceptibly, so it is common that the beginnings of the disease are noted only in retrospect. Ultimately, most aspects of intellectual ability become impaired. Early in the illness, though, difficulty remembering new information is the problem most commonly noticed by people with the illness, as well as their family and doctors. They may forget appointments or conversations that had taken place several hours or days before. They may have difficulty with tasks that require abstract reasoning, such as making financial decisions. They may have trouble handling problems at work or may not enjoy reading as much as they used to. Their personality may change, or they may become depressed. An examination by a clinician knowledgeable about the illness will reveal impairments in more than just the person's memory, but these may not yet interfere with their daily functioning.

> **At the beginning of Alzheimer disease, memory impairment is the problem most frequently noticed by the person with the disease and by their family**

In the second stage of Alzheimer disease, impairments in three areas become noticeable: language (speaking) abilities, doing everyday activities, and perceiving or visually processing the world. These symptoms are often not recognized until the person has had the illness for three or so years. Language impairment often begins with difficulty finding the right word, the use of incorrect words, or trouble understanding explanations. In the second stage of

Alzheimer disease, people also have increasing difficulty doing tasks that once were "automatic," like brushing one's teeth, using eating utensils, dressing, and writing.

Late in the illness, usually after six or seven years, the person becomes severely impaired, both physically and cognitively. Incontinence and inability to walk are common, and falls become frequent. The person may be unable to say more than one or two words and may recognize no one or only one or two people. They become unable to plan responsibly and often require care from family and friends or from professionals.

Alzheimer disease usually leads to death in about ten or eleven years, but it may progress more quickly (three to four years) or more slowly (more than twenty years). Occasionally Alzheimer disease progresses slowly for years and then more rapidly. Typically, though, the disease progresses slowly but relentlessly.

Dr. Alzheimer described two changes in the physical makeup of the brain that can be seen under a microscope at autopsy: large numbers of abnormal structures called *neuritic plaques* and *neurofibrillary tangles*. These structures indicate that there has been direct damage to brain cells and their connections. Plaques are made up of an abnormal protein named beta amyloid (sometimes amyloid beta). Tangles consist of a protein called tau. Until recently, the identification of these abnormalities by autopsy after a person's death was the only way a definitive diagnosis of Alzheimer disease could be made.

PET scans have been developed that can detect the abnormal amyloid and tau proteins in the brain (see Chapters 2 and 18). However, many cognitively normal people over age 70 have amyloid in their brains. As a result, amyloid PET scans by themselves cannot be used to make a definite diagnosis after age 70. However, *before the age of 66*, a positive amyloid PET scan and symptoms of dementia accurately indicate Alzheimer disease. After age 65, the presence of *both* beta amyloid and tau on a PET scan in people with cognitive impairment is diagnostic of Alzheimer disease. Several blood tests and spinal fluid tests that measure these abnormal proteins have been developed, but, at present, they are less accurate than PET scans. Advances in these diagnostic techniques are occurring rapidly, and new blood and spinal fluid protein tests are likely to be available over the next several years.

At present, though, the diagnosis of Alzheimer disease in a living person over age 65 is based on the types of symptoms the person has, the way the symptoms have progressed over time, the absence of any other cause of the symptoms, and a normal brain CT scan or brain MRI. Refinement of PET scan and protein measurement technologies will likely revolutionize the diagnosis of Alzheimer disease in the next few years.

Amnestic (Korsakoff) Syndrome

Amnestic syndrome, previously called Korsakoff syndrome after the Russian psychiatrist who first described it, causes impairment that is limited to memory. Other aspects of thinking are not affected. Because amnestic syndrome affects only one area of mental function, it is not a true dementia.

Cerebral Amyloid Angiopathy

The beta amyloid protein that is found in Alzheimer disease can also be deposited in the walls of blood vessels. This weakens the blood vessel walls and causes repeated episodes of bleeding into the brain (hemorrhagic stroke), thus leading to vascular dementia. This disease runs in families and usually begins before age 60 (see "Young or Early Onset Dementia" on page 304).

Chronic Traumatic Encephalopathy

People who experience multiple concussions are at increased risk of developing dementia. The most common finding during an autopsy of people who have developed dementia after multiple concussions is chronic traumatic encephalopathy (CTE), which is defined as the presence of tangles and tau protein in specific areas of a deceased person's brain. The tangles are located in different areas than in Alzheimer disease.

CTE has been most widely studied in people who suffered concussions during contact sports such as American football, hockey, and soccer. Soldiers exposed to high-energy explosions are also at risk of developing CTE. It is not clear whether helmets or other protective headgear lower the risk of CTE in athletes or soldiers, but their use is still recommended.

Corticobasal Ganglionic Degeneration

Corticobasal ganglionic degeneration, sometimes referred to as CBD, is a rare cause of dementia that is now included in the group of tauopathy dementias (see "The Frontotemporal Dementias" and page 303). Early symptoms include clumsiness of one arm caused by an apraxia—an inability to perform movements with the arm even though its strength is normal. People with CBD are also stiff and have impaired memory.

Depression

Infrequently, depression is a cause of dementia. Symptoms of depression are usually obvious, but must be asked about. People with depression-induced dementia are very slowed down physically and mentally but do not have changes in language or perception. More often, depression is the earliest symptom of dementia that is due to a brain disease, such as Alzheimer disease, stroke, or Parkinson disease.

Treating depression often helps the person who has dementia enjoy life and may reduce distressing behavioral symptoms

---

People with Alzheimer disease, Lewy body dementia, dementia of Parkinson disease, or vascular dementia may experience symptoms of depression after the onset of dementia. They usually have problems with language or perception, symptoms suggesting that they have both depression and a neurodegenerative cause of dementia. *Depression should be treated whether or not the person has an irreversible dementia.* Do not allow a physician to dismiss depression as an expected problem. Treating depression in people who also have an irreversible dementia often relieves the person's misery, helps them enjoy

life more, and improves their appetite. Treating depression may also reduce distressing behavioral symptoms. However, keep in mind that while the person's depression may improve, their memory problems may not.

The Frontotemporal Dementias

Approximately 5 percent of people who have dementia have brain cell loss and brain shrinkage that is limited to the frontal lobes (the parts of the brain behind the forehead) or the temporal lobes (the parts of the brain underneath the temples). On a PET scan and at autopsy, abnormal deposits of the tau protein are present. This form of dementia is referred to as *frontotemporal dementia (FTD)*.

Diseases in which the frontal and temporal lobes of the brain are affected are now considered to be a group of several different illnesses, all of which are characterized by abnormalities in the tau protein and are thus called tauopathies (see page 313). When the disease process is mostly in these specific lobes of the brain, these diseases are referred to as *lobar dementia* or *frontotemporal lobar degeneration (FTLD)*. Other sections in this chapter describe corticobasal ganglionic degeneration and progressive supranuclear palsy, two other diseases included in the tauopathy category.

Today, two common forms of FTD are recognized. The *behavioral form* begins with obvious changes in personality and behavior, and it is these symptoms that bring people to have an evaluation. Memory impairment is often minimal, especially at the beginning of the illness. As a result, the beginnings of the disease are often attributed to stress, a "midlife crisis," or the desire for a change in work or family situation. In the disinhibited form of behavioral FTD, socially inappropriate behaviors such as making sexually indiscrete remarks, arguing with authority figures, or shoplifting can be the very first signs of the disease. Other people with the behavioral form of FTD develop severe apathy as a first symptom—they seem to withdraw from life and from previously enjoyed activities.

In the *language forms* of FTD, people develop the symptoms of several types of aphasia (see page 303) at the beginning of the disease. They may lose their "dictionary" and not be able to come up with words. They may speak fluently but in a difficult-to-comprehend manner because they lose their grammar. They may also lose their ability to understand the meanings of words.

On average, FTD progresses more rapidly than Alzheimer disease. The average person lives six to seven years with FTD, but the range is wide: some people live only three years while others live more than fifteen years. About one-third of people with FTD have a strong family history of dementia, often beginning in family members in their 50s or 60s.

HIV/AIDS Dementia

AIDS (acquired immunodeficiency syndrome) first appeared in the late 1970s. It is caused by a virus, the human immunodeficiency virus (HIV), which disables the immune system and prevents the body from eliminating the virus and other infections. Before therapies for

HIV were developed, people with HIV/AIDS died from infections and cancers that their immune system previously had been able to ward off.

HIV is spread through sexual intimacy and contact with infected blood or other body fluids. A common source of infection was the use of hypodermic needles used by someone infected with the virus. Today, all blood used for transfusions is tested for the virus, so transfusions are safe. Those most at risk of contracting the disease are people with multiple sexual partners, intravenous drug users, and children born to infected mothers.

Before the development of drugs that eliminate HIV from the bloodstream, AIDS usually led to death within several years. Currently, however, treatments for HIV are so effective that life expectancy for people who continue on treatment is thought to be normal.

Before the development of antiviral medications, people with AIDS often developed dementia. Today, HIV-related dementia is uncommon. It occurs in people who cannot or do not take the antiviral medications and those who are infected with forms of HIV that are resistant to medication. Dementia occurs when HIV infects the brain or when people develop parasitic, fungal, bacterial, or other viral infections of the brain or a cancer that invades the brain.

The dementia caused by HIV causes mental and physical slowness and difficulty accessing memory. If a person has a brain tumor or brain infection in a certain area, the symptoms depend on the location of the brain damage.

Huntington Disease

Huntington disease (HD) is characterized by abnormal choreiform (from the Greek word for "dance-like") movements of the body that the person cannot control. It also causes dementia that is characterized by prominent mental slowness, impaired executive function (planning and mental flexibility), and a family history of a similar illness. The average age of onset is 45, but the disease can begin in adolescence or as late as 70 years of age. HD is caused by an abnormal gene on chromosome 4 that leads to a disordered form of the protein called *huntingtin*. The disease is inherited in an autosomal dominant fashion, which means that inheriting just one copy of the abnormal gene causes the disease.

Lewy Body Dementia

Dementia with Lewy bodies (DLB) accounts for 5 to 15 percent of all cases of dementia. The Lewy body is a microscopic abnormality found in brain cells at autopsy. Originally these abnormal structures were thought to be present only in people with Parkinson disease, but in the late 1980s doctors discovered that some individuals with dementia have Lewy bodies spread throughout their brain.

The symptoms of DLB are a mixture of those seen in Alzheimer disease and the dementia of Parkinson disease. While some doctors doubt that DLB is a distinct condition, there are features that distinguish it from both Alzheimer dementia and the dementia of Parkinson disease. About 85 percent of people with DLB experience visual hallucinations, often as a very early symptom. People with DLB may have mild symptoms of Parkinson disease, but these symptoms only minimally respond to the therapies for Parkinson disease that are usually very effective. Also, many people with DLB experience periods of drowsiness that last for days.

People with Lewy body dementia experience severe adverse side effects from antipsychotic medications. These medicines should be avoided or used in the lowest possible dose if they are needed to treat delusions or hallucinations. Reassurance about the visual hallucinations ("I know you see little people, but that is part of your illness" or "I know you are upset about those little people in the house, but I have the situation under control") can help the person feel less frightened.

Parkinson-like symptoms (called "parkinsonism") include stiffness, slowness, poor balance, and frequent falls. Protecting people from the negative effects of falls (for example, by removing low coffee tables with sharp corners and providing a rolling walker) is important. The cautious use of the medication L-dopa (Sinemet) may help lessen these symptoms.

Parkinson Disease–Associated Dementia

Parkinson disease is a brain disorder characterized by four symptoms: a rest tremor (rhythmic shaking of the hands when the hands are on a table or in one's lap), generalized body stiffness and rigidity, slowness of movement (called "bradykinesia") and thinking (called "bradyphrenia"), and poor balance. The dementia caused by Parkinson disease begins one or more years after the onset of these physical symptoms.

Slowness of thinking, difficulty with recall rather than true inability to remember, difficulties in problem solving, and diminished mental flexibility are the main aspects of the dementia. Visual perception is often impaired early in the disease. Speed of thinking and ability to organize thoughts may be improved by anti-parkinson medications.

Primary Progressive Aphasia

The first symptom of primary progressive aphasia (PPA) is a loss of the ability to express oneself with words. This is experienced by the person as a frustrating inability to find the words they want to say. The most common cause of PPA is the language form of frontotemporal dementia. As the disease spreads from the language area of the brain to other brain regions, symptoms such as impaired memory, perception, and judgment develop. PPA is occasionally the first symptom of Alzheimer disease. In PPA, MRI and glucose PET scans usually show abnormalities only in the left temporal lobe.

Progressive Supranuclear Palsy

People who have progressive supranuclear palsy (PSP) have a rigid body posture and difficulty moving their eyes. The ability to move the eyes upward is often impaired or lost at the beginning of the illness.

The word *supranuclear* refers to the fact that the centers, or *nuclei*, that control eye movement do not function normally because the fibers that enter those nuclei from above ("supra") are not working properly. As a result, people are unable to look up, down, or sideways when asked.

The dementia of PSP is characterized by mental slowness and inflexibility. Memory is usually relatively normal at the beginning of the disease, but executive function (planning and mental flexibility) is often impaired. The rigid posture and poor balance of people with PSP often cause them to fall.

Traumatic Brain Injury (Head Trauma)

Trauma to the head can destroy brain tissue by directly killing brain cells, by impairing the nerve bundles that connect brain cells to one another, or by causing bleeding within the brain that then kills brain cells. Automobile and motorcycle accidents are common causes, but the repeated head traumas of contact sports can lead to traumatic brain injury (TBI) as well. Soldiers and marines exposed to improvised explosive devices (IEDs) can experience brain trauma even though the head is not penetrated by shrapnel. Presumably this is due to brain damage caused by the pressure wave of the explosion.

The symptoms of traumatic brain injury depend on where the damage occurs. Cognitive impairment, personality change, and behavior change can occur, especially after repeated concussions. Head trauma can also trigger Alzheimer disease and possibly frontotemporal dementia.

Head trauma sometimes causes bleeding to occur outside the brain but inside the skull. This can cause a large collection of blood to form between the lining of the brain that is attached to the skull and the brain. This is called a *subdural hematoma*. Because the skull is hard and does not expand under pressure, a subdural hematoma puts pressure on the brain. This can directly damage brain cells or push the brain downward through the small opening in the base of the skull that leads to the spinal cord. This can lead to death if not treated as an emergency. Even mild falls can cause such bleeding in older people. Subdural hematomas are treated by surgical removal of the blood clot.

Vascular Dementia

The word *vascular* refers to blood vessels. Vascular disease causes dementia when brain blood vessels clot off (called infarcts), burst (called hemorrhage), or become inflamed. Each of these events kills brain cells, and the cumulative effect of multiple small strokes leads to dementia. Brain vascular disease may also make a person more likely to develop Alzheimer disease, but we do not yet understand how this happens. Some people may independently have both Alzheimer disease and vascular disease.

The symptoms of vascular dementia depend on what areas of the brain have been damaged. Common problems include impairments in memory, coordination, and speech.

> The symptoms of vascular dementias depend on what areas of the brain have been damaged

Some vascular dementias progress as time passes, but others do not get any worse for years. Sometimes, the progression of vascular dementia can be stopped by preventing further strokes and by treating the disease causing the blood vessel inflammation.

The treatment of stroke has advanced significantly in recent years. Clots can be dissolved or removed surgically if discovered early enough. If the source of blood clots or the cause of inflammation is identified, treatment can prevent new strokes from occurring. By preventing further brain damage, these treatments can lower the risk of dementia and its progression.

Young or Early Onset Dementia

Different illnesses cause dementia in people under age 60. Between the ages of 40 and 60, half of the people who develop dementia have Alzheimer disease and a little less than half suffer from frontotemporal dementia. Other diseases explain about 10 percent of cases. In people younger than 40, dementia is likely to be due to an autoimmune disease that attacks the brain's blood vessels, an infection of the central nervous system, or a rare inherited disease.

The care issues in young onset dementia are often different than in people over age 65. Most individuals under age 60 are working, and many have children at home. These responsibilities raise care challenges that can be particularly difficult. The behavioral and psychiatric symptoms discussed throughout this book can also be especially upsetting in younger people who have dementia, particularly because these individuals may not have developed the long-term family relationships that link them with a caregiver. Disability regulations have been changed to make it easier for younger individuals with dementia to obtain Social Security Disability status, but financial challenges are still very common and difficult to overcome.

Other Brain Disorders

There are several diseases that impair thinking but are not dementias.

Delirium

The term *delirium* describes a set of symptoms that includes changes in the level of concentration and alertness in addition to difficulty thinking. Like the person who has dementia, the person who has delirium may be forgetful, disoriented, or unable to care for themselves, but unlike a person who has dementia, the person with delirium is drowsy, less alert, inattentive, and easily distracted. Delirium usually begins suddenly, while dementia, unless due to brain trauma, develops gradually over months or years. Other symptoms of delirium include misinterpretations of reality, false ideas, hallucinations, incoherent speech, wakefulness at night, and increased or decreased physical (motor) activity. The symptoms of delirium tend to vary throughout the day.

Delirium usually begins suddenly. Dementia usually develops gradually over months or years.

Delirium has many causes and is usually reversible if the cause is found. Medication side effects, infection, and dehydration or fluid overload are common causes. Constipation and urinary tract infections can cause delirium. Too much medication or drug interactions can cause delirium, even weeks after the medication was begun. When an older person is ill or hospitalized and becomes confused, the physician must address any possible cause of delirium before making a diagnosis of dementia.

People who have dementia are more likely than other people to develop delirium. The sudden worsening of a person who has dementia should raise delirium as a possible cause.

Delirium is often treatable and usually reversible

Irritability, drowsiness, incontinence, agitation, and fearfulness may all be due to delirium—one of these symptoms may be the only noticeable indication that there is a problem. You may notice an increase or decrease in activity, a decreased level of alertness, or an increase or decrease in the amount of movement or motor activity. Visual hallucinations are common in delirium.

Stroke and Other Localized Brain Injury

Sometimes damage to the brain may be limited to one area, or "localized." This damage can be caused by brain tumors, strokes, or head injuries. Even though is it localized, such damage may affect more than one mental function. The symptoms can tell a neurologist just where the damage is. A localized injury is called a *focal brain lesion*. When the damage is widespread ("generalized"), the symptoms may indicate dementia.

> **Many people who have had a stroke improve significantly with rehabilitation**

Major *stroke*, which causes such symptoms as sudden paralysis of one side of the body, drooping of one side of the face, or speech problems, is an injury to part of the brain. Strokes can be caused by a blood clot blocking vessels in the brain or by the bursting of a blood vessel in the brain that leads to bleeding within the brain. Immediate treatment is important. Sometimes the brain cells are injured or impaired by swelling but can recover when the swelling goes down. Recovery may also occur when other parts of the brain gradually learn to do the jobs of the damaged sections of the brain.

Many people who have had a stroke can get better. They need to have rehabilitation training, which increases the likelihood of recovery and makes the remaining impairment less severe. Recovery can continue to take place over several years. The chance of having another stroke can be reduced by good medical management.

Transient Ischemic Attack

A transient ischemic attack (TIA) is a *temporary* impairment of brain function that is due to an insufficient supply of blood to part of the brain. The person may be unable to speak or may have slurred speech. They may be weak or paralyzed, dizzy, or nauseated. These symptoms last only a few minutes or hours and then totally resolve (go away) on their own. This is in contrast to a stroke, which has the same symptoms but results in long-lasting impairments. Improvements in brain MRI techniques have shown that permanent brain damage might occur even when the symptoms fully resolve.

TIAs should be regarded as warnings of stroke. Getting to an emergency room when the symptoms begin is crucial since "clot-busting" drugs are effective only when administered within twenty-four hours of the start of symptoms. Doctors will also search for a cause for the TIA since knowing the cause can significantly lower the risk of future strokes.

> **TIAs should be regarded as warnings of stroke. Prompt medical attention is essential.**

Transient global amnesia is a type of TIA in which a person has a brief (up to several hours) period of confusion. Even if there is full recovery, the person should be taken to an emergency room for immediate evaluation.

CHAPTER 18

Research in Dementia

We have reached an exciting point in dementia research. Not long ago, most people assumed that dementia was an expected result of aging, and only a few pioneers were interested in studying it. In the past forty years, that situation has changed. We now know the following about dementia:

- Dementia is not the natural result of aging.

- Dementia is caused by specific, identifiable diseases.

- Different protein abnormalities are the causes of each of the neurodegenerative dementias.

- Diagnosis is important to identify treatable conditions and guide treatment.

- A thorough evaluation is crucial for guiding the management of diseases that are not currently curable.

Today, research is focused on identifying causes and treatments of the specific diseases that cause dementia (see Chapter 17). Newly developed tools have allowed a much clearer look at what goes on in the brain during usual aging and during disease. Because of better public understanding, the demand for solutions is growing.

This chapter is more technical than earlier chapters in the book. We suggest that you read it when you are relaxed, or skip it if you wish.

Research is being carried out throughout the world. In the United States, research is primarily funded by the National Institute on Aging (NIA), the National Institute of Neurological Disorders and Stroke (NINDS), and the Department of Veterans Affairs (VA). The NIA has funded Alzheimer's Disease Centers, which pull together talented researchers, and much exciting work is taking place in these centers. Additional research funds come from individual donors, foundations, and pharmaceutical companies. Unfortunately, many potentially productive research projects go unfunded each year.

Understanding Research

The increased public awareness of Alzheimer disease has been accom-panied by an ever-increasing number of announcements of "breakthroughs" and "cures." Some of these are important building blocks in the search for a cure, but each breakthrough, in itself, is but one small step in the direction of a cure.

Understanding the therapeutic implications of the research can challenge scientists and families alike. Here are some things you need to know about research to help you understand what you read:

- Research scientists need to make their findings public, and the public wants to know what researchers are finding. The enthusiasm of the press in publicizing these findings plays an important role in maintaining public support for research funds. And yet, families are discouraged when the press makes announcements of "breakthroughs" that turn out to be disappointing.

- Science must go down some blind alleys. For a while, something will look like a good lead, and families and scientists will be excited. Then the trail will go cold. This is frustrating, but each time we rule out something, there is one less avenue to investigate. Many clues, like the pieces of a jigsaw puzzle, will eventually fit together to form the answer, but the pieces often do not go where we thought they would.

- Conditions like Alzheimer disease are different from infectious diseases, such as diphtheria, chickenpox, and polio. Each infectious disease has one cause, a specific infectious agent, leading to one outcome. Alzheimer disease has several, and perhaps many, causes.

In this way it is a family of diseases, like cancer. This explains some of the variability of the disease from one person to another. It may take a combination of several triggers for a person to develop the disease, and the disease is likely to have different triggers in different people, but in general the multiple causes lead to similar symptoms. As a result, researchers will have to track down several causes and treatments.

- It is essential that studies eliminate the influence of other factors. Sometimes when a new technique or drug is tried, the patient seems to improve. Sometimes families who participate in drug studies believe that their family member got better while taking the treatment, but when a well-designed study is done, it is found that people who received a placebo or sham treatment had the same amount of improvement. There are many reasons why this happens, from wishful thinking on the part of the researchers doing the study and on the part of the families, to cheering up the patient by giving them hope, to temporarily brightening the patient's thinking because of the added attention that comes with a research study or the prescription of a new therapy. This is called the placebo effect, and it is quite common, even in studies of surgery. Good studies of drugs and other therapies must be carefully designed to eliminate the possibility that other factors cause improvement.

- Preliminary treatment trials are usually carried out on small groups of people. The small size of the sample of patients increases the chances that extraneous factors not related to the treatment will confuse the outcome, but safety concerns require that only a small number of people be exposed to an untested treatment at the start of its development. If you hear of exciting results from a small-group study, remember that these results may or may not be confirmed by tests on a large group of people or by tests done by another researcher.

- Just because two factors occur together does not mean that one causes the other. Both A and B might be found in the brains of people who have dementia, but this does not mean that A caused B. A and B might both have been caused by an unknown factor, C. It may be years before the relationships among these disease factors are understood.

- The medications being developed that target the brain of a person who has Alzheimer disease are likely to cause serious side effects throughout the body. Sometimes research on such drugs must be stopped because the potential damage to other organs outweighs their therapeutic value.

- Animal research allows scientists to learn how the brain works and to test the safety of drugs in animals before they are given to humans. Studying animal species that age faster than humans provides answers more quickly than studies in humans. The federal government has strict laws to ensure that animals will be treated humanely. Researchers who work with animals take into account the ways in which the animals' reactions to treatments are similar to human reactions and the ways in which they are not. Giving large doses of a chemical to an animal with a short life span magnifies the chances of seeing a relationship, if one exists, between the chemical and a disease. Computer models help, but they do not replace animal research.

- The NIA and the Alzheimer's Association release reports on major breakthroughs and on highly publicized claims. These reports are available on their websites and are intended to provide families with accurate information. An excellent source of information about research breakthroughs is the National Institute on Aging's website on Alzheimer disease and related dementias (www.alzheimers.gov).

Bogus Cures

Some unscrupulous individuals promote "cures" that can be expensive, dangerous, or ineffective. These unfairly raise hopes. The Alzheimer's Association has a list of some of the fraudulent products and treatments and can advise you about which treatments are generally believed by doctors to be of little or no value. If a treatment makes a claim of benefit or cure that exceeds what the National Institute on Aging or Alzheimer's Association says is possible, we urge you to check it out thoroughly before considering using it.

Research in Vascular Dementia and Stroke

Multiple strokes are the second most common cause of dementia. Stroke frequency has decreased worldwide by 30 to 50 percent in the past half century, and this drop in the number of strokes may have contributed to a declining rate of dementia in some countries. If even better ways can be found to prevent strokes and blood vessel disease, many thousands of people will benefit.

> Rehabilitation therapy generally maximizes the amount of recovery that occurs after stroke. Recovery after stroke can continue for several years.

The risk factors for stroke include high blood pressure, high cholesterol and low-density lipids, obesity, diabetes, diets high in animal fat and salt, smoking, and heart disease. These factors also increase a person's vulnerability to vascular dementia. Direct treatment of these risk factors has been shown to lower the risk of stroke. Physical exercise has also been shown to lower the risk.

Researchers are also studying the changes in brain chemistry that take place during and immediately after a stroke. The hope is that drugs that block the release of destructive chemicals can lessen the amount of brain tissue that is destroyed. Researchers are also learning how, when, and to what extent specific rehabilitative training helps the brain reorganize more effectively to reverse the brain damage. It now seems clear that recovery from stroke can continue for several years, and there is accumulating evidence that rehabilitation therapy maximizes the amount of recovery that occurs.

Scientists have found that depression is common after a stroke, even when there is minimal physical impairment. This is important because this depression has been shown to respond to standard therapies for depression, such as medication and psychotherapy.

Research in Alzheimer Disease

Structural Changes in the Brain

When Alois Alzheimer looked at tissue taken from the brain of a woman who had the behavioral symptoms of dementia, he saw microscopic changes called neuritic plaques and neurofibrillary tangles. Similar structures are found in much smaller numbers in the brains of older people who do not have dementia. Scientists are analyzing the structure and chemistry of these plaques and tangles for clues to their formation and their role in the disease.

Brain Cells

The brain is made of billions of neurons, or nerve cells. These connect with other cells near and far, and these connections carry out the tasks of thinking, remembering, feeling emotions, and directing body movement. Other types of cells in the brain support and maintain the function of the neurons, fight infection, and repair injury.

One of the intriguing aspects of the different degenerative diseases such as Alzheimer disease, frontotemporal dementia, Parkinson disease, Huntington disease, and progressive supranuclear palsy is that each disease starts in a different set of nerve cells in a single different site in the brain and then seems to spread. For example, scientists have known for many years that a small area deep in the brain called the hippocampus loses many of its cells early in the course of Alzheimer disease. As the disease progresses, cells in other areas die in a predictable pattern that parallels the progression of the symptoms of the disease.

Neuroplasticity

The term *plasticity* is used to describe the ability of the nervous system to change. One of the great discoveries of the twentieth century was the demonstration that the brain can make new cells, even in old age. Prior to that discovery, it was thought that no new brain cells formed after brain development was completed early in life.

Equally important is the finding that brain cells can make new connections throughout life. This offers the hope that people can recover from dementia, even if some brain cells have died. Learning how new connections and new cells form in the brain is a major focus of research.

Neurotransmitters

Chemicals in the brain called *neurotransmitters* pass messages from one nerve cell to the next. These neurotransmitters are made, used, and broken down within the brain. There are many different neurotransmitters for different types of cells and probably for different kinds of mental tasks. In some diseases, there is less than the normal amount of certain neurotransmitters. For example, a person who has Parkinson disease produces abnormally low amounts of the neurotransmitter dopamine in an area of the brain called the substantia nigra because cells in that area die. The drug L-dopa increases the amount of dopamine and can dramatically improve the symptoms of Parkinson disease.

Scientists have found that people who have Alzheimer disease have deficiencies in several neurotransmitters, particularly acetylcholine. Somatostatin, norepinephrine, serotonin, corticotrophin-releasing factor, and substance P may also be deficient. It is likely that different people have deficits in different neurotransmitters. This may account for the variation in symptoms among people who have Alzheimer disease. One way that scientists have attempted to reverse Alzheimer disease is to find medications that increase the amount of acetylcholine and the other deficient neurotransmitters in the brain. However, this cannot cure the disease because it only replaces what is missing and does not stop the process that is killing brain cells. The same is true in Parkinson disease.

Electrical Signaling

Brain cells also communicate with each other through electrical signals, especially over long distances in the brain. Some scientists are exploring whether more direct electrical stimulation can enhance brain function and recovery from injury.

Abnormal Proteins

Proteins are one of the main components of the cells that make up the human body. The body takes food, breaks it down into amino acids, and then builds the proteins that it needs. The microscopic abnormalities of the brain that are characteristic of many of the diseases that cause dementia are made up of altered proteins. These include the plaques and tangles of Alzheimer disease, the Pick body seen in the brains of some people with frontotemporal dementia, the Lewy body found in Parkinson disease and in dementia with Lewy bodies, and the prion of Creutzfeldt–Jakob disease. If the deposits of these abnormal proteins are the cause of any or all of these diseases, then the removal or prevention of these protein deposits might treat or prevent the disease.

Researchers are exploring the possibility that it is the abnormal folding of these proteins that triggers or causes each of these diseases. For example,

abnormal deposits of a protein called beta amyloid are found in the brains of people who have Alzheimer disease. The microscopic neuritic plaques characteristic of Alzheimer disease have beta amyloid at their center, and some people who have Alzheimer disease have deposits of amyloid along blood vessels in their brain. If abnormal protein folding leads to the structural abnormalities seen in each disease, then the prevention of this folding or the removal of the abnormally folded protein might be an effective treatment or prevention. We know that the production of beta amyloid is controlled by a gene on chromosome 21, but the function of this protein is yet to be determined. The possibility that it is part of the body's immune response to foreign invaders is discussed below.

One theory that has received a lot of attention is that some people produce a breakdown product of the beta amyloid protein that the body cannot dispose of normally. The process of breaking down and disposing of amyloid is controlled by several enzymes that naturally occur in brain cells. Since one enzyme cuts the amyloid into pieces that can be removed and another enzyme cuts the amyloid into a piece that cannot be removed, the theory is that people who accumulate the non-removeable pieces go on to develop Alzheimer disease. Many of the drugs being tested to treat or prevent Alzheimer disease aim to do one of three things: remove the undesirable pieces of the amyloid protein, decrease the production of the undesirable protein, or increase the production of the desirable protein.

Abnormal Proteins within Brain Cells

Brain cells contain proteins that act like highways for chemicals to travel along. Some people who have Alzheimer disease appear to have abnormal forms of these proteins. Among these are tau protein and MAP (microtubule-associated protein). Many researchers believe that these abnormal proteins form after the amyloid protein abnormalities discussed above appear and must somehow be caused by them. These proteins are the basis of the microscopic neurofibrillary tangles that are present in the brains of people who die from Alzheimer disease.

Abnormal tau proteins are also found in frontotemporal dementia and progressive supranuclear palsy. Some people who have frontotemporal dementia inherit abnormal forms of several genes on chromosome 17 that are involved in the production of tau. This knowledge about the genetic component of the disease has led to research into drugs that remove the abnormal forms of the protein.

In Parkinson disease, the abnormal protein is called synuclein, and it collects in abnormal structures called Lewy bodies. Genetic changes have been found in a number of different genes in approximately 60 percent of people who have Parkinson disease. Some of these gene changes occur after birth, because it is uncommon for Parkinson disease to run in families. It is hoped that studying these different genetic abnormalities will lead to findings that are relevant to all people who have the disease.

Nerve Growth Factors

Cells within the brain and the spinal cord (as well as nerve cells outside the central nervous system) develop in specific patterns that are directed by proteins called nerve growth factors. It has long been known that nerves outside the central nervous system (called peripheral nerves) can regrow or regenerate after an injury. Since the recent discovery that new cells form and new connections are made in the brain throughout life, scientists have been studying whether the nerve growth factors that direct this process might become deficient and lead to dementia. They are also studying whether the nerve growth factors can be used to stimulate the replacement or regrowth of damaged brain cells and whether this would lead to new connections between cells in the brains of people who have different causes of dementia.

Infection

For many years, a small group of researchers has been studying whether bacteria, viruses, or fungi might trigger Alzheimer disease. There has been little support in the research community for this idea until recently. This skepticism has diminished since the discovery by several researchers that the amyloid protein might be part of the body's early immune response to foreign invaders such as bacteria. This suggests that the deposits of amyloid in the brains of people with Alzheimer disease begin when the amyloid surrounds the invading organism. Another theory being considered is that after the infectious organism has been contained by the amyloid for many years, it escapes the control of an aging immune system and then triggers further deposition of amyloid that continues to destroy brain tissue over time.

Prions

Prions (*proteinaceous infectious parti-cles*) are abnormal forms of a normally occurring small protein that have been shown to cause several rare dementias, including Creutzfeldt–Jakob disease, kuru, and bovine spongiform enceph-alopathy (or "mad cow" disease). It has previously been suggested that these particles or something similar might be a cause of Alzheimer disease or that the mechanism by which prion diseases spread throughout the brain might be similar to the way protein abnormali-ties spread in other neurodegenerative dementias. It now seems quite unlikely that prions are directly involved in Alz-heimer disease.

There have been many efforts to determine whether Alzheimer disease is infectious, that is, whether it can be transmitted to another person. At pres-ent there is no evidence to support the idea that Alzheimer disease is caused by a slow-acting virus, prion, or any other infectious organism.

However, what has been found is that the beta amyloid protein and the synuclein protein, when injected into animals, can cause the formation of other toxic amyloid and synuclein proteins. These altered proteins then damage other healthy cells. This is sim-ilar to the way prions spread through-out the brain. Scientists studying this process hope that treatments can be developed that would stop this method of spread and so prevent the death of brain cells in these diseases.

Brain (or Stem) Cell Transplants

The possibility of replacing damaged brain cells by transplanting new cells has generated much excitement in recent years. Since many dementias begin in a very specific area of the brain and initially affect a single type of cell, scientists believe it may be possible to replace and regrow the cellular systems specific to each disease. Work in ani-mals has shown that certain cells grown in the laboratory will reproduce and make neurotransmitters when they are transplanted into animals with brain damage. Some of these cells have been derived from stem cells, a type of cell that has the potential to form many dif-ferent types of cells. For example, skin stem cells are what replace damaged or dead skin cells.

Several experimental studies are un-derway to assess whether this will work in people who have Alzheimer disease. However, many experts are doubtful that transplanting brain tissue will re-verse the damage caused by Alzheimer disease after it has become widespread. It may be possible and even desirable to take cells from a living person and "reprogram" them to replace the spe-cific cells in the person's brain that are abnormal or have died. Whether such cells would replace damaged brain cir-cuits remains to be shown.

Metals

Aluminum has been found in larger-than-expected amounts in the brains of some people who have Alzheimer disease, and for years there was concern that it might be a cause of Alzheimer disease. Other metals, for example, manganese, are known to cause other forms of dementia. It now seems most likely that the presence of aluminum is a result of whatever is causing the dementia rather than being a cause itself. People sometimes wonder if they should stop taking antacids, cooking with aluminum pans, or using deodorant (all sources of aluminum). There is no evidence that the use of these items is a cause of dementia. Studies of people who have been exposed to much larger amounts of aluminum indicate that exposure does not lead to Alzheimer disease. Treatments that promote the elimination of aluminum from the body do not benefit people who have Alzheimer disease, and some of these treatments have serious side effects.

Immune System Defects

The immune system is the body's defense against infection. Studies show that some of the proteins the body uses to fight infection are present in the brain around the neuritic plaques that characterize Alzheimer disease.

Sometimes the body's defense system, which is designed to attack outside organisms such as bacteria and viruses, goes awry and attacks the person's own cells. One theory proposes that an initial abnormality, such as deposits of the beta amyloid protein, triggers an inflammatory reaction that then causes further brain damage. This "cascade theory" suggests that the progression of Alzheimer disease could be slowed or stopped by interrupting the inflammatory response and thereby

stopping this cascade, even though the initial damage is still occurring. So far, anti-inflammatory medications have not been found to halt or slow down Alzheimer disease once it has started, but it remains possible that specific aspects of the body's immune system have to be targeted to prevent or delay the onset of dementia.

Head Trauma

It has been known for almost a century that some boxers develop a dementia similar to Alzheimer disease and have tangles, but not plaques, in their brain at autopsy. The condition was called "punch-drunk" syndrome or *dementia pugilistica*. Today this form of dementia is referred to as chronic traumatic encephalopathy and is linked to repeated concussions (see page 299).

Drug Studies

Hundreds of drugs are being studied for their effect on Alzheimer disease and other dementias. Most of them are quickly found to be ineffective or to have toxic side effects. A few make the news because of preliminary evidence that they reduce symptoms.

Several drugs have been developed that slow or prevent the breakdown of acetylcholine (one of the neurotransmitters that is deficient in the brains of people who have Alzheimer disease). These drugs (donepezil, galantamine, and rivastigmine) temporarily improve cognitive function, but the disease appears to continue progressing at the same rate. These three drugs have been available for many years. They are equally effective but differ in their side effects. Another drug, memantine, is thought to work by blocking the toxic effects of another brain neurotransmitter called GABA. However, there is no evidence that any of these drugs prevent the death of brain cells or slow down the process that causes the disease.

Since these drugs do not slow down or reverse the damage that causes dementia, scientists have shifted their focus to removing or preventing the formation of the abnormal proteins that characterize Alzheimer disease as well as those that are found in frontotemporal dementia and Lewy body dementia. One drug, aducanumab (Aduhelm), which removes one of the proteins thought to cause the disease, has been approved by the FDA to treat mild cognitive impairment and early Alzheimer disease (see pages 293–94).

Epidemiology

Epidemiology is the study of the distribution of diseases in large groups of people. Studying the epidemiology of illnesses that cause dementia can identify links between a disease and factors in the environment. So far, Alzheimer disease has been found in all groups of people whose members live long enough to reach late life. Being older is the strongest risk factor for developing dementia and Alzheimer disease. Many epidemiological studies suggest that being a woman, having less education, having higher blood pressure in midlife, having diabetes, and having a family history of dementia increase the likelihood that a person will develop Alzheimer disease. Having depression earlier in life and being hearing impaired are other possible risk factors for developing dementia. This does *not* mean that people who have these risk factors will get the disease, only that they are more likely to get the disease than a person without those factors. Some epidemiological studies have found that people who have more education and have been more physically active are less likely to develop dementia. None of these findings proves that these factors are causative. Rather, they are clues that must be followed up—such linkages need to be either proved or disproved by other scientific approaches.

> The likelihood that a person will develop Alzheimer disease is higher for women and those with less education, higher blood pressure in midlife, diabetes, and a family history of dementia

Down Syndrome

People with Down syndrome, the most common genetic cause of intellectual disability, develop plaques and tangles identical to those of Alzheimer disease before they reach their 40s. Many people with Down syndrome develop dementia before age 60. Down syndrome is caused by having an extra chromosome 21 or an extra piece of this chromosome. This fact along with the finding that the gene that makes the amyloid protein is located within the area of chromosome 21 that causes Down syndrome has reinforced the importance of the role of the amyloid protein in the development of Alzheimer disease.

Aging

Living into old age is the greatest risk factor for developing Alzheimer disease. Why this is so remains one of the great mysteries of the disease. The risk that an adult will develop Alzheimer disease in the next year is about one-quarter of a percent per year at age 65, and this risk doubles every five years thereafter. As a result, at age 80 the risk of developing Alzheimer disease in the next year is 4 percent. Even at age 80, though, statistics show that 70 to 80 percent of people have normal or nearly normal intellectual function.

Heredity and Dementia

Some of the most stunning advances in dementia disease research have been in the area of genetics. Families often worry that this disease is inherited and that they or their children will develop it. As you learn about the genetics of Alzheimer disease, keep in mind that genes work in two general ways.

Some genes *directly cause disease* in everyone who inherits that gene. If you inherit that gene you will develop the disease if you live long enough. For Alzheimer disease, three such disease genes have been identified. These genes, located on chromosomes 1, 14, and 21, account for about half of the people whose illness began before age 60. Because it is uncommon for people to develop Alzheimer disease this young, these genetic abnormalities account for less than 2 percent of all cases of Alzheimer disease. By studying these rare cases, scientists hope to discover disease processes that may be responsible for the majority of the cases of Alzheimer disease.

For frontotemporal dementia, three other genes cause about one-third of cases, while several others cause a small percentage of cases. All people with Huntington disease inherit an abnormal form of a gene located on chromosome 4. For Parkinson disease, only a small percentage of cases are caused by inherited abnormal genes.

The second way that disease genes work is to *increase the risk* of developing the disease. "At risk" means that the person is more likely than other people to develop the disease, but it does not mean that a specific person will get the disease. "At risk" does not mean "for sure."

Inheriting an "at-risk" gene increases the chance that you will develop a disease but does not guarantee it

---

People who know they are at risk of developing a disease, even if it is an increased genetic risk, may be able to take steps to reduce the likelihood of getting that disease. For example, blood cholesterol and low-density lipids (LDL) are under strong genetic control. If you have a blood test and learn that you have high blood cholesterol or high LDL, you are at increased risk of having a heart attack or stroke. Changing your diet and/or taking medication can lower your cholesterol and LDL, and thereby reduce your risk of having a heart attack or stroke.

Scientists are identifying the genes that are involved in Alzheimer disease. One gene on chromosome 19 influences the likelihood that an individual will develop Alzheimer disease but does not cause the disease. This gene, the APOE gene, is by far the best studied. It exists in three forms: epsilon 2, epsilon 3, and epsilon 4. These are normal variants of the APOE gene. Since everyone inherits one copy of each gene from each parent, we all have two copies of each gene. That means each of us has a combination of two of the epsilon 2, epsilon 3, and epsilon 4 forms of the APOE gene.

People who inherit one copy of the epsilon 4 form of the gene have a two to three times greater likelihood of developing Alzheimer disease. Those who inherit two copies of the epsilon 4 gene, less than 5 percent of the population, have a twelve to fifteen times increased risk. People who inherit the epsilon 2 form of the gene are protected against Alzheimer disease.

A helpful way to understand this complex inheritance is to consider the risk of developing Alzheimer disease by age 80, when the overall population risk of developing the disease is 20 to 30 percent. An 80-year-old who has *one copy* of the epsilon 4 form of the gene has a 40 to 45 percent chance of having Alzheimer disease. Those *without* a copy of the epsilon 4 form of the gene have a 15 percent chance of having the illness.

Genetic tests that help trace your ancestry can identify which forms of the APOE gene you have inherited. You should consider whether you want to know this before taking such a test.

Another forty genes have been identified that increase the risk of developing Alzheimer disease, each by less than 1 percent. Researchers hope that discovering *how* these genes increase the risk will lead them to potential treatments.

> **If you decide to have genetic testing, meet with a genetic counselor first so you understand what the tests can and cannot tell you**

In frontotemporal dementia, gene abnormalities on chromosome 17 explain about one-third of cases. In Parkinson disease, 60 percent of cases have been linked to genetic abnormalities, but it is not clear whether these abnormalities are inherited or occur after birth.

All cases of dementia due to Huntington disease are caused by a genetic abnormality on chromosome 4. Everyone who inherits one copy of the abnormal gene will develop the disease unless they die of some other condition before the disease begins.

We recommend that individuals with a strong family history of dementia or Alzheimer disease contact a research center if they are concerned about their own risk. People undergoing genetic testing should meet with a genetic counselor before the testing is done to make sure they understand the implications and limitations of the genetic tests.

In the past, genetic factors and environmental factors were considered to be totally distinct. Scientists now recognize that they interact with each other in ways that are yet to be understood. Prevention of dementia is likely to involve addressing the contributions of both types of factors.

Sex

It is now clear that a greater percentage of women have Alzheimer disease than men at every age. The reason for this higher rate is not known.

Neuropsychological Testing

Neuropsychologists use standardized questions, tasks, and observation to evaluate people and determine whether they have experienced a decline in cognitive ability and to identify the level at which the person is currently able to function. They use these tests to identify the kinds of mental skills a person has retained and those that the person has lost. This information can help family members and clinicians come up with plans to help a person with dementia use their remaining skills and place fewer demands on their diminished abilities. Information from neuropsychological testing can help family members understand why a person is unable to do some things but successfully do similar activities. Neuropsychological testing can also confirm a diagnosis when there is doubt about whether a person has actually experienced a decline in their abilities.

It has long been known that different parts of the brain carry out different mental tasks (remembering, moving an

Standardized questions, tasks, and observation are used by neuropsychologists to identify the mental skills that are impaired and those that are still intact

arm, talking, experiencing fear, and so forth) and that still other parts coordinate these mental activities. By identifying what areas of the brain are afflicted most severely, neuropsychological evaluations and brain scans give researchers information about the disease and give clinicians and families information about how to provide good care.

Brain Imaging

CT (computerized tomography) scans, also called CAT scans, use multiple X-rays to visualize the tissue of the brain. MRI (magnetic resonance imaging) visualizes the tissues of the brain by briefly generating a very strong magnetic field. MRI can also be used to assess blood flow in the brain and to examine how brain cells are working.

PET (positron emission tomography) scans provide pictures of the working brain in two ways. First, they can show how much oxygen or glucose (blood sugar) brain cells are using and pro-

vide a picture of how well areas of the brain are working at rest and when stimulated to carry out specific mental activities. Second, PET scans can be performed with radioactive tracers that identify normal and abnormal proteins in the brain. In recent years tracers have been developed that identify beta amyloid and tau in the brain. They are being used to diagnose Alzheimer disease (see page 299) and to determine if experimental therapies decrease the amount of the abnormal proteins in the brain.

Keeping Physically and Mentally Active

People often wonder if remaining mentally, socially, and physically active prevents dementia (see Chapter 16). Many studies have found that people who do not have dementia were mentally and physically more active than people of the same age with dementia. This does not prove that activity was the factor that held off dementia for a time, though. It is possible that the lower levels of physical, social, or mental activity in the people with dementia were the earliest symptoms of the disease, symptoms present even years before the disease itself was recognized. Nonetheless, even without absolute proof that keeping mentally or physically active prevents or alters the course of Alzheimer disease, it is clear that physical and mental activity help maintain general health and improve one's quality of life.

A number of studies have shown that people with more education are less likely to develop dementia, but it is unclear whether this is because dementia is harder to detect in better-educated individuals. Similarly, some studies have found that those who retire are at greater risk of developing dementia than people of the same age who do not retire. Further study has shown that some individuals retire because they are in the early stages of dementia.

Continuing to exercise after Alzheimer disease develops may slow the progress of the disease and help a person remain active longer (see "Exercise" in Chapter 5).

The Effect of Acute Illness on Dementia

Sometimes people appear to develop dementia after a serious illness, hospitalization, anesthesia, or surgery. The evidence that any of these factors induces Alzheimer disease or alters its course is weak. Close examination usually shows that the dementia had begun, but was unrecognized, before the person had the surgery or illness. However, stroke and other diseases that directly affect the brain can trigger or further worsen a preexisting dementia. The most likely reason that people develop sudden cognitive worsening after a serious illness, hospitalization, anesthesia, or surgery is that people who have dementia are at high risk of developing a delirium (see page 305). By making the person's thinking temporarily worse, delirium can cause a mild dementia to become noticeable for the first time. Preexisting brain impairment due to mild dementia also makes recovery after an acute illness or surgery more difficult.

> **Even mild dementia can make recovery after an acute illness or surgery more difficult**

Many people report the onset or worsening of dementia after anesthesia. This is an active area of research, but the evidence that anesthesia is a cause of dementia appears minimal. Many studies have found that people undergoing heart surgery are at increased risk of developing dementia five or ten years after the surgery. It now appears that this increased rate of dementia is due to the vascular disease that led to the surgery rather than to the surgery or anesthesia itself.

Research into the Delivery of Services

Studies that tell us how to help people who have dementia live comfortable, satisfying lives despite their disease and studies that tell us how to assist the families who care for them will remain important until all types of dementia can be prevented or cured. This research has already shown how to improve the quality of life for people who have dementia and help them remain as functional as possible. This research has influenced many of the ideas we present in this book. For example, research has shown that people who had previously paced, screamed, and struck out became relaxed and had fewer distressing and disrupting behaviors when they participated in enjoyable activities.

We know that families need help: day care, home respite, support groups, and other assistance can make a positive difference. Researchers are studying how best to reach families, what things families need most, how to encourage families to use respite services, and the most cost-effective ways to provide respite. While it may seem that the answers to these questions are obvious, different kinds of families have different needs, and people do not always do what researchers predict they will do. Careful study will prevent people from wasting money on unnecessary services and keep services from going unused because families do not know about them.

> **We improve the quality of life in people who have dementia by helping them function as well as possible, reducing their anxiety and fear, and helping them enjoy their lives**

Protective Factors

Prevention is the ultimate goal of medicine. Identifying environmental, physical, and genetic factors that lower the risk of dementia might lead to strategies for both individuals and populations that prevent dementia from ever developing. Among the areas being explored are diet; physical, social, and mental activity; avoidance of stress; reversal of hearing loss; more aggressive treatment of blood pressure, diabetes, excess weight, and undesirable blood lipids; and treatments that enhance protective genetic factors. Several studies suggest that low cholesterol, small amounts of alcohol, and the use of protective headgear when doing activities that carry a risk of head injury might protect against or delay the onset of Alzheimer disease. Drug approaches to prevention include studying drugs that remove or prevent the formation of the abnormal amyloid and tau proteins that characterize the brains of people with Alzheimer disease. It may be that people who are genetically susceptible to Alzheimer disease will be able to lower their risk if they adopt preventive strategies to modify their environmental triggers. Good research is the only way to find out whether any of these approaches can prevent or delay the onset of the diseases discussed in this book.

One Disease or Many?

Although we often discuss Alzheimer disease as if it were a single disease, it clearly has multiple causes. As we discussed in this chapter (see pages 317–18), three different gene abnormalities cause Alzheimer disease in every person who inherits one of those genes, and at least forty other gene variants increase the risk of developing Alzheimer disease. Together, these genetic causes explain 40 to 70 percent of the risk of developing Alzheimer disease. This means that 30 to 60 percent of the risk is caused by environmental factors or by interactions between the environment and genes. Even though Alzheimer disease has multiple causes, one or several approaches might prevent or treat the disease no matter what the original trigger. It is also possible that each different cause will require its own therapy. While we wait for science to answer these important questions, the approaches described in this book can improve the well-being of both people with dementia and their caregivers, no matter what the cause.

Index

neuritic plaques, 290, 298, 310–11, 312, 315, 317; neurofibrillary tangles, 292–93, 298, 310–11, 312, 313, 317; neuroplasticity, 311; neurotransmitters and, 311–12, 314, 315–16; Parkinson disease, 41, 136, 300, 302–3, 311, 312, 313, 318, 319; primary progressive aphasia, 303; prion diseases, 312, 314; progressive supranuclear palsy, 303, 311, 313; transient ischemic attacks, 306; vascular dementia, 5–6, 100, 288, 299, 300, 304, 310

brain (or stem) cell transplants, 314

brain chemistry, 310–11

brain imaging, 13–14, 291, 299, 303, 306, 320

brain injury/damage: alcohol abuse and, 155; antioxidants for prevention, 291; behavioral symptoms, 20–24, 160–61; brain (or stem) cell transplant treatment, 314; as brain disorder cause, 295; dementia symptom fluctuations and, 43–44; inflammation and, 315; localized (focal brain lesions), 305–6; rehabilitative training, 306, 310; sexual behavior and, 142; traumatic (head trauma), 100, 292–93, 299, 303–4, 315; vision problems and, 108–9. *See also* stroke

brain tumors, 301, 305

bruises, 75, 92, 98, 100, 101, 109

burn injuries, 54, 62, 64, 68

caffeine, 68–69, 160, 236

cancer, 73, 115, 226, 308

canes, 82–83, 92

cardiovascular disease. *See* heart disease

cardiovascular risk factors, for dementia, 289

caregivers, 192–207; abusive, 224–25; age of, 259; alcohol or drug abuse, 222, 226, 236; caring for yourself, 24–25, 32, 57, 183–84, 202, 226, 232–43; children of, 57, 208–11; counseling for, 18, 222, 237–39, 297; death of, 120, 171–72; death of person cared for, 115–21, 220–21; depression in, 219–20; emotional reactions, 212–24; family criticism of, 144, 145, 201, 206, 214; family support for, 205–6; as final decision maker, 199–200, 202, 206, 218; giving up job, 207; giving yourself a present, 234; illness in, 169–71, 172, 183–84, 226; isolation, 222–23, 234–35; marriage, 200; need for friends, 219, 230, 232, 233, 234; need for privacy, 144; new romantic relationships, 230–31; recognizing warning signs in, 235–37; "shadowing" of, 143–44; substitute, 170–71, 173–74. *See also* family; spouses, of persons with dementia

caregiving, 10; breaks from, 24–25, 32, 144, 201,
205, 206, 210, 217, 232, 233; division of responsibility, 198–200, 202, 205–6; effect on mental health, 235–39; effect on family, 57–58; as family conflict cause, 192–93; general suggestions, 24–27; by out-of-town family, 204–5, 206; parent–adult child relationship, 196–97; planning for the future of, 228–31

care plans, 275

CARF (Commission on Accreditation of Rehabilitation Facilities), 263

catastrophic reactions, 28–32, 122, 135, 140, 145, 146–47, 149, 150, 156, 160, 161; accidents and falls and, 60, 63, 92; anger and, 150, 157, 158; about bathing and dressing, 28–29, 31, 80–81; caregiver's response, 31–32; combativeness, 33; communication problems–related, 35; complaints and insults, 144, 145; to exercise, 76, 160; about lost items, 30–31, 138; management, 18, 29–32, 33, 129, 134, 160, 161; to medication use, 106; in nursing homes, 274, 282; in public places, 146–47; repetitious actions and, 142; sexual behavior and, 140; sitter's response, 151; sleep disturbances and, 134, 135; sundowning, 137; triggers, 29–30, 35, 76, 77, 111, 137, 282; violent, 157, 158; wandering and, 127, 130

catheters, urinary, 89, 176, 276–77

Catholic Charities, 239

Catholic Family Services, 186

CBC (complete blood count), 13

CBD (cortico-basal ganglionic degeneration), 299–300

CCAH (Continuing Care at Home) programs, 261

CCRC (continuing care retirement communities), 261, 263–64

cemetery plots, 172, 253

Centers for Medicare & Medicaid Services, 284

cerebral amyloid angiopathy, 299

certificates of deposit, 252

certified nursing aides (CNAs), 266

chairbound persons, 93–94, 101

chairs, 87, 92; exercise in, 75; Geri Chair, 93, 133–34, 276; getting in and out of, 41, 63, 87, 91, 275–76; restraints or "lap buddies," 93, 133. *See also* wheelchairs

children, 57, 137, 192, 202, 208–11; adolescent, 209, 210–11; inappropriate behavior towards, 140–41; relationship with parent with dementia, 196–97; support groups, 241; visits to nursing homes, 282; of young persons with dementia, 304

choking, 72–73, 85, 102, 180
cholesterol level, 289, 310, 318, 323
cholinesterase inhibitors, 294
choreiform movements, 302
chore services, 188
chronic brain syndrome, 4–5
chronic traumatic encephalopathy (CTE), 293, 299, 315
Citrucel, 104
clergy, 56, 116, 117, 147, 252; as caregiver/family support, 121, 173, 210, 217, 219, 238; visits to nursing homes, 275, 282
clinging, 143–44
clock reading, 42
closets: hiding things in, 138; lighting, 109; locks and latches, 132, 138, 139; rummaging in, 139; urinating in, 86, 87
"clot-busting" drugs, 306
clothing. *See* dressing/clothing
clumsiness, 8, 40, 51, 61, 82, 87, 100, 299
clutter, 25, 30, 61, 62, 63, 96, 138
coconut oil, 292
cognitive function testing, 14–15, 319–20
cognitive impairment: fluctuations, 40, 43, 44; hospitalization and, 112–13; normal aging–related, 288–89, 290; in Parkinson disease, 303; preventing and delaying onset, 289–94; "senior moments" and, 288–89; in traumatic brain injury, 303; in vascular dementia, 304. *See also* intellectual impairment; memory loss
cognitive stimulation programs, 290–91
collections, of valuable items, 253
combativeness, 33
Commission on Accreditation of Rehabilitation Facilities (CARF), 263
commodes, 82–83, 87, 88, 134
communication, of persons with dementia, 25, 34–36; behavioral symptoms and, 23–24; comprehension problems, 23, 34, 36–39, 78, 109, 278, 280; cursing, 23, 35; distraction reduction during, 96; handwriting, 39, 54; intercom systems, 133; making oneself understood, 34–36; nonverbal, 27, 36, 38, 78, 88, 161, 282; in nursing homes, 281; by social media, 54; by telephone, 39–40, 54, 95, 205, 281; ways to improve, 37–39. *See also* hearing loss; reading skills; speech and language problems; written lists or instructions
companions: paid, 176, 187. *See also* sitters
competency: for medical decision making, 278; to write a will, 253–54
complaints, 144–47, 190, 281; about health, 154;

against nursing homes, 285–86. *See also* accusations
complete blood count (CBC), 13
comprehension problems, 23, 34, 36–39, 78, 109, 278, 280
computerized tomography (CT) scan, 13, 14, 299, 320
computer-based memory stimulation activities, 290, 291
concussions, 292–93, 299, 303, 315
confidentiality, 17–18
conflict: within family, 192–93, 197–200, 201–4, 259; with person with dementia, 214
confusion, 1–4, 60, 62, 98, 164, 184, 295; catastrophic reactions to, 28, 30, 122, 129, 160; clinging and, 143; comprehension problems–related, 23; dementia-related *vs.* delirium-related, 5, 16; depression-related, 6; eating behaviors and, 43, 69; exercise and, 76, 160; during hospitalization, 111–12, 113; incontinence-related, 86; living alone and, 56; medical and dental problems–related, 85, 98, 102, 103, 107, 306; medications-related, 104–5, 131, 135–36; in nursing home residents, 277; sexual behavior and, 286; suspiciousness and, 9, 165; vision problems and, 62, 134; visitors and, 77; wandering and, 129
conservatorship, 256–57
constipation, 67, 85, 89, 100, 103–4, 105, 305
Continuing Care Accreditation Commission, 263
Continuing Care at Home (CCAH) programs, 261
continuing care retirement communities (CCRC), 261, 263–64
contractures, 93
convulsions. *See* seizures
cooking, 79; aluminum pans, 292, 315; by caregiver, 66–67, 196; stove safety, 27, 47, 54, 55, 62, 64, 132, 135, 159
coordination problems, 8, 39–42, 60, 78, 91–94; driving ability and, 51; evaluation, 14–15, 40–41; in vascular dementia, 304
"cope notebook," 170–71
coping: with alcoholic person, 155; with behavioral problems, 24–27, 215–16; role changes and family conflict, 197–99, 201–4. *See also* counseling
cortico-basal ganglionic degeneration (CBD), 299–300
corticotropin-releasing factor, 311
costs: food, 245; funerals, 171; legal fees, 245; moving to new residence, 264

costs, of care: assisted living, 260; help, 245; long-term care, 270; medical care, 245; nursing homes, 244–46, 260, 273–74; planning for, 244–50; respite care, 245; tax-deductible, 250. *See also* financial issues; paying for care

coughing, 72, 99, 102, 295

counseling, 24; for caregiver/family, 237–39; for children, 210, 211, 241; finding, 238–39; marriage, 231; pastoral, 239; sexuality, 228; from social workers, 18

counselors, 154, 202, 204, 231; genetic, 319

COVID-19 pandemic, 102–3

Creutzfeldt-Jakob disease, 312, 314

crime, towards persons with dementia, 54–55, 133, 163, 176

criticism, 52, 144, 145, 201, 206

crying, 79, 100, 154, 220, 236–37

CT (computerized tomography) scan, 13, 14, 299, 320

CTE (chronic traumatic encephalopathy), 293, 299, 315

cursing, 23, 35

dancing, 75

debts, 196, 251, 253

decubitus ulcers (pressure sores), 82, 83, 93, 94, 98, 100, 101, 266, 277

dehydration, 70–71, 74, 87, 101–2, 115, 284, 285, 305

delirium, 4–5, 6, 98, 305; dementia and, 5, 16, 305, 321; hallucinations in, 150–61, 166–67; during hospitalization, 112; pneumonia and, 98; symptoms, 305

delusions, 166–67

demanding behaviors, 8, 148–50

dementia, 1–10, 296–304; age factors, 175, 296, 304; alcohol use disorder–related, 297; Alzheimer disease–related, 5, 296, 297–99, 304; behavioral and neuropsychiatric symptoms, 20–44, 122–52; causes, 5, 6, 7, 9, 13, 295–306; concealment of, 7–8; definition, 4–9, 296; delirium and, 5, 16, 305, 321; depression-related, 6, 8, 292, 300; diagnosis, 9, 11, 16, 45, 307, 320; economic cost, 7; HIV/AIDS, 301; lobar, 300; mild cognitive impairment, 7, 24, 27, 45–46, 68, 69, 261, 295–96; misdiagnosis, 7–8; moderate, 7, 24; normal aging *vs.*, 5, 6; onset, 7–8; Parkinson disease, 302–3; prognosis, 9; progression, 7, 8, 45, 296; pugilistica, 315; research studies, 307–23; reversible, 13, 15; risk factors, 289–93; tauopathy, 299–300; young or early onset, 304. *See also* fronto-temporal dementia (FTD); Lewy body dementia; vascular dementia

dementia care units, 260, 266–67

dementia centers, 16

dementia support agencies, 185

denial, 7, 28, 29, 47, 54

dental care/problems, 85, 100, 107–8, 175, 264

dentures, 69, 71, 84, 85, 103, 175, 246; lost or misplaced, 107, 108, 138, 164–65

depression, 7, 73, 153–54, 159; in caregivers, 32, 184, 207, 219–20, 222, 225, 236, 241; dementia and, 6, 8, 292, 300, 316; diagnosis, 14, 153; stroke-related, 310; suicide and, 155; symptoms, 154; treatment, 14, 46, 105, 153, 154, 268, 276, 300

depth perception, 108

diabetes, 13, 66, 70, 87, 101–2, 292, 310, 316

diagnosis, of dementia, 9, 45, 307, 320; accuracy, 11, 16, 24; conflicting, 9, 16

diapers, 90–91, 245, 246, 249

diarrhea, 99, 101–2, 103

diet: caffeine, 68–69, 160, 236; constipation and, 67, 103, 104; fiber, 67, 103, 104; high-calorie, liquid, 72; Mediterranean, 291; protective against dementia, 323; pureed, 69; to reduce dementia risk, 291–92; snacks, 69–70, 71, 111, 277; stroke risk and, 310; supplements, 66, 69, 72, 291–92, 297. *See also* fluid intake; nutrition; vitamins

disability benefits, 48, 188, 245, 252–53, 304

disability insurance, 252

discouragement, 223, 232–33, 235, 238; counseling for, 222, 238; depression and, 153, 154, 222, 236; suicide and, 155

disorientation, 5, 8, 96, 126–27, 134, 305

distractibility, 143, 305; noise-related, 30, 31, 96, 97, 110, 130, 132, 160, 228, 277

diuretics, 68–69, 101–2

dizziness and light-headedness, 2, 102, 105, 110, 295

DNR (do not resuscitate) order, 116, 118

dolls, 78

domiciliary care (board and care) facilities, 246, 261–62, 271

donepezil (Aricept), 294, 315

do not hospitalize order, 118

do not resuscitate (DNR) order, 116, 118

doors: safety issues, 63–64, 65, 97; locks and alarms, 62, 63, 95, 132

dopamine, 311

Down syndrome, 317

drawers: hiding items in, 138, 251; labeling, 28; locks, 61, 132, 139; rummaging in, 63, 139 dressing/clothing, 2, 8, 39, 79, 83–84, 143, 181–82, 183, 188, 248, 262, 298; catastrophic reactions to, 80; ill-fitting or uncomfortable clothes, 100, 140; inappropriate removal of clothes, 139, 140, 286; incontinence and, 87, 88; at night, 135; of nursing home residents, 275

driving, 65, 125, 218, 223, 224; by caregiver, 177, 196, 214, 241; evaluation, 50–52; refusal to give up, 46, 50, 52–53

drug abuse, 155, 226, 236

durable power of attorney, 240, 254–55; for finances, 251, 255; for health care, 117, 118, 255

Dycem, 68, 82–83

dying and death, 115–21, 220–21, 231; of caregivers, 120, 171–72; cause of, 115; deciding when treatment should end, 117–19; dying at home, 115–16, 117, 119, 176; end-of-life care, 74, 117–21, 255, 277; hospice/palliative care, 116–17; in hospital or nursing home, 117–19; memories of deceased loved ones, 162–63

eating: assistance with, 277–78; choking during, 72–73, 85, 102, 180; coordination problems and, 40, 68, 77; cues for, 67; denture use and, 85; dishes and utensils, 67, 68, 77–78, 82–83; distractions during, 143; hiding or hoarding food, 69–70; of inappropriate items, 61, 62, 70; nibbling, 70; problem behaviors, 69–70; refusing or spitting out food, 70; in restaurants, 67, 77–78; spoon-feeding, 69; swallowing problems, 71, 72, 93, 231, 278; of toxic or inappropriate substances, 61, 62, 70; tube feeding, 73–74, 119, 120, 265, 278; while living alone, 54

Eating Together programs, 67

educational level, 292, 316, 321

EEG (electroencephalogram), 13

Eldercare Locator, 176

electroencephalogram (EEG), 13

emailing, 54

embarrassment, 6, 40, 87, 216–17; of adult children, 197; about incontinence, 89; about sexuality, 226; of teenagers, 210

emergencies: 911 calls, 92, 116, 117, 169, 170; caregiver's illness, 169–72; death at home, 115–16; death of caregiver, 120, 171–72; in nursing homes, 276. See also falls

emotional overreaction. See catastrophic reactions

emotions: of caregivers, 193, 212–13, 231; of children, 208–10; expression, 212–13, 231;

memories of, 22, 156–57; mood symptoms and, 153–68; of persons with dementia, 7, 8, 20, 23. See also mood symptoms; and specific emotions

end-of-life care, 74, 117–21, 277; tube feeding, 73–74, 119, 120, 265, 278

Ensure, 72

environment: calm, 130, 131, 143, 159–60, 233; changes in, 44; during mealtimes, 67, 71; nursing homes, 277; safety issues, 60–64. See also home

epidemiology, 316

estate planning, 254

executive function, 303

Exelon (rivastigmine), 294, 315

exercise, 74–76, 79, 127, 134, 156, 226; in chair or bed, 75–76, 275; effect on dementia risk, 289–90, 316, 321; mental, 79, 290–91; in nursing homes, 275; recommendations for, 290; for restlessness reduction, 129; as stroke preventive, 310

expectations, 17, 194, 197–99, 200, 201, 244

Extra Help program, 249

eyeglasses, 28, 30–31, 109, 138, 175

falls, 62, 82, 135; caregiver's safety and, 92; dizziness-related, 110; at home, 63, 91–92; injuries caused by, 100–101, 304; Lewy body dementia and, 302; medication-related, 93, 104–5, 135–36; at night, 88, 135; in nursing homes, 274, 285; outdoors, 63–64; progressive supranuclear palsy and, 303; seizures and, 114

false ideas and beliefs, 122, 160–61, 305

familiar items and possessions, 27–28, 113, 278, 281–82; loss of, 56–57, 158

family: adjustment after loved ones move to nursing home, 283–84; advocacy by, 99, 233, 242–43, 272; conflicts among, 192–93, 197–200, 201–4, 259; division of responsibility, 198–200; failure to recognize dementia, 125; financial assistance from, 271; as help for primary caregiver, 173, 186, 205–6, 223, 237–38, 241; impaired person moving in with, 57–58; impaired person's inability to recognize, 141, 161–62; out-of-town, 204–5, 206; as paid caregivers, 188; physicians' interactions with, 17–18; as primary care caregivers, 183; psychiatric and psychosocial evaluation, 14; quality of life, 10; role changes, 46, 194–99, 201–3; sitter exchange arrangements, 186. See also caregivers; children

family conferences, 202–3, 210, 259

grief (*cont.*)
    as obstacle to nursing home visits, 283–84; sharing of, 24

grooming. *See* personal care and hygiene

guardianship: of person, 74, 118, 256, 257; of property, 251, 252, 256–57

guilt, 196–97, 205, 217–20, 235, 258–59

hair care, 8, 13, 33, 61, 78, 82, 84, 246, 282

hallucinations, 8, 96, 99, 102, 105, 122, 127, 134, 160–61, 166–67; in delirium, 167, 305; in Lewy body dementia, 302; medications for, 167; medications-induced, 166

handrails, 39, 63, 64, 92, 108, 274

handwriting, 39, 54

"hardening of the arteries," 5. *See also* heart disease

headaches, 99, 104, 105, 113

headphones, 95, 144, 234

head trauma, 100, 292–93, 297, 299, 303–4, 315

health insurance, 18, 83, 106, 116, 179, 245, 248, 252; long-term care, 187, 246–47, 260, 271. *See also* Medicaid coverage; Medicare coverage

health maintenance organizations (HMOs), 116, 248

hearing aids, 97, 109–10, 161

hearing loss, 37, 51, 95, 109–10, 161, 316, 323

heart attacks, 115, 169, 289, 290, 291, 318

heart disease, 66, 99, 101–2, 180, 310

heart surgery, 322

heat stroke, 55

Heimlich maneuver, 72–73

help, 173–91, 207, 322; in case of caregiver's illness or death, 170–71; costs, 245; family exchange arrangements, 186; family's feelings about, 172; finding sources of, 174, 184–86, 206, 217, 233, 235–42; from friends and neighbors, 173–74, 182, 186, 223, 233, 237–38, 241, 270; home care services, 176–77; kinds of services, 175–80; for living independently, 56; paying for, 176, 187–89; rejection by person with dementia, 180–83; short-stay residential care, 179–80; tax deductions for, 250; telephoning for, 39–40. *See also* adult day care; home care; sitters

helplines, 123, 239, 240, 242

hematoma, subdural, 303–4

heredity. *See* genetic factors

hiding items, 9, 49, 138–39, 164, 166, 240, 251

highway safety, 65

hippocampus, 290, 311

history taking, 12, 14

HIV (human immunodeficiency virus), 13, 301

hoarding, 55, 69–70, 138–39

hobbies, 77, 78, 222, 229, 230, 231, 281, 291

home: clutter reduction, 25, 30, 61, 62, 63, 96, 138; dying at, 115–16, 119, 176; as financial asset, 249, 252, 265; lighting, 62, 67, 88, 95, 108–9, 133, 134; low-cost repair programs, 175; making changes, 94–97; safety devices, 95–96, 245; safety hazards, 60–64; selling of, 256; trying to get back to, 168

home care, 176–77, 243, 259–60; hidden costs, 203; Medicare coverage, 248; paying for, 187–88, 203, 246, 249; planning for, 180, 245; quality, 179; rejection by person with dementia, 180–83

home care workers, 164

home health aides, 176, 187

homemakers, 176

homes for the aged, 261–62

home visitor programs, 76

hopefulness, 223–24, 308

hormones, 136–37

hospice care, 116–17, 118, 176, 246, 268

hospitalization, 111–13, 129, 130, 219, 321; of caregiver, 170–71; discharge from, 247–49, 260, 269; dying during, 117–19; Medicare coverage, 247–48; move from nursing home to, 276; move to nursing home from, 248–49, 260, 269, 279; of nursing home residents, 276; VA hospitals, 268

hot drinks, 68

hot meals, 53, 67, 175, 250

hot water temperature, 62, 81

housekeepers, 56, 152, 164, 177, 181

housework, 55

housing costs, 245

human immunodeficiency virus/acquired immune deficiency syndrome (HIV/AIDS), 13, 301

humor, 25, 178, 202

hunting, 65–66

Huntington disease, 302, 311, 318, 319

hygiene. *See* personal care and hygiene

identification (ID) bracelets, 25–26, 105, 128

identification cards, nondriver, 53

illness: acute, 321–22; behavioral effects, 23, 31; in caregivers, 169–71, 183–84, 226; as dementia cause, 13, 20–21, 46–47; influenza, 102–3; monitoring for, 98; pneumonia, 1, 73, 98, 102, 115, 119, 120, 248; signs of, 99–100; stress-related, 213. *See also* infection

immune system, 301, 311, 312, 313–14, 315

income: as long-term care financing source, 271, 272; loss of, 245

income tax, 55, 57, 125, 175

incontinence, 86–91, 99; bowel, 86, 89–91; cleaning up, 89–91; drug-related, 87; management in nursing homes, 276–77; medication-related, 104–5, 135–36; at night, 87–88; supplies, 90–91, 245; urinary, 9, 86–89

incontinence wear, 90–91, 245

independence, 45–59; decision about living alone, 53–59; driving, 50–53; during early stages of dementia, 46–47; evaluation for, 46; giving up job, 47–48; loss of, 46–47, 144–45, 197, 218; mild cognitive impairment and, 45–46; money management, 48–50; supervised, 56

infection: as Alzheimer disease risk, 313–14; of caregiver, 91; central nervous system, 13, 304; as death cause, 115; as delirium risk, 305; HIV/AIDS, 13, 301; laboratory tests for, 13; lab testing for, 13; oral, 107; tube feeding and, 73–74; urinary tract, 87, 89, 149, 305

inflammatory response, 315

influenza, 102–3

information and referral services, 186, 189, 206, 254; Alzheimer's Association and National Institute on Aging, 16–17, 224, 240, 309; for children and adolescents, 211

information processing impairment, 7, 8, 23, 288–89, 298

informed consent forms, 14, 74

ingestion injuries, 62

inheritances, 203, 218, 253, 318

injuries, 100–101; anger-related, 157; broken bones, 98, 100; bruises, 75, 92, 98, 100, 101, 109; burns, 54, 62, 64, 68; in caregivers, 169; head trauma, 100, 292–93, 297, 299, 303–4, 315; myoclonus and, 115; seizures and, 114. *See also* accidents; falls; safety concerns

instructions, 42; step-by-step, 30, 84, 85; for substitute caregivers, 170–71; understanding, 14–15. *See also* written lists or instructions

insults, 144–47; to sitter, 151–52

insurance: disability, 252; fire, 252. *See also* health insurance

intellectual activity, 290–91

intellectual disability, 295, 296

intellectual function, aging and, 317

intellectual impairment, 5, 6, 296; evaluation, 14–16. *See also* cognitive impairment

intercom systems, 133

Internal Revenue Service (IRS), 125, 250, 251

irritability, 7, 8, 23, 122, 157–58, 159, 274; alcohol use–related, 297; in caregivers, 158, 236; illness-related, 31, 99; incontinence and, 87; management, 105, 158

IRS (Internal Revenue Service), 125, 250, 251

isolation, of caregivers, 222–23, 229–31, 234–35

jellyfish fluorescent protein, 292

Jewish Family Services, 186, 239

jobs: benefit programs, 252–53; giving up by caretaker, 207; giving up by person with dementia, 245

joy, 10, 220

judgment impairment, 7, 14–15, 55, 60, 133, 295, 296

kidney disease, 13

Korsakoff (amnestic) syndrome, 291, 299

kuru, 314

labeling items, 28

laboratory tests, 13, 15, 248

"lap buddies," 93, 133

laughter, 25, 26, 178, 202, 220

lawn mowers, 64

laxatives, 104

L-dopa (Sinemet), 302, 311

lead exposure, 292

learning impairment, 12, 22, 26, 40, 42, 60, 92, 95, 109, 125, 127, 149, 215, 306

legal issues, 253–57; advance directives, 45, 118, 277; competency for medical decision making, 279; financial assets protection, 247; guardianship of property, 251–52, 256–57; guardianship of the person, 74, 118, 256, 257; legal fees, 245; planning for future, 229; sexual behavior in nursing homes, 287; wills, 45, 171, 203, 253, 255–56. *See also* attorneys; durable power of attorney; power of attorney

Lewy bodies, 312, 313

Lewy body dementia, 293, 295–96, 300, 302, 312, 313, 316

licensing/accreditation: continuing care retirement communities, 263; driver's license, 52, 53; family and social service agencies, 19; home care, 176; long-term care facilities, 272; nursing homes, 265, 272; respite care services, 189–90

life care facilities. *See* continuing care retirement communities (CCRCs)

life insurance, 246, 252

life plan communities. *See* continuing care retirement communities (CCRC) life-sustaining treatment, 74, 117, 118, 119, 255, 277

lighting: glare, 97, 108, 277; at mealtimes, 67; motion-detector, 133; at night, 62, 88, 108–9, 134; in nursing homes, 277; vision problems and, 95, 108–9

listening, 38, 103, 281

listlessness, 8, 26, 156

lists. *See* written lists or instructions

liver disease, 13

living arrangements, 229, 258–87; adjustment to, 58–59; adult foster care, 245, 261, 262; board and care (domiciliary care), 246, 261–62, 271; Continuing Care at Home, 261; continuing care retirement communities, 261, 263–64; decisions about living alone, 53–59, 126, 193; dementia concealment and, 125; family disagreement about, 259; living alone, 46; living with relatives, 57–59, 203; moving with a person with dementia, 264–65; planning for future, 58, 228–29; retirement communities, 56, 261, 263–64; senior citizens' apartments or condominiums, 261, 263; subsidized housing, 261; waiting lists, 186, 260, 261, 269, 270. *See also* long-term care; nursing homes

living wills, 118, 277

locks, 132; for automobiles, 65; childproof, 61, 62; on doors, 62, 63, 274; on windows, 135

long-term care: admission, 269; COVID-19 in, 102–3; diversity of populations served by, 262; end-of-life care, 119; finding, 269–78; guidelines for selection, 269–70; paying for, 270–72; planning for, 260, 261; quality of care, 260, 261–62, 263, 264, 269, 272, 284, 285; sources of information about, 240, 269–70; staffing, 242; waiting lists, 260, 261, 269, 270. *See also* assisted living facilities; nursing homes; skilled nursing facilities (SNFs)

long-term care insurance, 187, 246–47, 260, 271

loss: of familiar places and possessions, 56–57, 158; family's feeling of, 283; of friends, 230; grief as reaction to, 196–97, 220; of independence, 46–47, 56, 144–45, 197, 218; of responsibility, 46, 47, 196, 197; of sense of time, 42–43, 149. *See also* memory loss

lost: feeling of being, 23, 283. *See also* getting lost

lost or misplaced items, 9, 28, 30–31, 46, 138, 159, 164–65, 182

love, 10, 78, 102–3, 121, 192, 212, 219, 220, 223, 268, 282; of children, 209; between spouses, 200, 202, 215, 221, 227, 228

low-density lipids (LDLs), 310, 318

lumbar puncture (LP), 13, 14

Lutheran Family Services, 186

Lyme disease, 13

magnetic resonance imaging (MRI), 13, 290, 299, 303, 306, 320

malnutrition, 70–71, 115

manganese, 315

MAP (microtubule-associated protein), 313

marijuana use, 236

marriage, of caregivers, 57, 198, 200, 228, 229, 231, 240; same-sex, 198. *See also* spouses, of persons with dementia

marriage counseling, 231

masturbation, 140, 168, 286, 287

MCI (mild cognitive impairment), 7, 24, 27, 45–46, 68, 69, 261, 295–96

meal preparation, 66–67, 79, 137, 176, 195, 265; costs, 245; home-delivered meals, 53, 67, 175, 250, 261. *See also* cooking; eating; food

Meals on Wheels, 53, 67, 175, 250

mealtimes, 102, 171, 180; Eating Together programs, 67; environment for, 67, 68, 127; infection prevention during, 102; scheduling of, 25, 71, 137; snacks, 69–70, 71, 111, 277. *See also* eating

Medicaid coverage, 278, 284; applying for, 272; boarding homes, 261; care supplies, 83; eligibility, 247, 249, 260, 265, 271–72; family responsibility law for, 247; home care and day care, 187–88; hospice coverage, 116; long-term and nursing home, 250, 260, 265, 271–72, 273; Medicare dual-eligibility, 249; memory care units, 267; PACE program, 248

Medi-Cal, 271

medical care, 11–19: access to, 265; in assisted living facilities, 262; at continuing care retirement communities, 264; coordination of, 11; costs, 245; for dementia, 17–19; in nursing homes, 276; in residential living facilities, 262; resources for, 11–19; tax deductions for, 250. *See also* paying for care

MedicAlert bracelets, 26, 128

MedicAlert Foundation, 131

medical evaluation, 12–17, 149; brain imaging, 13–14, 291, 299, 303, 306, 320; components, 12; discussion with doctor, 15; EEG, 13; finding someone to perform, 16–17; history taking, 12, 14; lab tests, 13, 15, 248; mental status examination, 12–13; neuropsychological testing, 14–15, 297, 319–20; occupational therapy evaluation, 14, 40–41, 125; physical

monitoring devices, 95–96, 133, 177

mood symptoms: agnosia, 109, 161–62; alcohol or drug abuse, 52, 155, 222, 226, 235–36, 297; anger and irritability, 157–59; anxiety, nervousness, and restlessness, 158–59; apathy and listlessness, 156; in caregivers, 232; complaints about health, 154; delusions and hallucinations, 160–61, 166–67; depression, 153–54; false ideas, 122, 160–61, 305; having nothing to do, 167–68; remembering feelings, 22; suicidality, 155, 237; suspiciousness, 8–9, 50, 55, 105, 156, 161, 163–65, 274

motion detectors, 132–33

moving: costs, 264; to new residence, 56–59, 205, 264–65; to residential care, 259–60, 263, 264–65, 278–79

MRI (magnetic resonance imaging), 13, 290, 299, 303, 306, 320

muscle weakness or stiffness, 41, 76, 91, 104–5, 300, 302

music, 21, 50, 75, 77, 95, 144, 156, 177, 178, 275, 281; calming effect, 89, 135, 156; as distraction, 143; singing, 3, 4, 77, 78, 281, 282

mutual funds, 252

myoclonus, 115

nail care, 84

Namenda (memantine), 294, 315–16

naming problems, 1, 4, 6, 8, 34, 234, 289

naps, 134, 137

National Adult Services Association, 176

National Citizens' Coalition for Nursing Home Reform, 272

National Consumer Voice for Quality Long-Term Care, 284, 285

National Institute of Neurological Disorders and Stroke (NINDS), 307

National Institute on Aging (NIA), 66, 123, 307; website, 16–17, 224, 240, 309

nausea/vomiting, 99, 101–2, 105, 110, 295

neighbors, 125, 221, 281; concerns, 55; explaining dementia to, 133, 146, 147, 174, 216–17; false accusations toward, 165; help from, 53, 56, 173–74, 182

nerve growth factors, 313

nervousness, 112–13, 158–59

neuritic plaques, 290, 298, 310–11, 312, 315, 317

neurocognitive disorders, 4–5

neurodegenerative diseases, 311

neurofibrillary tangles, 292–93, 298, 310–11, 312, 313, 317

neuroleptic drugs, 41

neurological examination, 12, 14

neurologists, 11, 17, 305

neuroplasticity, 311

neuropsychological testing, 14–15, 297, 319–20

neuropsychologists, 11, 23–24, 319, 320

neurotransmitters, 311–12, 314, 315–16

night-lights, 88, 108–9, 134

NINDS (National Institute of Neurological Disorders and Stroke), 307

noise distractions, 30, 31, 96, 97, 110, 130, 132, 160, 228, 277

norepinephrine, 311

nurse practitioners, 18

nurses, 11, 118, 120, 150, 190, 272; advanced practice, 18, 238; hiring, 18, 187; hospice, 116; in hospitals, 112, 113, 130; incontinence management, 89; licensed vocational (practical), 18; in nursing homes, 33, 274, 276, 285; psychiatric, 238–39; visiting, 94, 116, 176, 245

nursing homes, 56, 99, 258–59, 265–66; activities, 275, 277, 281, 285; adjustment to, 278–84; behavioral management, 266, 274, 275, 276, 279, 285; care and services, 275–77, 284–85; cleanliness and safety, 274, 285–86; complaints against, 285–86; contracts with, 273; costs/paying for, 188, 203, 244–45, 244–46, 250, 260, 265, 270–72, 273–74; decision to use, 56, 57, 174, 199, 200, 257, 258–59; discharge of residents, 273, 286; dying in, 117–19; end-of-life care, 118; family adjustment, 283–84; family visits, 230, 266, 269, 270, 273, 278–79, 280–84; fire safety, 190, 262, 273; guidelines for selection, 272–78; hospice care, 268; incontinence management, 276–77; licensing, 265, 272; meals and nutrition, 71, 102, 270, 277–78, 282; Medicaid coverage, 260, 265, 271–72; medical care, 260, 276, 285; Medicare coverage, 247, 260, 265–66, 271, 273; Medicare law regarding, 248–49; medication errors, 107; medication management, 276, 285; meeting regulations, 273; mental health care in, 268; moving to, 259–60, 263, 264–65, 278–79; ombudspersons, 186, 190, 268, 277, 285; physical environment, 277; problems in, 284–86; quality of care, 265–66, 269, 273; residents' privacy, 275, 277, 282; residents' rights, 278; respectful treatment of residents, 277, 285; sexual issues, 286–87; sources of information about, 240, 269–70; staff, 274–75, 277, 279, 283, 285; tax-deductible costs, 250; terminal care policies, 277; transfer from hospital to, 248–49, 260, 269, 279; transfer to hospital from, 276; use of restraints, 275–76 nutrition, 66–76; choking and, 72–73, 85, 102, 180; denture use and, 85, 107; end-of-life, 119, 120; malnutrition, 70–71, 115; meal preparation, 66–67; in nursing home residents, 71, 277–78; problem eating behaviors, 69–70; tube feeding, 73–74, 119, 120, 265, 278; weight loss, 71–72, 73

nutrition programs, 175–76

obesity/overweight, 69, 71, 100, 289, 290, 310

occupational therapists, 11, 14, 18, 41, 50, 61, 76, 245

occupational therapy, 248, 275; evaluation for, 14, 40–41, 125

office on aging, 18, 56, 67, 179, 185–86, 190, 240, 269, 285

Older Americans Act, 175

ombudsperson programs, 186, 190, 268, 277, 285

ophthalmologists, 109

oral health and hygiene, 82–83, 84–85, 99

osteoporosis, 100

outdoor safety hazards, 63–66

overreacting. See catastrophic reactions

PACE prescription drug plan, 248

pacing, 8, 57, 66, 71, 74, 77, 100, 126, 127, 130, 142, 159, 277

pain, 94, 98, 159; after falling, 92, 99, 100; behavioral effects, 23, 31, 99; catastrophic reactions, 31; constipation-related, 99, 103, 104; end-of-life care–related, 119–20; exercise and, 75; oral, 70, 85, 99–100, 107

pain management: end-of-life care, 120; hospice/palliative care, 116, 119; medications, 104, 120, 155, 236; in nursing homes, 265, 266

palliative care, 116–17, 121, 268

panic, 2, 3, 4, 29, 32, 46, 63, 127, 129, 130, 164. See also anxiety

paranoia, 8–9, 55, 163, 164. See also suspiciousness

parent–adult child caregiving relationship, 196–97

Parkinson disease, 41, 136, 252, 300, 302–3, 311, 312, 313, 318, 319

parkinsonism, 91, 302

Pastoral Counseling, 239

paying for care: financial issues, 187–88; home or respite care, 176, 177, 180, 187–88, 203, 246, 249; hospice care, 246, 268; legal responsibility, 203; long-term care, 188, 260, 270–72; memory care units, 267. See also Medicaid coverage; Medicare coverage

PEG tube. See tube feeding

personal care and hygiene, 54, 79–85, 84; by adult children, 197; care supplies, 82–83, 90–91; changes in, 54, 55. See also bathing; dressing/clothing

personal care homes, 261–62

personal care services, 176, 181–82, 188

personal history boxes and scrapbooks, 281–82

personality changes, 4, 8, 20–21, 54, 99, 125, 149, 295; alcohol use–related, 297; in Alzheimer disease, 4, 298; evaluation, 12; in frontotemporal dementia, 300–301; in traumatic brain injury, 303

personal loans, 253

PET (positron emission tomography) scan, 13, 14, 299, 300

pets, 78, 106, 132, 275, 282

pharmacists, 19, 70, 83, 103, 105, 106, 107, 170, 173

phenylketonuria (PKU), 293

physical examination, 12, 14

physical therapists, 11, 14, 18, 41, 75, 76, 92, 94, 176, 245

physical therapy, 2, 91, 248, 275

physical therapy consultations, 41, 93

physicians, 11, 17, 154, 214; conferring with family, 112, 206, 217; at continuing care retirement communities, 264; driving cessation interventions, 52–53; in end-of-life care, 118, 119, 120; incontinence management, 86–87, 88–89; medical evaluation by, 12–17, 193; Medicare coverage, 248; nursing home care and, 276, 285; primary care, 11, 18; specialists, 11, 17; visits to, 110–11, 276

physician's assistants, 18, 276

Pick bodies, 312

PKU (phenylketonuria), 293

placebo effect, 308

planning, 228–231: costs of care, 244–50; death at home, 115–16; dementia care, 9; end-of-life care, 117–19, 120–21; future disability, 253–54; home care services, 180; long-term care, 260, 261, 269; medical evaluation–based, 14; moving, 58

planning ability impairment, 8

pneumonia, 1, 73, 98, 102, 115, 119, 120, 248

poisons, 62, 122, 146, 166

Posey restraints, 133

positron emission tomography (PET) scan, 13, 14, 299, 300

power of attorney, 255; health care, 117, 255, 256; limited, 254, 255

preferred provider organizations (PPOs), 248

stimulation, 26, 27, 96, 97; overstimulation, 137, 159–60; social and intellectual, 290–91

stock certificates, 252

stove safety, 54, 55, 62, 64, 135

stress, 53, 128, 179, 277, 280, 323; caregiver/family, 57–58, 76, 131, 137, 149, 169, 170, 200, 206, 236, 237; catastrophic reactions, 31, 32, 137; combativeness and, 33; dementia misdiagnosed as, 7–8; effect on mental health, 235–39; as illness cause, 213, 300–301; sundowning and, 137; wandering and, 127, 213

stroke, 13, 91, 115, 290, 318; as brain damage cause, 6, 21, 305–6, 310; in caregivers, 169; choking prevention, 72; effect on language and speech, 35, 176, 306; hemorrhagic, 299; prevention/risk reduction, 66, 304, 310; treatment, 304

stubbornness, 29, 31, 79, 150–51

subsidized housing, 261

substance abuse, 155; in caregiver, 222, 226, 236. *See also* alcohol use/abuse

substance P, 311

suicide, 155, 237

sundowning, 136–38

supervision, 55, 56, 91, 175, 176, 179, 185, 188, 189, 261, 262, 265; medical, 104, 236, 276

Supplemental Security Income (SSI), 48, 188, 249, 252, 262

supplements, dietary, 104, 291–92, 297

support groups, 9–10, 32, 46, 123, 180, 200, 202, 206, 216, 222, 234, 239–41, 246, 322; excuses for not attending, 240, 241–42; for teenagers, 241. *See also* Alzheimer's Association

surgery, 321–22

suspiciousness, 8–9, 50, 55, 105, 156, 161, 163–65, 274; accusations of stealing, 8–9, 49, 145, 161, 163–65; delusions, 166–67; hiding behaviors, 9, 49, 138–39, 164, 240, 251; of sitters, 151–52, 165, 181

Sustacal, 72

swallowing problems, 70, 71, 72, 93, 231, 278; choking due to, 72–73, 85, 102, 180; in medication use, 106; tube feeding for, 73–74, 119, 120, 265, 278

swelling, 75, 92, 99, 101, 306

swimming pools, 64, 133

symptoms, of dementia and Alzheimer disease, 5, 7–9, 43–44, 296; Alzheimer disease, 290–91, 297–98; behavioral and psychiatric, 153–68; fluctuations in, 43–44. *See also* behavioral and neuropsychiatric symptoms; mood symptoms

synuclein, 313, 314

syphilis, 13

tauopathies, 300

tau protein, 298, 299, 300, 313, 320, 323

Tax Guide for Seniors, 250

tax issues, 245, 249, 250, 251, 252, 253, 254, 264

TBI (traumatic brain injury), 292–93, 299, 303–4, 315

telephone calls, 54, 205; forgetting, 148; to nursing home residents, 281

telephones: emergency use, 170; helplines, 123, 239, 240, 242; locator apps, 26, 128, 133; recording devices, 95

television, 27–28, 43, 77, 95, 96, 133–34, 167–68, 179, 275, 283; as distraction, 30, 31, 67, 110; during mealtimes, 43, 67, 137; in nursing home, 275, 280

temper, loss of, 8, 31–32, 217, 224–25, 236

testamentary capacity, 253–54

thermometers, 99

thyroid disease/disorders, 5, 13

TIA (transient ischemic attack), 306

time, loss of sense of, 42–43, 149

toileting: in nursing homes, 276; schedule, 88, 134

toilets, 82–83, 87

toothbrushing, 82–83

touch, 32, 78, 142, 167, 227, 282, 286

toxic substances: exposure, 292, 295; safety procedures, 61, 62, 70

toys, stuffed, 78

tranquilizers, 41, 222, 236

transient ischemic attack (TIA), 306

transportation, 175, 236, 261, 273; to adult day care, 179, 185, 188; costs, 188, 203, 245; to Eating Together programs, 87; in retirement communities, 263, 264, 265

traumatic brain injury (TBI), 292–93, 299, 303–4, 315

tremors, 41, 302

trust accounts, 253

tube feeding, 73–74, 119, 120, 265, 278

tuberculosis, 13

turmeric, 292

uncooperativeness, 150–51

urinary incontinence, 9, 86–91

urinary tract infections, 87, 89, 149, 305

US Department of Housing and Urban Development (HUD), 261

US Department of Veterans Affairs (VA), 268, 271

VA (US Department of Veterans Affairs), 268, 271

vacations, 205, 206, 226, 233

vascular dementia, 4, 5–6, 100, 288, 289, 292, 299, 300, 304, 310

VDRL test, 13

videos, 96, 102–3, 177, 181–82, 184, 205

vision problems, 51, 67, 108–9, 134, 161, 303

visits: behavioral responses, 278–79, 280–81; by children, 282; day care centers, 129; dementia care units, 267; by in-home care providers, 176–77, 180, 182–83; nursing homes, 230, 266, 269, 270, 273, 277, 278–79, 280–83; by out-of-town family, 205; by physicians, 276; to physicians, 110–11, 276; to select long-term care facility, 269, 270; special visitors, 174

vitamins, 13, 67, 72, 291, 297

volunteers/volunteering, 188, 200, 235, 242

walkers, 87, 92, 95, 302

walking, 285; as exercise, 75, 104, 275, 290; for restlessness reduction, 129

walking problems, 8, 41, 51, 104–5, 185; falls due to, 91–92; gait apraxia / shuffling, 8, 39, 93; home safety and, 91–92; inability to walk, 93–94; in nursing homes, 273

wandering, 54–55, 63, 105, 168; causes, 126–27; ID bracelets and, 25–26, 128; management, 25–26, 64, 127–34, 127–36; at night, 126, 127, 132, 134–36, 225, 228, 262; in nursing homes, 274, 276; tracking devices and, 25–26

Wandering Support for a Safe Return, 131, 133

water heaters, temperature of, 62

weight loss, 71–72, 73, 99–100, 154, 290

wheelchairs, 82–83, 84, 94, 95, 245, 277

wills, 45, 171, 203, 253–54, 255–56

windows: automobiles, 64–65; glare from, 97, 108; locks and alarms, 63, 95, 132, 135

word-finding problems, 6, 7, 23, 27, 34, 35–36, 119, 279, 289, 298, 301. *See also* speech and language problems

worry, 25–26, 35, 42, 158, 159, 193, 205, 222, 223, 235; about developing dementia, 317; by children, 208, 209

writing problems, 8, 14–15, 39, 54

written lists or instructions, 7, 27, 28, 30, 42, 46, 113, 125, 127–28, 165, 181, 280

More Books in Dementia Care and Aging from Hopkins Press

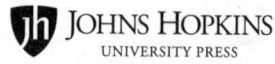
JOHNS HOPKINS
UNIVERSITY PRESS

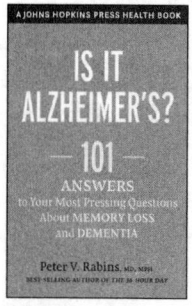
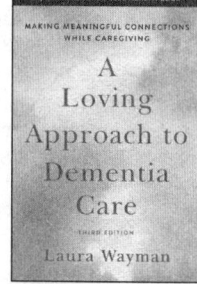
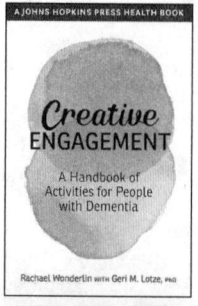
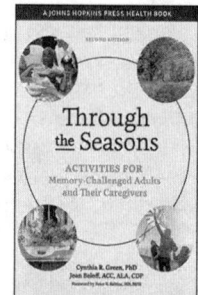

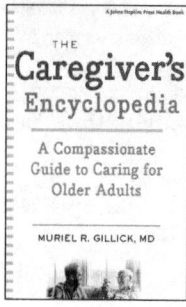
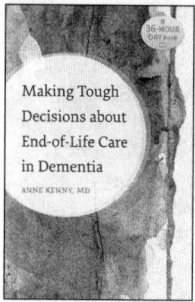
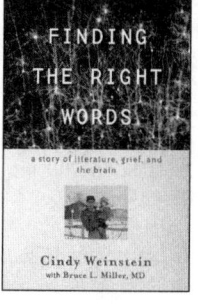
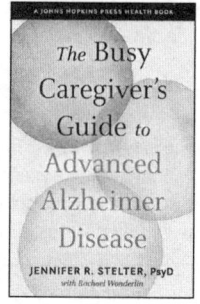

Is It Alzheimer's?
101 Answers to Your Most Pressing Questions about Memory Loss and Dementia
*Peter V. Rabins, MD, MPH,
best-selling author of* The 36-Hour Day

A Loving Approach to Dementia Care
Making Meaningful Connections while Caregiving
third edition
Laura Wayman

Creative Engagement
A Handbook of Activities for People with Dementia
Rachael Wonderlin
with Geri M. Lotze, PhD

Through the Seasons
Activities for Memory-Challenged Adults and Their Caregivers
second edition
*Cynthia R. Green, PhD,
and Joan Beloff, ACC, ALA, CDP*
foreword by Peter V. Rabins, MD, MPH

The Caregiver's Encyclopedia
A Compassionate Guide to Caring for Older Adults
Muriel R. Gillick, MD

Making Tough Decisions about End-of-Life Care in Dementia
Anne Kenny, MD

Finding the Right Words
A Story of Literature, Grief, and the Brain
Cindy Weinstein
with Bruce L. Miller, MD

The Busy Caregiver's Guide to Advanced Alzheimer Disease
Jennifer R. Stelter, PsyD
with Rachael Wonderlin

 @JHUPress

 @JohnsHopkins
UniversityPress

 @JHUPress

For more Dementia Care and Aging books, visit press.jhu.edu